Improbable Journeys

From Crossing the Himalayas on Horseback
to a Career in Obstetrics and Gynaecology

A Medical Memoir

Dr. Bernard A. O. Binns
Ron Smith

W0006974

Rock's Mills Press
Oakville, Ontario
2020

Published by
Rock's Mills Press
www.rocksmillspress.com

Photographs included in the book are from Bernard Binns' personal collection.

For information about this book, please contact the publisher at
customer.service@rocksmillspress.com
or visit us online at www.rocksmillspress.com.

For Elaine

Contents

Foreword

Seldom do our dreams unfold as we expect them to. A small distraction here, a moment of misunderstanding there, and we enter the accidental world of serendipity. For Dr. Bernie Binns, whose story this book unfolds, life has been a matter of chance, of the unpredictable, not because he is unfocussed or indecisive, but because he has always been open to need and possibility. Perhaps this is a family characteristic. Many of his family, he says, embraced happenstance, his father in particular. Kismet or karma, whatever the case, they have repeatedly enjoyed the gift of good fortune or luck.

The first time I heard one of Bernie's anecdotes we were enjoying a cold beer on a hot summer's afternoon, shortly after we had become next-door neighbours. I think it might have had something to do with his birth in Port Stanley on the Falkland Islands. I had probably asked him where he was from, assuming he would name some quaint countryside village in the English Midlands. I was confident I recognized his accent. But he surprised me. I'd never met anyone born on the remote archipelago that lay five hundred kilometres east of Argentina in the Atlantic Ocean. Until that moment those wild and stormy islands had mythical status in my imagination. He then announced proudly and somewhat optimistically, I thought, that he had started to write a book about his life.

We were now familiar enough to talk 'over the fence', although in this case the fence was a solid wall of granite, loose stones, brambles, dozens of foxgloves, a few trees from what I imagined a Tom Thomson landscape would look like, and a broad patch of moss and lichen.

His claim that he had started to write a book reminded me of a story I had heard about an encounter between Margaret Laurence, the gifted author of *A Jest of God*, *The Stone Angel* and *The Diviners*, and a surgeon who had told her now that he had retired from his medical career he was going to take up writing novels. Oh, she replied, that's an interesting coincidence, now that I've written my last novel I've decided to take up brain surgery. Whether or not this conversation had actually taken place, I loved the delicious irony of her response, probably undetected by the retired surgeon.

Bernie continued to tell me personal stories over the following months and years, every so often reminding me of the volume he was amassing, at one stage mentioning he was well over two hundred thousand words. At night, when I went out for a walk, I could see him encircled by light in his 'crow's nest' study slaving away on his computer, but I assumed he was solving Sudokus or playing chess with one of his many opponents from around the globe, not writing!

Then one day he asked me if I would be willing to read what he had written. While I had been bracing myself for this question, I hadn't expected him to arrive on my doorstep with a manuscript of well over eight hundred typed pages. It was a massive stack of paper, more than half-a-foot thick. Literally a lifetime's work. And when I began to read it I was horrified. I asked my wife if she would give the manuscript a cursory look and perhaps do a quick copy edit? After a short while she emerged from her study, looking haggard, and asked me what I expected her to do? "The writing is dreadful," she said, "extremely repetitive, chaotic, ungrammatical, vague, unfocussed. And *the spelling*!" she muttered.

Her response was not unexpected. And yet, from Bernie's oral presentations I knew the stories themselves were informative and provocative; sometimes brooding, sometimes gripping; occasionally adventures in time, casting us back into a past through cultures that hadn't changed in centuries, other times pulling us into the future through scientific research. But what, I wondered, had happened in the transition from the spoken to the written word?

When I approached Bernie, with a degree of apprehension, to tell him his book needed extensive revision, he was surprisingly receptive. In fact, he seemed relieved and grateful. I was dumbstruck. His reaction was almost furtive. And I felt as though I were a participant in some sort of jiggery-pokery. His behaviour was abnormal! Most writers, no matter what their skill level, are thin-skinned, if not defiant, when it comes to defending their precious and hard-won words. Bernie was not the slightest bit fractious. I was puzzled.

Then he asked if I'd be willing to edit the manuscript, to which I agreed. I set to, but realized early on that minor changes were not going to be enough. After months of revision, I came to the disturbing insight that I had taken on the 're-writing' of his life. I was making changes from diction to sentence to paragraph. The challenge was to retain the authenticity of his voice.

"I have a mild form of dyslexia," he told me apologetically, "didn't I tell you? I'm sorry, I should have mentioned it. And I'm almost blind in one eye. I need help. I've always relied on my visual memory or verbal interpretations rather than written descriptions to learn. Whilst I love the written word, I understand things much more thoroughly from exhibits in museums, drawings, or paintings in galleries. From demonstrations. From doing dissections or experiments in labs. From examining bottled samples."

This confession explained a lot. Having had a major stroke recently, I knew the brain can compensate for loss or damage in a multitude of ways. And words, whether spoken or written, can make up the distance between the senses, the space between understanding and not understanding, whatever the language and whether presented as letters or pictograms.

I had always found Bernie's memory for events and their details extraordinary, perhaps a result of adapting to his dyslexia. And when he remembered episodes from his life orally, his language was spontaneous, filled with hope that he would be heard, and, most importantly, his life celebrated. That seemed a noble and worthy goal. His dyslexia had given him the strength and aptitude to speak the truth of his story in his way. Based on his spoken words, I have tried to help him put his story into a written form, one that traverses space and time and perhaps hints at a life as it has been lived, fully and in the present. The seer seeing. The moment lived with depth, I believe, is what gives our existence duration and substance.

My hope is that the reader will read with joy. The story, of course, is Bernie's; the book a collaboration. When I first read the extremely rough draft of his memoir I was amazed by the range of events he had experienced and witnessed, and the places to which he had been. All

"Lives" are comments on the world the narrators have lived through as well as a revelation of their own engagement with it. Bernie's is no different. As his story recounts, he *has* been a fortunate man.

RON SMITH

Improbable Journeys

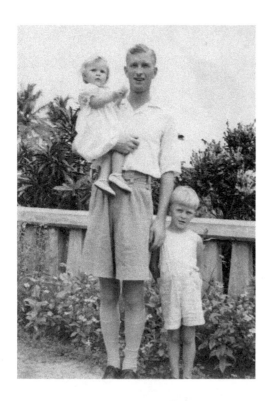

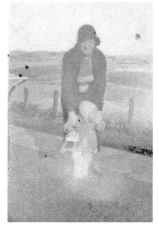

Above: Bernard and Mother in the Falkland Islands.
Left: Father, Marjory and Bernard in India.
Below: Bernard swimming in the Indian Ocean.

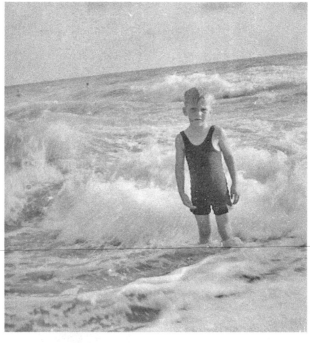

Chapter 1
The Falklands and Pre-War India

My early life began in the Falkland Islands, where I was born, took me to England, and then to India and Chinese Turkestan—but my memories of this time only consist of fragments, scraps of memory dredged up from childhood images and family tales spun around the kitchen table.

In 1933, my father was working as a house surgeon at the Royal Chesterfield Infirmary in Derbyshire. After breaking up with his fiancée, a brave thing to do, he started a new relationship with the Theatre Sister, also a midwife, who worked at the same hospital. A few months later, after meeting and courting the woman who was to become my mother, he suddenly found himself needing to find another job—his rotation was coming to an end.

He considered going into general practice locally, but those prospects were limited. With the depression in full swing, employment opportunities were rare and a lot of young men were looking for work overseas, which in those days usually meant taking up a post in the British Colonies, as a part of the Foreign Service, ideally in either Australia or Canada. So he approached the Colonial Office in London about positions around the Commonwealth. They came up with two suggestions—either a job in Nigeria, commonly known as the "White Man's Grave," or a post in the Falkland Islands, which, for the most part, nobody had heard of before Prime Minister Margaret Thatcher announced the invasion of the islands by Argentina in 1982.

The Colonial office had a rule that they only sent single men to the Nigerian jobs and married men to the Falklands.

Armed with this information my father returned to Chesterfield and asked my mother if she would marry him. She told me she had no idea where the Falkland Islands were but she assumed they were probably somewhere north of Scotland. She always added, with a wry smile, that knowing their location would not have made any difference to her accepting my father's offer of marriage.

They started the trip to the Falkland Islands from Southampton on a large trans-Atlantic liner bound for Montevideo and Buenos Aires. When they arrived at the docks in Montevideo, where they had to change ships, my father was on deck talking to the purser. He turned and asked him if he knew the SS *Lefonia*, which was to take him and his new wife to Port Stanley in the Falklands.

"Oh yes! It's over there." And he pointed to a small boat tied up at the next dock.

"She's not very big, is she?" my father noted. "How's she behave?"

"You'll likely have a pretty rough trip down to the Falklands," the purser said. "The seas down there are the roughest in the world, but she's been sailing them for many years and I've never heard of her having any trouble. I'm glad it's you, though, and not me making the trip. I'm told that even the crew get seasick on some trips!"

"Well," my father replied, "I don't get seasick myself, but my wife, Ada, may not be so lucky. She's been feeling a little queasy, even on this large liner."

This statement was a harbinger of bad news for my mother who was so seasick over the next twelve days that she wouldn't have cared if the boat had gone down. As she described it, the seas were so rough that the boat 'corkscrewed' its way all the way to Port Stanley.

Two days into the trip my father went below to the galley looking for breakfast. As he approached the serving hatch, he realized that talking to the cook could only be done by standing with his feet spread to correct for the ship's motion, and even then they could only talk when they both came to the vertical.

"Good morning, sir ... what are you doing ... down here?"

"I thought ... I would like some ... breakfast. What have you ... got today?" asked my father.

"Oh!... What would you ... like?"

"Anything that's ... going."

"Will some ... coffee and ... toast do? It's too rough to cook."

"Yes, ... that will be fine."

The only other person to come below for breakfast was the captain, who was another of those lucky people who didn't get seasick. He told my father that this was one of their worst trips in some time for weather and rough seas. Apparently it took my mother several days to get over the voyage. During her recovery she realized she was pregnant, which later she felt had something to do with the terrible nausea she had experienced on the boat.

I was born in Port Stanley on the second of April 1934, although my parents were based a sea-journey away at Fox Bay, which is on the West Island. My father was the only doctor on the island and our nearest neighbour was a sheep farmer half a mile distant, on the other side of the bay. To get to the neighbour's my parents had to go a mile upstream before being able to cross the creek that fed into the bay. In those days the only form of transport was by horse or small boat. Communication was achieved through a communal telephone line with a system of long and short rings to identify who the call was for. When the doctor's number came up everyone would pick up their phones to 'listen in' to see what was happening and the whole phone system would give out for lack of power.

Years later Mother told me my birth had been unusually difficult. First of all, I was premature by several weeks; second, I presented hand and arm first, waving frantically from her vagina, as if departing rather than arriving; third, I was an awkward forceps birth; and fourth I broke my collar bone and several ribs during the procedure. The attending doctor and midwife were so concerned I wouldn't survive the ordeal, they placed me in an incubator and waited twenty-four hours before telling father, who had remained behind in Fox Bay, of my arrival. When he finally heard he had a son he was, in his usual manner, quietly relieved.

At the centre of the island was a fairly high peak of 2,297 feet surrounded by a peat bog. This inhospitable terrain meant that to travel to the other side of the island one had to follow the coastline. These distances were often long and the treks arduous. My father told the story of receiving an urgent call about a young man with abdominal pains, suggestive of acute appendicitis. At this time, appendicitis could be fatal if not treated quickly. The patient and his family lived at the north end of the island and the medical team immediately set off on horses. Falkland horses were taught to trot and therefore were changed every four hours at specific sheep stations along the route. This trip took twelve hours to complete. My father reflected that "they don't change the riders, though, and after twelve hours of trotting there isn't a bone in your body that doesn't ache. And your rear end will likely be in even worse shape." Luckily, in this situation, the patient's condition had improved when they arrived and they didn't have to do anything except rest and recuperate from the journey.

Over the years I was told only a few stories about my birthplace. It was not discussed much, but Mother said that she remembered a few striking things. One of these was the wind. It was always blowing hard. There was no protection from it; no trees. The land was as barren as the moon. During her two years there she specifically remembered two days which were clear and calm; they stood out as exceptional. The winters were cold and the islands often received a light dusting of snow. On one occasion Mother heard a knock on the door and when she opened it there stood a neighbour who asked if she was trying to "harden me off." I was blithely crawling around in the snow. The wind had been so strong it had blown over the pram in which Mother had carefully placed me.

Many years later, when I was a medical student, my mother told me that the Falkland Islands were the most depressing place she had ever lived.

Penguins, albatrosses and Canada geese were frequent visitors to Fox Bay while seals, sea lions, walruses, foxes and other small mammals managed to scrounge out an existence amongst the coastal rocks. The main occupation for people on the Falklands was, and still remains, sheep farming, and my parents soon learned a lot about it. Mutton, of course, was the only easily available meat and I gathered, from what my parents said years later, that a steady diet of it sat heavy in the stomach. I have few recollections of their ever eating mutton or lamb. It was not a popular dish in our house, even after their return to England in 1946.

4

When my father accepted the job in the Falkland Islands he had been told that he would receive relief breaks, holidays and one month a year in the city of Port Stanley. These contractual benefits, which mattered if you lived in an isolated posting, did not materialize. After two years and many conversations with the Colonial Office about the importance of relief and holidays, my father took a rather bold step and told them what they could do with their job. He quit. Technically he was breaking his contract and, therefore, had to pay for all the tickets he needed to get his family back to England.

Regrettably, I have no personal recollections of these events and images and have not managed to return to the Falklands to see what it's really like as a place to live. I gather that now there are some primitive roads for 4x4 vehicles, but that nothing else has changed much. What did surprise me was my anger when I heard that Argentina had invaded the Islands in 1982. No matter how irrational my attachment now seems, this violation brought home to me how important one's birthplace is and how sensitive people can be about it.

On arrival in England my father quickly found work as an assistant in general practice. He worked in Mansfield and Liverpool and was offered a partnership after two years. Partnership required that you invest in the practice and at the time the fee was £4,000. My father arranged to take a loan through the British Medical Association office in London and travelled there to finalize the transaction.

On his arrival in the London office, the clerk had all the papers ready but told my father there would be an additional £10 stamp duty on the cost of the loan. Stamp duties had been introduced into Europe in the 1600s. In the 1930s they remained as a government tax attached to many kinds of legal documents, including financial transactions such as cheques and loans. A physical stamp had to be placed on the documents to show that the duty had been paid before the document was legally effective. This practice is still in effect in many places around the world. The question of who was responsible for paying the stamp tax on the loan became an issue with my father. "This seems to be a bit unfair," suggested Father. "I would have thought your company should pay the tax."

"I'm sorry but my instructions are to charge the stamp duty to the customer," said the clerk. "I don't have any choice."

"What happens if I don't pay it?" asked my father, who was a principled man.

"We won't be able to arrange for the loan," said the clerk.

"Could you check that with your superior? Now, please!"

The clerk went into the back of the office, returning a few minutes later to confirm that my father would have to pay the stamp duty. This aggravated him so much that he said, "In that case, I'll not be taking the loan after all." And he stormed out of the office.

A few hundred yards down the road from the British Medical Association my father found himself standing opposite the India Office, which was the British government department responsible for administrative activities in India. These included the employment of civil servants who basically ran the country (district officers, teachers, nurses, medical staff, etc.) and the Indian Army. He stopped and wondered if they might have a job for him; after all, he reasoned, his elder brother was already working for them.

Impulsively my father entered the building and asked the clerk if there were any jobs for a doctor in India. The clerk gave him a short form to fill in. When my father had completed it the clerk took it to the back office. A few minutes later another man came through the door and asked, "Do you have any references on you?"

"No, but I could get some without any trouble."

"I notice that your name is Binns. Are you related to Bernard Ottwell Binns, in the British Foreign Service in India, by any chance?"

"Yes, he's my elder brother," replied my father.

"Ahh! Just a moment please. I'll be right back."

A few minutes later he returned and said, "If you want to go to India we could offer you a job in the Indian Medical Service as a commissioned officer. Would you be interested?"

"Yes," my father replied.

"Well, then, fill out these forms and send them back to us. We'll see what can be done." This was the story my father always told about his second impetuous job decision.

My mother, an easy-going person, was never critical of any of the decisions that my father made. She was brought up at a time when wives were expected to go along with their husband's decisions. Her only comment was that India was a long way away and she would miss the rest of the family.

In early 1938 we moved to India. Father went out on his own, ahead of us. Mother was expecting her second child and my parents decided it would be better if she stayed in England for the birth. My sister, Marjory, was born in April and we joined my father in Cannanore (Kannur) a few weeks later. The city was located in the province of Kerala on the southwestern coast of India. Although I have some vague recollections of living in Worksop, Nottinghamshire, with my grandfather before our departure, I don't remember much of the trip to India or the train ride to Cannanore. This is not surprising; I was only four years old.

My first vivid memory of India was of nearly drowning in the ocean. Boiling surf rushed over my head when I fell into a hole in the sand where I was paddling in the waves. I stood up, but could only see sunlight sparkling through the water that surged over my head. I didn't panic, even when I was knocked over by another wave. Once again I found myself rolling around at the bottom of the hole. I stood up again, but still couldn't reach the surface. I remember trying to crawl up the side of the pit. As I got to the edge, the sea receded and I was able to draw a gasp of air into my lungs. Then I was knocked over once more by a new wave and returned to the bottom of the pit. This time I remember clawing deep into the sand as I crawled back up the side of the hole. When I got to the top, I managed to use my hands to anchor myself to the sand and, although the sea continued to rush around me, this time I managed to stay half out of the hole. As the sea receded, I scrambled out the rest of the way, got to my feet and wheezed before being able to inhale a few deep breaths. Then I walked back to where Mother was sitting with my sister, fifty yards up the beach. "How did you get your hair wet, Bernard?" she asked me.

"One of the waves knocked me over," I told her.

"Were you frightened?"

"Not really."

"Where were you?"

"Just over there."

"If the waves are big enough to knock you over, don't go there."

"All right," I said and did not tell her about the big hole in the sand where I had been.

At the time, I was between five and six. I didn't appreciate the danger. I remember thinking that if I'd told my mother the full story I wouldn't have been allowed to paddle on the beach and that was something I liked doing.

In Southern India we had a spacious house with high ceilings and large windows through which cool breezes flowed. There was a veranda around three sides of the house and the circular drive led up to a porch at the front. The outside walls were white-washed, the doors and windows painted red, and the roof was corrugated iron. The expansive compound was surrounded by a solid, reddish-brown six-foot wall. In the front of the house, a typical tropical garden bloomed with bougainvillea, hibiscus, cosmos and other brightly coloured shrubs and flowers. Several exotic trees, including a flame tree, two coconuts trees, a clump of bananas, two large mangos and several paw paws, shaded the compound. The servants' quarters, a modest two-room building, stood behind the main house.

We didn't have electricity or running water and slept under mosquito nets. Suspended from the high ceilings in several of the rooms were what the Indians called *punkas*. These were made of a heavy carpet-like material set on a frame which hung from the ceiling. Attached to the frame was a rope and pulley system that allowed the *punka walha* to pull the *punka* back and forth from a location at the back of the house. The movement of the *punka* stirred the air and created a cooling breeze when the days became unbearably hot and humid.

Within the household we had a house boy, a cook, an *ayah* and a couple of garden boys who, when needed, also acted as *punka walhas*.

They all doted on my sister and me, keeping us out of trouble without being too strict. I don't remember seeing much of my father at this time. He used to leave for work early in the mornings and did not get back until 4:30 p.m. We were put to bed by 6:30 p.m when it started to get dark. On the weekends we were able to go to the club, which was located across the road from us.

My sister and I would play with other expat children while the adults were playing tennis, bridge, or billiards; or we would scamper to the beach next to the club and spend hours playing in the sand and water. My father didn't really like to socialize, but he did go to the club to play tennis. Mother was much more inclined to go to parties, which were held in the evenings when my sister and I were in bed.

India was a safe place to grow up. It was hard to escape the notice of my mother or one of the servants. One day, though, as we were preparing to go to a birthday party, the *ayah*, who was obviously very distressed, came running into the room where Mother was getting me ready.

"Miss Marjory is lost!" she cried.

"What do you mean, she's lost? I just dressed her for the party."

"I cannot find her," the *ayah* said.

"Get Kamara, Cook and the garden boy to help look for her. She can't have gone far."

For the next ten minutes the search for Marjory, who was only two years old, reached into every corner of the house and, as time went by, everyone became more frantic. At this point Father arrived home and took charge. "She obviously must have wandered out of the house into the compound or down the road."

He told Cook and the garden boy to go and look down the road and along the path to the beach. They ran out the front door and down the drive. Mother decided to search the house again and Father went out into the garden. I was alone in the front room when Kamara, the house boy, entered.

"What is the trouble, *chota-sahib*?" he asked.

"Marjory's lost and everyone's looking for her. Do you know where she is?"

"No, but I will go and look."

Several minutes later Mother, Father, the garden boy and Cook all came back empty-handed.

"Well," Father said, "this is becoming very serious. I think I'd better get hold of the police to see if they can help."

"She can't have gone far, and there are no holes or wells that she could have fallen into," Mother reasoned.

As we stood helplessly debating what to do, Kamara came into the room carrying a soaking wet Marjory. "I've found her!" he announced with a broad grin.

"Where was she?" asked Mother. "She looks like a drowned kitten! Just look at her party dress! It's ruined."

"She was in the big *chutti* in the bathroom," said Kamara.

Marjory told us she was too hot in her party dress. She had climbed into the large earthenware pot in the bathroom to cool down. Because there was no running water in the houses, these large pots were used to store water. The vessel stood about two feet high and had a wide opening. It was a bit of a mystery how Marjory managed to climb into the *chutti*, but luckily this story had a happy ending.

Life was comfortable for our family—we could afford to have three servants who looked after the house, cooking, garden and family. Father worked regular hours, Monday through Friday, and was with the family at the weekends. We adjusted to the heat, and apart from the occasional poisonous snake, there were few dangers. Malaria and other tropical diseases could be a problem and we were very cautious about what we ate. Father insisted we eat only hot-cooked food and that we never be tempted by anything that had been left to cool for too long.

However, in 1939 events in Europe changed our idyllic existence.

One evening, just before sunset, I was in the garden playing when I became aware of a strange noise in the sky. The noise came from behind me, but when I looked around, I couldn't see what was making the sound. As I listened, the rumbling grew louder. Suddenly there was a roar from beyond the trees and a large object, like a giant dragonfly, flew over the roof of the house. I stood still, holding my breath; I had never seen one before. The object, with its whirring propeller, continued to rise and flew straight out to sea. I remember watching it get smaller and smaller as it continued on its way. Just as it vanished from sight, Father arrived home from work.

"Daddy! Daddy! What was that big thing in the sky? It flew over the house and out over the sea and didn't come back."

"A plane," he said, "a two-seater bi-plane. It came from up north and is now on its way to Ceylon. It's a long way so the pilot had to stop here to get some more petrol."

"How can something as big as that stay up in the sky?" I asked.

"It's difficult to explain. It's a bit like a big kite. The engine drives the propeller that pulls the plane through the air. The wings are set at an angle and lift the plane into the sky." I must have looked confused because Father paused and said, "One day you'll learn more about how planes work. But for now, let's go and find your mother. I have important news."

We went into the house and found Mother in the sitting room. She immediately called Kamara the house boy.

"Yes, *Memsahib*."

"Could you bring the tea? Master is home." She turned to Father. "How were things at work today?"

"Well," he said, his lips taut, "there's some bad news. War has broken out in Europe."

"That's terrible. What'll happen to our families? Will they be safe? Will you have to return home?"

"I don't think so, at least not at the moment because I'm Indian Medical Service. It's a long way to send us. A lot will depend on how things go against the Germans and whether the war escalates and involves other parts of the world. If Japan joins in we could be affected here in India. We'll just have to wait and see."

"Will they want me and the children to go back to England?"

"I gather that some of the wives want to do that, but it could be dangerous and I wouldn't think it a good idea at the moment. You should be safe here. If I have to go to Europe, then you and the children might have to go back to England."

"Daddy, if you have to go, will you have to fight?" I asked.

"No, I'll be looking after the wounded, but I might have to go to the front line to pick them up."

"That could be very dangerous, couldn't it?" Mother asked.

"I suppose so, but war is dangerous for everyone involved."

In 1940 Indian troops were shipped out to the Middle East and Father had to go with them. He spent eighteen months supporting them in his role as a medical doctor. First he was in charge of the injured soldiers on the Ambulance Train that ran between Asmara and Cairo and then he took a position at the base hospital in Cairo where he gave anaesthetics. Here he became ill and was eventually sent back to India to recover his health.

Mother, my sister and I stayed in India. It was considered safer than England although we did not stay in our large house. We were moved to Bangalore and were put in a boarding house. There were several other service wives at this boarding house as well. I remember the house being very crowded and uncomfortable. I was nearly six, so Mother decided that it was time I went to school. I was sent to Ooty Command Boarding School, which was in the Nilgari Hills in South East India. The language of instruction was English and the subjects taught were the same as the ones in England. Ooty Command Boarding School was where all the British service families in the area sent their children.

To get to this new school a teacher accompanied me and a few other boys on a six-hour train trip from Bangalore to Ooty. I had no problem on the train and enjoyed seeing new things through the open window. There were several station stops filled with brash peddlers and brightly decorated station bazaars. Many of the peddlers came up to the train and tried to sell us tropical fruits, freshly cooked foods, trinkets, ice cream, and Indian sweets. They called us "Chota sahibs." We had been told not to buy anything, especially foods. To make sure we obeyed, all our pocket money was held by the teacher. Even so, the smells from the spicy foods were richly tantalizing.

Once off the train we all boarded a bus for the last part of the journey, which took us through tea and coffee plantations, to the Blue Mountains.

The air was dry, dusty and grey, but the clothes worn by the women were bright reds, blues, greens and purples mixed with white and brown. Their saris contrasted with the reddish brown soil; the grass; the flame, jacaranda, and banana trees; and other colourful shrubs—all of which were dwarfed by towering Banyan trees and coconut palms. Stray dogs, chickens, and monkeys scampered about freely, creating a pandemonium that was ubiquitous at these stations.

The bus trip started out on a fairly straight dirt road, the bald tires throwing out a great turbulence of reddish brown dust as we went along. After half an hour we started to climb into the hills and the road began to twist and turn. At first I felt a little queasy but as the bus continued to go up the increasingly winding road I was sure I was going to be sick.

I put my head out the window, but it didn't help. I vomited. The other boys on the bus thought it was a hell of a joke. It was the first time I remember being humiliated. This episode was a portent of things to come, and began a period of my schooling that turned out to be a total disaster.

Ooty Command Boarding School was a two- or three-storey Victorian building with red brick walls. The dormitories held up to fifteen boys and each of us had a bed with a wooden locker and shelves built into the wall at the head. The floors were bare polished wood. The classrooms held up to twenty school desks with chairs. There was a sparsely furnished common room and a single dining room that seated up to sixty boys on benches at long planked tables.

Within ten days I got the measles and spent the rest of the term quarantined in sick bay. The actual schooling I received was limited and I don't remember much about it. The next term I got whooping cough after a couple of weeks and again spent most of my time in sick bay. The third term was an improvement. I actually remember attending classes, but having missed the first two terms, I was woefully behind the other boys and was completely lost. I did enjoy the field days and sports, but I didn't participate in those as often as I would have liked. Once again I ended up in sick bay when I contracted tonsillitis twice during the term.

When I finally got home to Bangalore after this last term Mother decided Ooty Command was not good for my health. She would not send me back. She had a friend, a Mrs. Aston, whom we visited weekly for supper and whose husband taught at the Institute of Science. They lived on the beautiful Institute of Science grounds. They had two boys—Roger, who was my age, and Quentin, who was a few years younger. The boys were being given their lessons at home by private tutors, so Mother arranged for Marjory and me to join them. While I was at the Astons' I learned how to ride a bicycle, but not to read or write.

One morning I sensed an excited fluttering in the boarding house. Mother seemed particularly ruffled. She came to me and said, "Daddy is coming home today. I received a message this morning. We have to go and meet him at the station. Don't be surprised by how he looks. Your father has been very ill and that's why he's returning to India. You and Marjory must be strong and well behaved."

"Yes, Mother," I said, alarmed by the note of apprehension in Mother's voice.

Mrs. Aston took us to the station that afternoon to meet the train. The Bangalore Station was large with numerous platforms covered by a roof. The train came into the station puffing out clouds of smoke and steam. Although I had been on a train before, I had never been so close to an engine. I was frightened by it and all the people milling around on the platform.

"Let's move down," Mother said and motioned with the back of her hand. "I think your father is in the third carriage."

As we got nearer I could see a tall, thin, white-haired old man being helped down the steps by a soldier.

"My God, that's Pat!" exclaimed Mother to Mrs. Aston.

"You said he's been ill and the long trip will not have helped. He must be very tired," said Mrs. Aston, trying to reassure Mother.

"But he looks so old and his hair has gone white!"

It was then I realized the old man was my father. Mother recovered from the shock quickly and we edged closer. By this time Father had reached the platform. He turned round and saw Mother for the first time.

"Ada," he said, struggling for words, "how good to see you again." He put his arms around her and gave her a kiss.

After some moments Mother broke away, her face flushed, and said, "I brought the children to meet you. Here's Bernard, and the big girl there is Marjory."

Father hobbled to where we stood with Mrs. Aston, shook her hand, and gave each of us an awkward hug. "You two have grown up a lot since I last saw you."

"The Astons have asked us to stay with them for a while," Mother said. "They have lots of room at the Institute and Dorothy kindly drove us here to meet you. Have you got much luggage?"

"Just two small cases that Sam, my batman, is standing by over there. They should fit into the boot of the car easily."

During the next few weeks Father spent a lot of time at the hospital in Bangalore. Although nothing was ever said I suspect he was receiving treatment. Mother never told us what Father's problem was but he did gradually get better. I remember sitting at the breakfast table one day and seeing him curl up in pain as he tried to eat some toast. The spasm started in his face and was so bad that he went white and had to be helped back to his room by one of the servants and Mother. He was still very thin, but his strength returned as the weeks went by. Then one day, as he sipped his tea at breakfast, he became quite cheerful.

"What do you think of the idea of going back to Cannanore?"

"I would love that," said Mother.

"So would I," Marjory and I chorused.

"Well, rumour has it that this is where they will be sending me in a week or so, if I'm fit enough."

I was excited by this news because I had liked Cannanore and preferred it to where we were staying in Bangalore. The city was nicer, it was on the coast, and the climate was pleasant. But most important, as far as I was concerned, was that I would be free to run about on my own and go where I liked. Two weeks later we drove back to Cannanore in an old Vauxhall 14. We didn't get our old house but we got one that was similar. Happily we had the same *ayah* and servants.

I was now almost seven and spent a lot of time with the servants and their children in the compound behind our house. As a result I learned to speak the local language, Malayali. This was a help to Mother because I was able to translate all her instructions to the *ayah*, cook and garden boys who did not speak good English. Kamara, who was the official interpreter, could speak English although I noticed Father spoke to him in Urdu, which he had had to learn as part of his training in the Indian Medical Service. I asked Kamara if he could teach me to speak his language. He and the cook were more than happy to start daily sessions. Within a few months, I became quite fluent in Urdu. Like all children I soaked up new words with ease.

There were two beaches within walking distance of the house. One of them was quite shallow with gentle breakers rolling in. Father took me there several times and showed me how to use a surfboard. Although I still couldn't swim, I was at least able to keep my head above water.

Between the two beaches a small river flowed into the sea. An old wooden footbridge crossed the river just before it reached the sea and passed over a popular fishing hole. One of the garden boys was eager to teach me the secrets of bringing home a fish. Early one morning, we set out to catch some fish for breakfast.

"This will be the last day for fish," said the garden boy. "Monsoon come today."

"Don't be stupid," I said. "Look, there are no clouds and it's hot, just like yesterday."

"It will come. You see," he insisted. "Oh! I got one!" he shouted. "It's a big one, too." And he pulled in a ten- to twelve-inch fish.

As the fish flapped about on the bridge, I bent down to pick it up.

"Don't pick it up. It will sting you," he said.

He then put his bare foot on the fish to hold it down. He showed me where the fish had a ridge of sharp spines along its back and two on the underside. These spines, he told me, carried a poison.

"Can they kill you?" I asked.

"Oh, no. They are not that bad, but very painful for some days. There are some snakes in the sea that can kill you. They have many colours and are very beautiful, but do not get near them. They are more poisonous than the small snakes we have in the garden and they can kill you with one bite."

Snakes were a problem in Cannanore. My parents had warned us about them. There were two that were deadly and common, the cobra and the krait. The cobras hunted for lizards, frogs and toads in the garden and were quite easy to spot. I saw several while we were there and I would go and tell the garden boy who would then proceed to kill them. The krait was a small, thin viper which grew to about eight inches and came into the houses at night seeking warmth and sheltered spots like shoes and boots. The krait was also known to fall out of the rafters onto beds at night. This nocturnal habit was one of the reasons why we always had our mosquito nets up when we went to bed. I only saw one and took off as fast as I could because everyone had stressed how deadly they were.

I did see a python once, up a tree, down the road from our house. The garden boy said it was resting after eating and was not dangerous. This python probably measured ten feet long.

We were not overly fearful of these snakes. We knew what to do when we came across them and we knew where they were likely to be found. However, when you cornered one unexpectedly, you had to be careful to get out of its way without getting into the snake's striking range.

At teatime, I noticed some big clouds forming in the sky over the sea and pointed them out to Mother. "The garden boy says that the monsoon will come today. Do you think those clouds are the beginning of it?"

"It could be, but they look as though they are a long way off and being blown the other way."

"They could easily come this way in a few hours," said Father.

"What's a monsoon like?" I asked.

"Very wet and windy," said Father.

A few hours later I was wakened by a tremendous crash of thunder, accompanied by a powerful wind. I sat up in bed, looked out the window and saw flashes of lightning strike over the churning sea. Then I heard a few light pings on the corrugated iron roof. At first these sounds were scattered and quite loud. A metallic ring reverberated throughout the room. Then the pings came closer and closer together, reached a crescendo, and seemed to explode on top of us. There was another bright flash of lightning, followed immediately by a crash of thunder right over the house. This woke Marjory and she started to cry. The *ayah,* who slept on the veranda just outside our room, came in to comfort her. At the same time Mother arrived to see if we were all right. The noise on the roof increased and we had to shout to hear each other over the din.

"It's just a thunderstorm," said Mother. "It should get quieter soon."

"Rain will not stop for many days," the *ayah* informed us with certainty.

Marjory was put back to bed and I was told to go back to sleep. The noise of the rain on the roof made sleep impossible. The thunder and lightning continued. I sat up and looked out the window. Torrents of rain blew against the house, one blast after another. From our bedroom window I could see the corner of the driveway and saw that it was now a shallow lake. When the number of lightning flashes decreased and I tired of watching the rain, I lay down and fell asleep.

In the morning it was still pouring. I got up and put my shoes on. We were not allowed to go anywhere without our shoes on because of the risk of hookworm. I went out onto the veranda and saw a garden that was completely changed. The red dusty earth was red mud. The driveway was now a river of water inches deep, running into what had been a dry ditch at the side of the house. The water streamed towards a wider ditch on the other side of the wall that surrounded the house. The culvert under the wall was not wide enough to take all the water away from the house and garden, and a large pond had formed.

Dry leaves, grass, small sticks and other light debris floated on the pond. The veranda was soaking wet and slippery, but it was not cold. A damp musty smell saturated the air and the noise of the rain on the roof was continuous. The wind had subsided and the thunder and lightning had stopped. Kamara joined me on the veranda.

"You were right about the monsoon," I said. "How long will it rain for?"

"Up to six weeks."

"What? All the time?"

"Rain will come every day. Sometimes it will rain all the time for one or two weeks. Everything will get wet and it will be difficult to dry the clothes."

Mother and Father, still in their pajamas, came out to look at the rain.

"Kamara says it will rain all the time for six weeks," I said.

"Not all the time, I hope," said Mother.

"I'm afraid Kamara is right," said Father. "It will rain heavily every day for several weeks now. If we're lucky we may get the odd day with some sun, but most of the time it will be like this, dull and raining."

Surprisingly, we got used to the rain after a few days. The air temperature stayed warm and the rain was not cold, so getting wet was not that uncomfortable. I noticed many locals just walked around as if it were not raining. Some used umbrellas, but there were no rain coats or slickers to be seen.

Some weeks after the rains had ceased Father announced that we would be moving again, this time to Abbottabad in northern India (now Pakistan) where he had been posted by the Indian Army. The journey to Pakistan was a long one, taking over a week by car and train.

The train portion of our journey took us through Delhi and Raul-pindi. Our tickets required us to change trains, but we missed the connections at both stations and got our first taste of Indian hotels. In those days, hotels in India were opulent and the clientele were pampered. Because Father was an officer we travelled first class on the train. We had half a carriage to ourselves, which included some cooking facilities and a 'sitting room' separate from the sleeping area.

As we left the coast and travelled north, the landscape and people changed. I heard new languages in the stations and Kamara, who accompanied us on the journey, explained to me that there were over five hundred languages spoken in India. When we got closer to Abbottabad, there were more Sikhs with their turbans, long beards and flowing garments. I saw my first Holy Man at one of the stations and asked what he did. Kamara explained that he taught people about Allah. For the first time I realized people called God by different names.

When we arrived in Raulpindi we spent the night in a hotel. The next day we boarded a smaller train and Father explained that this was a narrow gauge train, like the one on which I had gone up to Ooty. Soon after we departed from Raulpindi, we started to climb into hilly countryside. The stations were smaller and more frequent. The railway tracks began meandering and I could hear the engine straining away at the front like an exhausted water buffalo. At times, the train slowed down to a crawl and it seemed on the verge of slipping backwards. For the first time, I saw fir or pine trees. At the stations I noticed the clothes people were wearing were again different and heavier. All the men wore turbans and the women wore veils. Kamara explained that the women were Muslims and in *purdah* (female seclusion). Eventually we got to Abbottabad and we were taken to the hotel in a small bus. We would be staying there for several months.

One morning after we arrived, we were sitting at breakfast when there was a lot of shouting from guests outside the dining room. "I wonder what that's all about?" asked Father of nobody in particular.

"It's something about a mad dog," I said. "I'm not sure what they're trying to do. My Hindi's not good enough yet. I think they're trying to shoo it away. They're frightened and have sent for a policeman."

The waiter arrived with toast.

"What's all the noise about?" asked Father.

"There is a mad dog outside. They have sent for the police to come and shoot it. You should all stay in the dining room until it has been killed," he said.

"Mummy, look, do you think that's the sick dog?" asked Marjory, pointing towards the front door of the dining room.

We all turned and stared at the poor dog that had just come in through the door. It was swaying slightly as it stood glancing about the room. Its eyes were dull and red, saliva dripped from its mouth, and it appeared as though it were going to fall over at any moment.

The waiter dropped the tray he was carrying and ran for the kitchen door. The people, who were seated nearest the dog, all got up and moved away. One or two climbed up on their chairs and two small children were lifted onto tables. With all the commotion the dog seemed to wake up and ran into the room with surprising speed. We didn't move as the dog darted about, as if performing a crazy circus trick. As it veered towards them, people shied away from it. Others followed the waiter through the kitchen door.

"Stop moving around or he may go for you!" shouted a policeman from the door. I saw that he had a revolver in his hand.

At the sound of the loud voice, the dog stopped in the middle of the room and peered around, rather bewildered. Then it lowered its head slowly. As it did this, more frothy saliva drooled onto the floor.

"You two behind the dog, move slowly to your right. I'm going to have to shoot it. I don't want you in my line of fire."

"Oh dear," said Mother. She picked up Marjory and held her firmly against her chest so that Marjory couldn't see what was going on. The policeman raised his revolver and shot the dog. I jumped. The dog fell to the ground, blood seeping from the back of its head.

"Good shot," said someone in the room.

"I think we'd better get out of here while they clean up the mess," Father suggested. "Don't go near the dog," he added.

"Why?" I asked.

"The poor dog was rabid," Father answered. "And rabies is fatal to humans."

While in Abbottabad I was sent to school for the second time in my life. It was an army day school and there were approximately twenty children attending it throughout the year. The students were of all ages and there was only one teacher who spent most of her time with the older children. Here I was introduced to the rudiments of reading, writing and arithmetic, which I did not enjoy. I felt out of place and could not make any friends. I got on much better with the servants' children at the hotel. Consequently my Hindi improved. Soon I was fluent. I also learned to fly a kite, a common pastime in Pakistan at certain times of the year.

One day, when I was home from school, Father told Marjory and me that he was going on a long trip and would be away for about three months.

"Where are you going, Daddy, not to the war again?" asked Marjory.

"No. It's not to the war, but to a place a long way north of here. It's the wrong time of year or we would all be going together. At this time of year it would be too dangerous for you and Mother to go. I'm going to come back in three months to collect you."

"Where is this place?" I asked.

"It's called Kashgar, in Chinese Turkestan. It takes a few weeks to get there if you have a full caravan. That's why I'm travelling lightly now, so I can get there before the rivers flood and become impassable. When I come back to collect you it will be autumn and the rivers will be lower and easier to cross. Leaving now will also give me a chance to get things ready for you and your mother."

"If you're not going to the war what job will you be doing there?" I asked.

"I'm being lent out to the British Foreign Service as a Vice Consul. They also need my skills as a doctor."

"When will you be leaving?" asked Marjory.

"Next week, if all the arrangements can be made—the sooner the better, I've been told. There's a large glacier and two mountain passes to be crossed and, if it gets too warm, we could be delayed for a long time by flooding." Father was a conscientious man and I knew he'd find a way to reach Kashgar, no matter the obstacles.

Early one morning, a week later, I was still in bed when I heard a heavy vehicle drive up to the front door. I sat up. Through the mosquito net I could see that an army truck had arrived. A soldier got out and came to the front door.

"Is Dr. Binns ready?" the soldier called.

"Yes," I could hear Mother answer.

"How much luggage is there?"

"Not much. It's out on the veranda, ready for you. Pat's just gone down to the hospital to see a couple of patients before he leaves. He told me to tell you to pack up the truck and he'll be back in about half an hour."

"Thank you, ma'am," the soldier replied and started loading the truck with Father's bags.

Quietly I tip-toed out on to the veranda to watch. Suddenly Mother was standing behind me.

"You're up early, aren't you Bernard?"

"The truck woke me. I don't want to miss Daddy leaving."

"Go and put some clothes on. He won't be back for a little while and he won't leave without saying goodbye. I'll get Marjory up."

Fifteen minutes later Father returned. "Is everything ready to go?" he asked, looking at his watch. "I should already be on the road."

By this time the family had gathered on the veranda. "Are you sure you have everything you need, Pat?" asked Mother.

"I think so. Warm clothing and my papers. I should have enough money to get me there. The Indian Army's paying the bills. All I need is some emergency funds."

"Remember to write us as soon as you get there," Mother said, and reached up to straighten Father's collar, as she was always doing to me, much to my annoyance. "We'll all miss you. The next few months are going to pass slowly."

"It'll be three or four weeks before I get to Kashgar and the mail back will take even longer. It's possible you won't hear from me until I get back in the autumn to collect you and the children. But I'll write as soon as I arrive. As far as I know, there's no other way of getting a message to you."

Father stepped over to me, bent down and gave me a hug. "Look after your mother and be a good boy while I'm away."

Then he picked up Marjory, gave her a hug and kiss. "Bye bye, Marjory. Be good. You'll be much bigger when I see you next."

He kissed Mother, said goodbye, and climbed into the truck. The driver ground the truck into gear and edged out onto the main road. Father leaned out the window and waved at us as the truck gathered speed. A cloud of dust and dry leaves swirled behind them.

My father's job in Kashgar had come about by chance. He was working as an anaesthetist for a surgeon who happened to be a colonel in the Indian Army. The colonel had been asked by his commanders to find a doctor to work for the British Consular Service in Kashgar and while operating over a patient he had asked my father if he would be interested. My adventurous father couldn't resist the temptation of going somewhere exotic. Later on, he admitted to me that he thought the experience would either "kill me or cure me," but he couldn't say no to the opportunity.

Mother, Marjory and I stayed in Abbottabad for the next three months. I continued to attend school during the mornings. Because of Father's army rank our family was allowed to use the army club facilities, which included a swimming pool. Mother decided that it would be a good thing for me to learn how to swim, so, several times a week, we all went to the pool after school. I was frightened of the water after what had happened to me in Cannanore, but with a lot of coaxing from Mother, I eventually lost my fear and put my head under. I learned how to dog paddle across the width of the pool. One day, one of the young men at the club took me out to the deep end and, to my horror, threw me in and left me to fend for myself. I remember I got to the side coughing and spluttering. Everyone thought it was a great achievement and I felt proud of myself, but I wasn't sure why.

By September 1943 we had been in Abbottabad for nine months and Father had been gone for three. One afternoon, when I got back from school, Mother announced, "We are moving to Srinagar the day after tomorrow. Remember to say goodbye to your school friends and the teacher tomorrow. Today you can decide what toys you want to take with you. Show me the toys you want to take, the rest we can leave for the servants' children. We don't want to take anything too big if we can help it."

"Why are we going to Srinagar?" I asked.

"Because it's nearer to the start of the trail to Kashgar," Mother explained. "We'll be leaving for Kashgar from Srinagar in two or three weeks. I got a letter from the Consular Service this morning. Your father is on his way down to pick us up there. Srinagar is one of the holiday stations for expats in India. A lot of people go there for local leave. There are some very beautiful lakes in the area, and other famous attractions. We may be able to see some of them while we wait. I've a friend there who will show us all the sights."

I was glad to be leaving school. I didn't like it very much, I was bored, and I hadn't made any friends.

We were driven to Srinagar in the luxurious Consular Service car. The trip took most of the day. We stayed at the consular houseboat on the river Jhelum, the largest of the many rivers in the Indian state of Punjab. Alexander the Great fought one of his last battles in the area. Staying on this houseboat on the river was one of the most pleasant three weeks I remember spending in India.

There were two houseboys and a cook to look after us. As part of my daily routine I used to go to the bazaar with the cook. To get there we paddled in a *shikari*, a flat-bottomed boat that was used on the rivers and lakes of Kashmir. The cook taught me how to paddle one properly and I found this useful years later when I had to paddle a canoe. The bazaar was filled with many treasures, from daggers to honey-coated treats. Here I learned to haggle over prices.

While we were in Srinagar, Mother's friend took us to see some of the famous sites. The three weeks seemed to go by very fast. Then, one morning as I clambered onto the houseboat from the *shikari*, I found a strange man sitting at the end of the gangplank. He was dressed in loose-fitting, white pajama-like trousers and jacket. His top was covered with a short-sleeved leather jacket and he had sandals on his feet. On his head he had a flat hat with a rolled circumference, like a beret. His face was broad, dark and weathered. His eyes were brown and there was a smile in them. When he saw me he got hurriedly to his feet. "You must be *Chota-Sahib* Binns. I am Suggi and I have come to take you, your mother and sister to meet Dr. Binns who has arrived from Kashgar. Where is your mother? I will explain everything to her," he said in English.

"I think she's gone out with her friend, but she should be back soon. Where is my father and why didn't he come with you?"

"He is one day away by truck, arranging for the caravan to go to Kashgar. There is not much time and he has to be there to get everything organised. We should be leaving tomorrow morning. It takes almost a whole day to get to your father. I have a letter for your mother explaining everything."

"She shouldn't be long because it's lunch time," I said. "You'd better come onto the boat and wait there. If you need anything you can ask the houseboy who is usually at the back near the kitchen."

Mother arrived for lunch. When I explained about Suggi, she said that she'd been expecting him and everything was ready to go. I called for Suggi and he gave Mother the letter. After informing us he'd get the bus to come for us in the morning, he left.

I could see Mother was both apprehensive and expectant. I'm sure she was eager to see Father again and to get settled in our new home. Our peripatetic existence had become wearing on all of us. While it would be a relief to be settled, a dangerous journey lay ahead; the next three years would take us on a journey into a totally mysterious world.

After Suggi was gone, I went back to my room to make sure all my things were packed, especially my only stuffed toy, a long-eared rabbit doll that I called Freddy. I remember sitting on the bed wondering what Mother had meant when she said she was not sure how things were going to turn out.

Chapter 2
Over the Himalayas to Kashgar

In the fall of 1943 my mother, sister and I began the journey to Kashgar in Chinese Turkestan. We travelled from Srinagar by bus with our servant, Suggi, to meet Father who was waiting for us at the start of the mountain pass. The route took us out of the forested area of Srinagar and into an open, flat, semi-arid landscape strewn with boulders of various sizes and intriguing shapes. As the day passed, the air became noticeably dryer.

Around noon we started climbing into the hills, which were covered by scattered grasses and a few stunted trees. A short time later we came to a river that we followed upstream. At first the river was quite wide, flowing fast over large rocks, creating white-water areas and large whirlpools. Small willows interspersed with birch, tamarisk and other smaller bushes grew along its banks. As we wound our way up river, the number of trees thinned and the volume of water rushing past lessened. Eventually the bus rounded a corner, slowed down and, to my surprise, drove straight to the water's edge and came to an abrupt stop.

The driver got up and came over to where we were seated.

"M'sahib, we have to cross the river here. It looks as if there is much water today. I think you and the children should get out and wait to see how it goes."

Looking around, I saw no people, no signs of habitation. Where the bus had stopped the river was quite wide with an island in the middle. There were no tire marks or other evidence of buses or trucks having gone through recently, but I presumed the driver knew where he was going and what he was doing. Suggi, who had been riding on the top of the bus, came over to us.

"There was a lot of water yesterday. The river was up by those trees behind us. I think we will get across today and not have to go back."

"If the bus gets over, how are we going to get across?" asked my mother.

"I will carry you so that you do not get wet, M'sahib," he replied.

"I think I may have to wade across myself. I will be far too heavy for you, Suggi."

"No, M'sahib, I am strong and can carry you easily."

"Well, let's see if the bus makes it first."

We stood on the shore and watched the driver edge the bus slowly into the river. As it moved on towards the island, the bus started rocking from side to side in slow motion. Halfway to the island it lurched sideways. Water now flowed over the top of the bus's wheels, almost tipping it over; then the current caught the back end and swung the vehicle round to face upstream. Shouting, the driver and his two assistants jumped out of the bus into the water and tried to hold it facing into the current.

"I will go and help," said Suggi, who ran off into the water.

The noise of the engine revving and the men shouting, heaving, and splashing continued for several minutes, but eventually they managed to get the bus back onto the shallower part of the ford. Once there, the bus was able to make slow progress onto the gravelly island, and then manoeuvre to the other side of the river without further trouble.

"I suppose it's our turn now," Mother said to Suggi.

"Yes, M'sahib. Who's going to be first?"

"Bernard, you go first, then Marjory. That way you can look after Marjory on the other side while I come across."

Suggi knelt down and I climbed onto his back. He stood up and waded across the ford. I was surprised by how sure-footed he was. "Do you have to do this often?" I asked.

"Yes. There are many difficult rivers to cross in Hunza and on the road to Kashgar."

Marjory came over next and seemed to enjoy her piggyback ride. Mother was not so happy, but Suggi was true to his word and he had no trouble carrying her across without her even getting her feet wet. There were three more fords to cross that afternoon, but we were able to stay in the bus as the water level had dropped markedly by the time we had to cross them.

In the late afternoon we rounded a bend and there, in front of us, was a small village of mud-walled huts. This was no ordinary village—there were hundreds of horses, donkeys, camels and a few yaks, all tethered to long heavy ropes that were, in turn, held to the ground by big wooden stakes. Caravan men looked after all the animals. They were fierce-looking people who wore long flowing robes, leather knee-length boots and ragged turbans. Some of them wore the same rolled woollen hats that Suggi wore. Most had whips and long knives stuck into their cloth cummerbund belts. The bus slowed down and drove through the mass of animals and men until it came to a small clearing in front of a stone building covered by a rusty corrugated roof. Someone had attempted to whitewash the walls at one time, but most of the paint had washed away or rubbed off. The building had a veranda along the front and standing on the veranda was my father.

As the bus came to a stop he climbed in.

"Welcome to Bandipura," he said, his hands making an awkward gesture, his voice wavering. "How nice to see you all again," he said, lifting Marjory out of her seat and giving her a hug. "I think there's some tea ready for you. How was the trip?"

"Not too bad," Mother said, "although the bus almost got stuck at the first ford and Suggi had to carry us across. We all got a bit dusty, I'm afraid, and could use a good washing. Can we get baths here?"

"It's a bit primitive but there will be some hot water in about an hour and we can all wash up then."

"How long will we be staying here, Daddy?" I asked.

"One or two days at the most. I think we've managed to select the horses and caravan men we need to get us to Gilgit. It'll take us about two weeks to get there. Then we'll stay at Gilgit for a few days while we hire another caravan to take us all the way to Kashgar."

"Why can't we take the same horses all the way?" I asked.

"The caravan men and horses here only go to Gilgit and Afghanistan. They're not used to the route through Hunza and into Chinese Turkestan. Some of them say it is too far and others are frightened

29

because of the difficult trails along the mountain cliffs and over the Batura glacier on the other side of Hunza." He paused and placed his hand on my shoulder. "Let's go and have tea. We can talk more about the journey then. It's not really as bad as all that."

Father had already done the trip twice and was clearly confident with what he knew about what we faced.

Tea was served on a rickety old table on the veranda, which overlooked the river about a hundred yards away. I could not see the caravan animals or the herdsmen from where we were sitting but I could hear and smell them.

"How many horses will we need?" I asked.

"They say sixteen. We have quite a bit of luggage with us. There will be a few more needed. The caravan men will be taking some of their own merchandise to sell in Gilgit. The men I've chosen are from that area and know the road well. Suggi and Izatu, the cook, both come from Hunza and speak the same language as the caravan men, which will make things easier."

"Do we all have to ride horses?" asked Mother. "Neither of the children has ever been on a horse before."

"I asked about that and the caravan men assure me they have some good riding ponies for Bernard and Marjory. Don't worry. They'll be led all the time. There shouldn't be any danger."

"I'm glad to hear that. How good a cook is Izatu, and can he speak English?"

"He's quite a good cook but doesn't speak much English. He seems to understand a lot more than he can say; I've not had any trouble getting him to understand how I want things cooked."

"But you speak some Urdu," said Mother. "That must make it easier."

"I think you'll find everything will work out, Ada. Suggi can always interpret if worst comes to the worst. Izatu is supposed to be one of the best cooks available in Gilgit and he is willing to go all the way to Kashgar. They have both been there before and know their way around. They can also speak Turkic, the language spoken in Kashgar. That will be a great help," said Father.

After tea I went for a walk through the small village and caravan campsite. The trees in the valley bottom were mainly willow, but further up the hillsides I could see some pines and other evergreens. The river was clear and fast running and flowed right past the caravan men's camp. As I walked around I counted several hundred horses and donkeys and a few camels. I had not seen camels before and was surprised to see how big and ungainly they appeared. They were also noisy. There was a strong smell of animal urine and manure. Many of the camels had rope muzzles over their heads and I learned later that this was to stop them from biting.

The horses were of two kinds. Most were small, powerfully built ponies. Many had scars on their backs where I presumed packs had been placed. Some had fresh sores that were red, weeping and covered with flies. The other horses were much bigger and more handsome. They didn't have any scars on them. As I was standing looking at the animals one of the caravan men came up to me.

"Do you like the horses?" he asked in Hindi.

"Yes, but the big ones look too big for me. I've never been on a horse."

"I will show you how to ride. You have a long way to go and you don't want to fall off in the mountains. That would be bad."

At that moment Father came over from the rest house. "What are you doing? Not bothering anyone, I hope."

The caravan man, who perhaps worried he'd done something wrong, shook his head.

"I was looking at the horses. The caravan man says he will teach me how to ride."

"We were going to do that tomorrow but the hot water for your bath won't be ready for another hour. Why don't you have a go now if you want to?"

"Father says you can start to teach me now if you want," I said to the caravan man in Hindi.

"That is a good idea. Come with me. I have a horse over there already saddled. It is a quiet animal for Memsahib to take his first ride. The one we have chosen for you does not have a saddle on at the moment," he replied. He guided Father and me to the far side of the camp, near some rather bedraggled tents. On the way we passed several groups of men speaking a language I hadn't heard before.

"Where do those men come from?" I asked the caravan man.

"They are from Afghanistan. They will be leaving in the morning and will be going by a different route from ours."

We arrived at the tents where ten to fifteen horses were tethered. These horses looked better cared for than the pack horses I had seen earlier. Two of them had on saddles and bridles.

"These are the riding horses. This brown mare is the horse for you to learn on. First we must get the stirrups set right for you." He threw up the leather side of the saddle so that he could adjust them. The saddle was deep, covered with sheepskin, and it had a handle in the front that I could hang onto. I was reassured because it seemed a very long way up into the saddle. After he had shortened the stirrups he tightened the girth, explaining that if this was not done the saddle would slip around the horse when I mounted it and cause me to wind up under the horse. I didn't like the sound of that. The whole idea of getting on the horse was a bit frightening.

"We need to find a big stone for you to stand on. Then I will show you how to get your foot into the stirrup and swing up into the saddle."

He led the horse to the edge of the camp, where the trail left the village. At the side of the track there were many large stones from which to choose. He selected one that was about two feet high and fairly flat on top.

"This is a good stone for you. You climb up onto it and I will hold the horse so that you can hold onto the saddle with your left hand and put your left foot in the stirrup. You can use your right hand to help guide your foot into place. Remember, keep the horse's head to your left as you face the saddle. If you do not do this you will end up facing the tail when you climb up. Everyone will laugh."

He led the horse around so that I could reach the handle of the saddle with my left hand. I did this and managed to get my foot into the stirrup. Just as I started to pull myself up the horse decided to swing away from me. I lost my balance and my grip on the saddle. I fell off the stone, rolled right under the horse on my back and found myself looking up between the horse's hind legs.

"Wowa!" shouted the caravan man. "Don't move, Chota-Sahib, or the horse may be frightened and kick you." Hearing his instructions, I rolled onto my side, and put my hands over my head and waited. The horse then stepped away, carefully avoiding me.

"Good. I told you she was a gentle animal. We will try again. This time, don't let go of the saddle when your foot is in the stirrup. Once you have got a hold of the saddle and your foot is in the stirrup, it does not matter if the horse moves away from you. Just hang on and pull yourself up."

My second attempt was successful and I found myself in the saddle. Immediately I became aware of how high up I was.

This unsettled me, which the caravan man must have noticed. "Just sit there and look straight ahead for a minute. It is not that far to the ground and, to start with, you can hang onto the handle in front of you."

I was already hanging onto the saddle with both hands for dear life. I thought for sure I was going to fall off. Luckily this didn't happen and after a minute or so I did get used to the height and felt more at ease.

"Now you can put your other foot into the other stirrup. Just slide it in gently or you will make the horse walk or run and you do not want that to happen until you are ready. At the moment, I am holding the horse's bridle so you do not have to worry."

After giving these instructions, he began walking the horse around the campsite. I soon got used to the feel of sitting on a moving animal and became confident enough to take one hand off the pommel. We had walked around for about ten minutes when he said, "I am going to move faster so the horse will start to trot. When this happens you will start to bounce. You will find it uncomfortable, so you have to sit up and down in time with the horse or you will get a sore bum."

When he did get the horse to trot I found it quite easy and began to enjoy the ride more. At this point my instructor got rather winded and we had to stop for a rest. "I think that is enough for today," he panted. "I will teach you some more basics tomorrow morning. You will not have any trouble with horses." Then he helped me dismount.

The next day Marjory and I had some more practice on the horses. The caravan man put me onto a small but well-behaved Kashmir pony. He taught me how to control the pony and I was allowed to walk it around the campsite and village on my own. On these rides I saw many stray animals and smelled the familiar aromas of Indian cooking. People asked where I came from and where we were going. When I told them we were going to Kashgar they were surprised. They said it was a long way, that the journey was difficult, and that the way there went up very high into the mountains.

Early the next morning we started for Gilgit. Our caravan consisted of eighteen pack horses and our four riding horses. The luggage had all been packed into crates and boxes about four feet long by two to three feet square. Each horse carried two crates or boxes. If the packs were thought to be light by the caravan men, they piled more things on top of the boxes. Some of the packs were made up of sewn gunny sacking and contained rolls of unknown merchandise. I asked Suggi about them. He told me they belonged to the caravan men and that they contained cloth and carpets from Afghanistan, which would be traded in Gilgit.

The first day the trail followed the river for about fifteen miles and continued up the valley that we had followed a few days before. Soon after we left the village the track started to climb and the terrain became more rugged. By lunch time the sun was getting hot so we stopped near a large pond surrounded by willows, distant from any villages. The caravan that had left before us was well out of sight. After lunch we lingered in the shade of one of the older trees.

"Did you know that Bernard can swim now, Pat?" Mother asked Father.

"No. When did this happen? How good is he?"

"He's been swimming several lengths of the pool in Abbottabad for months and recently dove off the top board."

"Bernard, would you like to show me how well you can swim? You can have a go in the pond here. I'm sure it's deep enough."

"You're sure it'll be all right? I won't upset the caravan men, will I?"

"No. We all had a swim on the way down the other day. The other caravan men probably went for a swim this morning when they came by. You'll find it a bit cold but it's not too bad. I'd like to see you swim."

I took off my clothes, dove into the water and swam across the pond. Father was right, the water was freezing. I didn't stay in for long and noticed that no one else seemed interested. Father clapped enthusiastically as I climbed out and congratulated me on my swimming.

As we followed the contours of the land, we rose, higher and higher into the hills. Now the sun set earlier and the temperature dropped quickly. When we arrived at our next stop, Izatu prepared an early supper.

"What did you think of the first day's trek? Are you and Marjory sore from sitting on a horse all day?" Father asked, after we had eaten.

"It was fun. The insides of my legs are a bit sore, though," I said.

"Most people get sore legs their first few days on horseback. The stiffness will wear off in a day or two. Try walking for a while every hour. That should provide some relief. Today was an easy day. Tomorrow our climb gets steeper. In three days we'll cross over the first big pass. It's called the Burzil Pass and isn't too difficult. You should find it exciting."

I asked Father what he meant by a 'pass' and he explained that it was a route through the high mountains. He went on to tell me that the Himalayan Mountains were a great watershed that drove rivers to flow either south into India or north to China. They were the highest and most rugged mountains in the world. We needed to cross over three passes and a glacier to get to Kashgar, he continued. The highest pass we would have to conquer was the Mintaka at just over 18,000 feet.

Our path followed one of the Silk Routes that had been used to take spices and cloth between India and China and then on to Europe. Marco Polo was one of the first Europeans to travel to China by land and his adventures in the northern part of the route, from Afghanistan to China, were documented in his book *Il Milione*. Marco Polo had stopped in Kashgar on his outward bound journey to China in 1271.

The route my family took linked present-day Pakistan to the northern Silk Road. The first leg followed one of the tributaries of the Indus River into the mountains. To get to Gilgit, the track climbed up over a saddle between two lower mountains of the range. This was the Burzil Pass.

During the next few days we continued following the river upstream, fording it when the terrain demanded. By now there was not as much water in the river, so crossing was not a problem for the horses. The caravan men told me that at certain times of the year there was so much water flowing downstream that the horses could not get across and they might have to wait several days for the level of the water to drop. This was especially true in the spring with the snow-melt. We averaged about fifteen miles a day of fairly easy travel. Each day we seemed to come closer to the clouds that circled the mountains and my lungs hurt whenever I tried to run. Shortness of breath did not appear to bother the caravan men or animals.

One evening Father told us that we would be starting early in the morning because we had to get over the Burzil Pass and down the other side in one day. We started at dawn. As usual, the caravan men and pack animals had gone ahead an hour or so earlier. To start with, there did not seem to be much difference in the trail but after an hour it left the river and ascended steeply. As we continued to climb, the track cut into the side of the mountain. While the track was wide enough, the mountain sloped away at a forty-five degree angle down to the river.

We soon emerged above the tree line and, looking back, caught our first clear view of the country we had travelled through during the past few days. The view was breathtaking. I hadn't realised how high we had come. Some of the distant peaks were capped with snow. Snow was new to me and I had to ask the man leading my horse what the white stuff was. He was surprised and tried to explain what snow was like. In winter, he told me, at least two or three feet of snow could fall and blanket the earth. He added that even in summer there were times when snow fell on the trail, but summer snowfalls were not usually deeper than a few inches and usually melted in a day or two.

At this point our progress slowed and the track became dangerous. The terrain grew rugged and turned greyish-red in colour. Where the sun lit the mountainsides, this colour contrasted starkly with the shaded areas below and the white snow above. Beyond the tree line, only scant grass, mosses and the occasional small bush grew. This late in the season, no flowers bloomed.

Shortly after coming out of the trees, the track went round the side of the mountain and I could see it continuing up towards peaks in the distance. Packhorses and caravan men spread out a mile or so ahead of us. The animals struggled and I could hear the men shouting at them. The sound travelled easily in the clear, rarefied air. It seemed a long way to the saddle between the peaks and I remembered that we had to go down the other side before getting to the next rest house.

"How long will it take to get to the top and down the other side?" I asked a caravan man.

"Oh, three or four hours to the top, and then about five to the rest house. It is a long day, but the weather is good so there should be no problems."

"What could go wrong?" I asked.

"Sometimes there are storms here with strong winds, rain and snow. Then we have to go back if we can. Sometimes, if we cannot go back, we have to camp on the side of the mountain. That is not good for the animals or for us. If they get frightened they can fall down the mountain and we lose the packs and the animals. Occasionally an animal will die because they are not used to the thin air in the high mountains. Then we have to reload the other animals. This is not easy to do farther up the trail, where it gets narrower. So, you see, many things can happen here. But today the weather is good and there should not be any trouble," he repeated to reassure me.

As we continued up the side of the mountain we stopped to look at the panoramic view of the rugged Himalayas, as if at a grand performance. Our height above the river was frightening. Although I could see the water breaking over the rocks in the river bed we were so far up I couldn't hear the river's rush. Such quietness was eerie.

Soon after midday we finally reached the Burzil Pass and I could now see the full extent of the mountain range as they extended north as far as the eye could see. Far below us there was another river and in the distance more snow-covered mountains. I couldn't imagine how we were going to get through them in the next few weeks.

"Rather a spectacular view, isn't it?" said Father who had stopped at the top and was waiting for us to catch up.

"They go on forever," said Mother.

"Once we get down to the river you can see in the distance there, the rest of the trip to Gilgit will be much like it's been for the past few days. Even so, it will take another week for us to reach the Indus River, which we have to cross to get to Gilgit. The next rest house is located back in the trees. It's quite quaint with a small mountain stream running past it. Since it's not too cold, and there's no wind, we'll stop here for lunch."

While we were eating our sandwiches, I studied the mountains we had to go through and wondered if any animals could live in this wild, barren land. During the past two weeks we had been through some villages and there were always a few people at the rest houses, but what I was seeing now looked very hostile. Not an easy place to live in at all. As we started the descent I was still thinking about this and asked the caravan man leading my horse, "Do many people live on this side of the pass?"

"Between here and the Indus there are three small villages. The biggest is Astor, which is ten days from here. We will stay there the day before we cross the Indus. Beyond that there is Chilas and Bunji before we get to Gilgit."

"What about animals? I haven't seen any in the past few days."

"That is because you do not know where or how to look for them. There are plenty of wild animals, but they are up in the mountains and are not easy to spot. Many of them do not come out in the day. There are some mountain sheep, which I will show you if I see some on the slopes. Wolves and a few snow leopards live here, but you do not see them often. Marmots live in the ground and there are plenty of them. You will see them as we go down the mountain today. When we get near the trees we may see some *chucours* and pheasants, which we eat if we can catch them. Near the villages there are sparrows, other small birds, crows and pigeons. There are migratory birds that come through twice a year—ducks, geese, ravens and some big hawks. The ducks and geese fly over the mountains and go to China and Russia, but they stop here in the valleys on their way north or south. In the trees you will see some squirrels, and there are mice and rats. So it is not as barren as it looks."

"Please tell me where to look when you see them."

It was late afternoon and the sun was just tucking in behind a mountain when he stopped my horse. "Look, up the slope to your left. Where the top is very rocky against the sky—there are some big mountain sheep."

I looked up to where he was pointing but could not see anything but rocks. Then as I continued to look I saw a movement and recognised the outlines of animals. There were eight mountain sheep about three-quarters of a mile away. Once I had seen them they were fairly easy to distinguish in the waning light. They stood very still, watching us, while we watched them.

"What do they find to eat up there?"

"They eat grass, mosses and small bushes. In the winter they come down from the mountains to the valleys where there is more food. They are very good climbers and can go almost anywhere in the mountains. They stay away from us. We hunt them for food when we can get near them."

We resumed our trek and were soon back into the trees. Reaching a small river, the trail turned, following the river downstream. Eventually it would join the Indus. As a crescent moon slipped into the sky, we reached the rest house where we stayed the night.

Most rest houses consisted of four walls and a mud floor. Inside were separate bedrooms with sleeping platforms on which we placed the bedding we had brought with us. There was a table and chairs for eating, but the kitchen was out the back in an area with a wood fire. The cooking utensils and most of our food were carried on the pack horses. We got our water from wells or took it directly from rivers. We had been buying fresh eggs and produce along the way, but Father warned us that there would be no more rest houses and no more fresh produce after the Mintaka Pass.

Two days later, as we rounded a bend in the trail, I looked up and saw a mountain that was much higher than any others near it. The sun shone on its peak making its snow cap brilliant against the blue sky. Although this mountain was still a long way off, it dominated the landscape.

"Does that mountain have a name?" I asked Father who was just ahead of me on the trail.

"Yes. It's called Nanga Parbat and is over 26,000 feet high. It's famous amongst mountaineers because of its difficulties and the superstitions that surround it. A number of people have tried to climb it and have failed. Some have lost their lives on that mountain. The locals say that it's impossible to climb, but I expect someone will find a way one day."

Nanga Parbat, the ninth-highest mountain in the world, continued to dominate the scenery for the next three days. The trail came quite close to its base. Here the mountain's size and magnificence were overpowering and overwhelming. Never before had I felt so tiny. So insignificant.

Days after leaving Nanga Parbat behind, we came to the Indus River, the largest river on the western subcontinent. Even as far up in the mountains as we were, the Indus was large and muddy, flooding through a gorge with high reddish-brown walls. We had to cross the river using a bridge that was suspended over the gorge. From a distance the bridge looked precarious, as if spun by a spider. When we reached the bridge we were met by a very old, white-bearded gatekeeper, who waited for us in a small room at our end of the bridge. In a large ledger, with a green cover, he kept a record of all the people who crossed the bridge

"Salaam, Dr. Binns. You are back with your family I see."

"Yes, Abdul. We are going all the way to Kashgar this trip."

"You must sign the book for all of you."

The gatekeeper brought the book out and Father signed us all in before looking through it to see if he recognised any of the names of previous travellers.

"This book goes back many years, Abdul. How long have you been in charge of the book?"

"Forty years!" he said with great pride. "You know, sahib, I have never seen any English children come this way before. Your son and daughter must be the first to cross over this bridge."

"That's interesting. We hope to come back this way in a year, so we will see you then," said Father as we moved out of the room to start the crossing.

"God willing," Abdul said.

Father, realizing the bridge did not look that secure, tried to re-assure us. "I know, this suspension bridge feels and looks rather rick-ety. Walking over it will feel unsafe because it moves, but it is not real-ly that scary once you get used to the movement. All will be well if you keep your balance. If you feel uneasy, don't look down at the water. That will only make you feel worse. Keep your eyes focussed on the end of the bridge. Suggi will carry Marjory and Izatu will hold Ber-nard's hand. I will help you, Ada," he said, taking my mother's hand.

We stepped onto the bridge and began our swaying walk over the Indus. The bridge was wide enough to take one laden packhorse, the surface made of wooden planks nailed to cross pieces that were lashed to cables. The entire bridge was suspended on two heavy cables which stretched the entire length of the crossing, about two to three hundred feet. These supporting cables were suspended from two large stone structures on either side of the gorge. The sides of the bridge were made up of gunny sacking and rope netting, which was held in position by ropes going vertically from the top cables to the floor structure. I could see easily through the sides to the fast moving water below, and immediately felt my legs weaken and begin to tremble.

The whole construction did not look safe to me. We had been told that it would be okay to ride over on the horses if we wanted, but Father thought it would be easier and safer for us to walk. At the beginning of our crossing, the bridge moved slightly, but as we got about a third of the way over, it started to sway from side to side and the floor began to undulate, making walking and keeping balanced precarious.

There was a rope hand-hold on one side of the bridge, but to use it you had to go over to the edge of the bridge which made the sight of the gorge and river far, far below even more terrifying. Falling into the river meant certain death. Izatu was a calming influence, although I don't ever remember gripping someone's hand that hard before. Marjory seemed comfortable on Suggi's back, but I noticed she had her eyes closed. Father, on the other hand, who had been over the bridge twice before, was not concerned, and made the mistake of gloating; while Mother, who appeared to take the crossing in her stride, was not at all pleased about the experience. When we reached the safety of the other side, she vented her fury.

"Pat, if you had told me about this bridge, I would never have come with you! Are there any more bridges like that one?"

"There are a couple more, but they're not as long and they don't sway quite as much," my Father reassured her, not daring to smile.

"Well, I suppose we'll get used to these things as we get more experience," she replied, composing herself, while attempting to set a brave example for Marjory and me.

The closer we got to Gilgit, the more people and small villages we saw. Gilgit was bigger than any of the villages or stops we had passed through since leaving Srinagar. The main street was lined with Indian *duchas* or shops which sold every kind of merchandise, many of them highly scented. The smell of perfumes and incense mingled with the distinct aromas of Indian foods, which were cooked and sold in the open. The street bustled. Suggi and Izatu explained that Gilgit was the main trading centre before going north to China, west to Kabul in

Afghanistan, via Peshawar, or southwest to India. We had come from the southeast. In total, four major caravan routes met in Gilgit.

We spent five days at the rest house in Gilgit, on the edge of the town, near a small river, surrounded by willow, popular, mulberry and apricot trees. It was the end of summer and the apricots were ripe. We ate them right off the trees. Suggi took Marjory and me into town several times to meet and see all the people who had travelled from so many different places. Many of the things on sale I had never seen before. There were brilliant coloured silks and cottons from China. There was one shop that sold only knives and I must have spent an hour there. In his best tradesman style, the shopkeeper showed me knives from as far away as Egypt and southern China. Another shop specialised in carpets from Morocco to Tibet.

Marjory and I were forbidden, by our parents, from eating any local foods; they felt they were not safe. Nonetheless we sampled all the foods we were offered and I suppose it was a combination of luck and acquired immunity from living in India that saved us from the ravages of dysentery, cholera, and other problems.

During our short stay in Gilgit, Father hired a new caravan of twenty horses driven by Turki caravan men. Suggi told us the next phase of our journey would be longer and more dangerous than the trip from Srinagar. Father disagreed; it wasn't any worse, only longer.

Our first few days back on the trail reminded me of our travels up the left bank of the Hunza River. On the fifth day the valley narrowed and the river danced and swirled much faster. There were a few villages whose terraced fields and fruit orchards stepped up the hills that skirted the mountains. As the day wore on the track moved away from the river and etched a fine line into the mountainside.

As we rounded a corner a single mountain loomed up before us, as if its image were cast on a massive cinema screen, presented suddenly, rising from the banks of the river, straight up into the sky, reaching for something beyond the mist and clouds. The gods, perhaps. Layers of green vegetation and willow trees changed into bands of conifers, before becoming bare rock. Craning my neck, I could see glaciers and the snow-covered peak against the sky. It was magnificent, almost other-worldly, the way everything else seemed to rest against it. And rely on it for definition.

This was the most dramatic vista I had ever seen (including all the mountain ranges in Europe and America I would see over the next seventy years).

"Does *that* mountain have a name?" I asked Father.

"I think it's called Rakaposhi. It's very famous because the mountain starts at 6,000 feet, by the river there, and is 25,555 feet at the top. There's no other mountain whose face rises as abruptly, so high and steep."

"How close do we get to it?"

"We go past the base tomorrow. Then we are into the rugged and chiselled Karakoram Mountains. Baltit, the capital of Hunza, is a few days away yet."

During the next four days the Hunza River became a gorge. We climbed up the side on a track that was cut out of the rock face, exposing a sheer drop in places on our right of several thousand feet. The silent river glistened at the bottom like a skein of silk. The track was barely wide enough for two laden horses to pass. In fact, in some of the higher sections, which were several miles long, I wondered if such a manoeuvre would even be possible.

"What do you do when another caravan comes the other way?" I asked the man leading my horse.

"It does not happen very often, but when it does, one caravan comes to a stop and the horses are held close to the rock face so there is enough room for the others to go by. Sometimes, if a horse gets excited, it will fall over or cause another to go over the edge to the bottom. When this happens there is a great palaver because someone has to pay for the loss. Do not worry, Sahib, we will not let you ride when we pass other horses."

Even in this bleak land our caravan passed through pockets of people living in small villages. Most were situated on tributaries of the Hunza River. When we arrived all the villagers would come out and stare at us. Mother, Marjory and I attracted particular interest because they had probably never seen a white woman or children before.

Our arrival in Baltit (Karimabad), the capital of Hunza (an independent princely state until 1974, now governed by Pakistan), was obviously expected. A large crowd of people had gathered to greet us. At the head of the crowd stood a platoon of soldiers in ceremonial dress.

"The Mir of Hunza, Mohammad Ghazan Khan the Second, is expecting us," Father explained. "I met him on the way down. He has asked me to stay a day or so to see some patients. We will have a chance to rest and clean up before we start the next stage of our journey. The rest house here in Baltit is especially comfortable. The Mir is an educated man. He attended university in Oxford and speaks very good English. He'll probably invite the adults up to the palace for a meal. I don't think you children will be expected to attend, but I will ask."

Mother immediately panicked, worried about what she would wear, but Father reassured her that casual dress would be fine. I sensed that Mother wasn't fully convinced. Nonetheless she didn't pursue the issue.

When we reached the crowd and the platoon, the officer in charge marched over to us, came to a halt and saluted. "His Royal Highness, the Mir of Hunza, welcomes you. He has ordered me to take all of you to the rest house and then to escort the doctor to the Palace for a meeting with His Highness. Please follow me." Then he about-faced and marched back to the platoon. When we got to the platoon, it divided in two; half marched in front of us and half behind. In this distinguished manner, we were escorted to the rest house, which was built next to a small tumbling stream that overlooked the valley a hundred feet below.

The town of Baltit was built on a flat plateau on one of the larger tributaries of the Hunza River and had been inhabited for centuries. At the back of the town I could see terraced fields that were larger than any we had seen so far. These fields went up both sides of the valley, getting smaller with each step, until the mountainsides became too steep to be terraced. The lush green fields ended where the river emerged from a gorge, about a mile away.

To my surprise, apple, pear, apricot, peach, and cherry trees as well as an abundance of mulberry bushes grew around the town. Standing amongst these, taller pines and firs provided some shade.

Baltit was a large township, but it was not as big as Gilgit. The houses were small, made from stones held in place with a mud-straw mixture. The roofs were thatched. As we wound our way into town I was taken aback by how many people came to their doors to greet us. Everyone smiled. Many looked very old—the state of Hunza was said to include some of the oldest people in the world. After a quick wash and change of clothes Father was escorted off to see the Mir.

Father and Mother were invited to the Palace the next evening for a meal. Marjory and I were introduced to the Mir at the beginning of the evening but were not allowed into the Palace dining room. While my parents ate dinner, we were looked after by one of the Mir's *ayahs* and met some of his children with whom we passed the evening.

After three days, we set out on the trail again. Beyond Baltit the route narrowed as we once more clambered away from the river, on what looked like a threaded line, into the jagged mountains. The track was less travelled and I felt hemmed in, almost claustrophobic, by the mountains towering over me. That evening, over dinner, Father made the following announcement.

"Tomorrow we have the Baturia Glacier to cross. The glacier is long but only a couple of miles wide. Our crossing will be slow as the track goes over bare ice, snow and rocks. There will also be a couple of ice streams to cross. They can be tricky. They fill up later in the day and turn into roaring torrents so we will have to start early in order to get across them safely. I have arranged for some yaks to carry us over the glacier. They are more sure-footed than horses. The caravan will leave before us so we won't be bothered by the pack horses and men."

"Is there any danger in crossing the glacier?" asked Mother.

"Not if you do what the guides tell you. Just watch where you put your feet when they ask you to walk."

"What's a yak, Daddy?" asked Marjory.

"It's a sort of mountain cow with long hair. They have big, gently curved horns with sharp points. Originally they came from this part of the world and there are still wild yaks roaming about. The ones used as pack and riding animals are docile, but they are very sure-footed and good for the sort of terrain we'll be going through tomorrow. The caravan men will put the packs on the yaks when they cross the glacier so that the horses can get across safely."

We rose at dawn the next day. After a couple of hours, we got our first sight of the glacier. Large boulders and irregular rocks lay embedded in ice, partly covered with shale. This mass of rock and ice extended to the horizon. The entire prospect was what I imagined the surface of a comet might look like.

"How are we going to get across this?" I asked the caravan man.

"We go up the trail here on the left for about a mile and there we will put you onto a yak. There are two paths across. You and your family will be taken over the glacier on the lower path on the backs of the yaks especially here to do that. I will have to take the horses two miles further up to where they can get across. There are more yaks on the higher path to carry the packs across. The horses are led across without their loads," he explained.

"Why don't we all go that way?" I asked.

"You could, but there is a deep ford to go over and the water is very cold. We cannot see the river here because it is under the ice, but you will hear and see it when you cross it on the ice bridge over there," he said, pointing out over the mass of rocks and ice.

We continued up the trail, with the glacier on our right, for half an hour before arriving at a small clearing that contained a few huts and the yaks.

As Father had said, they did resemble longhaired cows and their long horns looked ominous. Their legs were much shorter than the horses' legs and their long, matted hair hung down to within a few inches of the ground. Four were greyish and two had some dark brown in their coats. There was a man with each animal which he controlled with a rope that was passed through a hole in the animal's nose. Each man carried a stout stick. The yaks were already saddled; everything was set for us to start our trip across the glacier.

Because they were shorter, mounting a yak was easier than getting on a horse. My yak preferred to keep his head lowered, making me wary of his horns. I asked about these and my caravan man assured me there was no danger from the horns. The narrow track across the glacier wound its way between large rocks and boulders, some of which were bigger than houses. Between the rocks there were expanses of jagged ice and pools reflecting the electric blue sky. Small rivulets trickled down the glacier. The combination of translucent ice, greenish-blue water and bright sun produced a ghostly picture. Once we had gone a hundred yards or so onto the glacier, I could no longer see the small village we had just left, nor could I see across to the other side of the glacier. I just concentrated on staying on the yak's back.

We had been making our way for over an hour when the man leading my yak looked back at me. "Can you hear that noise, Sahib?"

"Yes. What is it?" I had noticed a slight rumbling sound a few minutes earlier, but had no idea where it came from.

"It is the underground river. It is quite big this year. You will be able to see it as soon as we get to the other side of the ice-bridge."

During the next quarter of an hour the noise gradually swelled until it became almost deafening.

"We are over the moving water now," shouted the man. He pointed down. "You cannot see it but it is there."

A few minutes later we edged around a jagged shard of ice. Over to my right I could see an enormous fountain of water rising, ten to twenty feet into the air, before crashing down onto some rocks and forming a large whirlpool that vanished into an emerald green, cavernous hole. The uproar silenced us. We all stopped to gaze at the grand spectacle before moving on.

Shortly after leaving the river behind, my yak balked at one of the many steams we had to cross. I assumed it wanted to drink. The yak man tried to urge the animal on, pulling on the nose rope. In response, the yak jumped the steam, stopping suddenly on the other side. I flew over its head, barely missing its horns. I somersaulted, landed on my rear end and lay still on the ice. The yak man hurried over to me, saw that I was not hurt, and helped lift me back onto the yak.

"Very sorry, Sahib, yaks like cats, they stop before they jump."

I'm not sure why the yak decided to jump over that particular stream rather than walk through the water. Happily it did not jump again. Once off the glacier, we transferred to the horses and continued to the next village and rest house.

That evening, after supper, we sat on the veranda overlooking another small river and my parents discussed the days ahead.

"This is Misgar, the last big village in India," Father explained. "Tomorrow we'll have a longer day than usual. The next rest house is fairly isolated and will probably be the last house we stay in until we reach Kashgar. The following day we'll cross the Mintaka Pass, which is 17,500 feet high, and then enter Chinese Turkestan."

"How much longer do we have to travel? I'm beginning to think we'll never get to Kashgar." Mother was definitely tired of travelling on horseback. I think she was fed up with pack animals, caravan men, the food, the hard beds, and longed for the company of other women.

"We've been travelling for nearly four weeks and we still have two and a half weeks to go, so we are about two-thirds of the way there. Once we get over the Mintaka Pass the trail is not as rough. Riding will be easier. There are no rest houses, though. We'll have to use our tents. If we're lucky we'll be able to stop at Kurgiz camps."

"What are Kurgiz?" asked Marjory.

"They're nomads who, at this time of year, leave the steppes for higher ground in the mountains. They herd sheep and yaks and go where there's grass. If we cross paths we should be able to stay with them. Originally they came from Mongolia. They speak their own language and are completely different from the Indians you've been with for the past few years."

Two days later we reached the summit of the Mintaka Pass. We had risen early to cross the border ahead of the rest of the caravan. At the top there was a notice standing beside a large cairn of rocks.

"What's that say?" I asked Father.

"It says we're leaving India and entering China. This is one of the borders. We're in a unique part of the world here. Within a few miles of this spot there are two other borders. We're standing at the junction of India, Chinese Turkestan, Afghanistan and Russia. Fortunately, we don't have to cross the other two or we'd have had to get visas. And they're very difficult to get at the moment."

"If this is the border why aren't there some guards here to stop people from crossing when they're not supposed to?" I asked.

"There are few travellers," Father said, "and we're at 17,500 feet, where no one can live. The border guards live at the bottom of the pass, in the valleys below." He pointed back down the winding path which seemed to disappear into space. "The Indian guards were stationed at the same rest house we stayed at last night."

Father had checked in with them, but they hadn't asked to see anyone else. He wasn't sure what the guards on the Kashgar side would require but he knew they were expecting us.

"What will happen if they won't let us through?" asked Mother.

"I suppose we'd have no alternative but to go back," Father laughed. "But they know about me and I told them I was coming back with my family when I was here a month ago. Hopefully crossing the border will not be an issue."

We looked back at India for the last time and started our descent into Chinese Turkestan. The rounded mountains to the north were dwarfs when compared to the awe-inspiring formations we had travelled through for the past four weeks. I was surprised at how quickly the change occurred.

Three hours later we reached the floor of a river valley where we met Chinese border guards. Their small hut stood at the side of the trail and there were six of them all dressed in the quilted khaki uniforms of the Chinese Army. They were armed with rifles and looked sullen. They offered us tea, looked at Father's papers, and then advised us that there was a Kurgiz camp only three hours away. They definitely didn't want us to stay with them, even though we were willing to put up our own tents. By this time the rest of the caravan had caught up to us. After much discussion we decided to go on to the Kurgiz camp.

In time we emerged onto a large plateau. Behind us we could still see the Karakoram range of mountains. Ahead of us there was a vast expanse of rolling, rounded hills that went on and on as if the horizon had been erased. What a spectacularly contrasting sight this relatively horizontal world made to the vertical world we'd survived.

"This is also what the steppes of Central Asia look like but they are on the other side of the Gobi Desert, much further north and east of here," said Father. "If you look over to your left you can see where we'll be stopping tonight. We should be there in half an hour or so. The Kurgiz are very kind people and will insist on looking after us."

When we reached the camp about forty women and children came out to greet and stare at us. Like the villagers along the caravan trail, they had never seen a white woman and children before and were curious. I also noticed a few men watching discreetly from a distance. When we had dismounted, Suggi came over.

"The Kurgiz are going to put up another yurt for you, M'Saib, and the children. Everyone is in camp today and the other yurts are crowded."

"What's a yurt?" I asked.

"It's one of those round shelters over there. The Kurgiz live in them. They're like tents. One can be put up in an hour. To keep them warm they put an open fire in the middle. There's no wood here so they burn dried yak and horse dung. It gives off a good heat and does not smell too bad. You will see a big hole in the top of the yurt to let the smoke out. When it gets very cold, they can pull a felt cover over the hole to make it smaller. Then it smells bad. You'll see how they put one up."

"Where's it going to go?" my Father asked Suggi.

"Over there," he pointed, "next to the bigger one. That one belongs to the chief. He has asked if you will come and eat with him tonight," replied Suggi.

"Will you thank him for us and tell him we'll be ready in about an hour?"

"What will we get for supper? And will it be safe for the children to eat?" Mother asked.

"The main meal will be some sort of pilau, with rice and mutton or possibly yak," Father said. "They have chickens but rarely eat them. You'll see them running about, free range, in the morning. We'll also be given unleavened bread and sour milk, cheese, and some white jelly stuff. I'm not sure what it is, but it's served with a hot, red chilli sauce. Treat this sauce with respect and be careful how much you try. As far as safety is concerned I didn't suffer any ill effects on my two previous occasions and you know how sensitive my stomach is. I would stick to the cooked food and avoid the cold stuff as much as possible. Just to be safe."

For a moment I had the impression he was about to say more, but then he gazed towards the chief's yurt and said, "It looks as though they're about to put up our yurt."

Half-a-dozen men dragged out a number of large pieces of felt and stacked them to one side. Three others shaped sections of wooden trellising. These sections were about four-and-a-half feet by ten feet. Several sections were put together to make a twenty-foot circle. The roof was made up of a number of flexible, single, long poles. The "chimney" at the top of the yurt consisted of a single strip of wood which had been bent into a circle about six feet in diameter. The roof poles were lashed to this with hide strips and then raised to the top of the trellising. One man, in the centre, held the "chimney" up with a Y-shaped stick until all the pieces were in position. When they had been lashed into place the frame was remarkably stable and stood about fifteen feet high at the centre. After the frame was up, the felt pieces, which were approximately twelve feet square with ropes attached to the corners, were pulled up over the frame using the ropes. Then the ropes were tied down to stakes in the ground. In this way, the frame was covered with one or two layers of heavy felt, making the whole structure windproof. The entrance was made up of two flaps of felt which could be tied down quite easily.

Once the yurt was up, the men put some Kurgiz carpets on the floor and around the inside walls to keep out the cold. The result was a cozy circular tent.

We spent the rest of the evening dining and sharing stories with the chief, before retiring early. While everyone was friendly and hospitable, we had to rise at dawn the next morning, pack up and resume our journey.

During the next two weeks we travelled west along the northern edge of the Pamir range of mountains. Each day we travelled greater distances as the footing became easier for the animals and men. Except for the occasional Kurgiz camp, there were no people or villages along our route. Most nights, during this part of the trek, we had to put up our tents.

As we travelled north-west, the weather got warmer. As usual we were following rivers, but now we were proceeding downstream. As soon as we had crossed the Himalayas, all rivers flowed towards the north. One morning, when we were about to start, Father said, "This will be our last day on the trail. We should reach Tash Kuergan tonight. With any luck, the Consular truck will be waiting to take us to Kashgar tomorrow. The luggage, Izatu, and the caravan will take another week to get there. Suggi will come with us, in the truck."

Towards the end of the day we came out of the hills. In the distance I could make out some trees and square buildings. This was the first village we had come to in Chinese Turkestan. As we got nearer, I could see that the buildings were completely different from the villages we had stopped at in India and in the state of Hunza.

Tash Kuergan was situated beside a river in a flat, semi-desert landscape. The trees were mainly poplar and willows but there were also some fruit trees. The houses were square with flat roofs and were made out of a reddish, mud-straw mixture. Around the village there were fields of maize, melons, millet and green vegetables.

As our caravan approached the village, I noticed an old half-ton Ford truck parked outside one of the buildings.

"We're in luck. Mohammed and the consular truck made it," Father announced to Mother with a smile. Mother nodded but, like Marjory and me, she was paying more attention to the hubbub in the street.

Everywhere I looked, people were busy. I expect they knew we were coming and saw us as customers. Many of the men wore small skullcaps and knee high boots. Some of the men rode on donkeys, and were curiously perched over the hind legs. Later, Suggi told me this was the most comfortable way to ride a donkey. The people, who had Mongolian features, were gaily clothed, reminding me of strings

53

of fluttering prayer flags. They were happy and very curious about us. They spoke Turki, a language I couldn't understand. Subsequently I found out that Turki was similar to the language spoken in Turkey, but ethnically the groups were distinct.

We spent the night in a dusty, cobwebbed building. The next morning, after packing some of our belongings into the truck, we squeezed into the cab and started out for Kashgar. The drive took most of the day and was mainly through desert. It was boring country, especially when compared to our trek through the mountains on horseback where every twist and turn on the icy trail had presented us with the thrill and threat of multiple dangers; where every foothold held the possibility of being swallowed by a crevasse or plunging down sheer walls into a river at the base of a gorge. Life risking death.

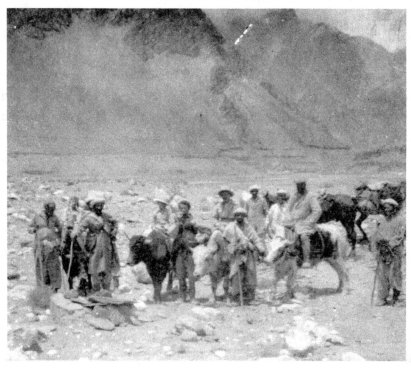

Above: Crossing the glacier in the Himalayas en route to Kashgar.

Chapter 3
The War Years in Chinese Turkestan

"You can see Kashgar in the distance over there," said Father, pointing through the windscreen of the Ford truck towards a brownish mound barely visible through the haze. "It's a walled city with a population of about ninety thousand people."

I think we were all relieved to be at the end of our six-week trek. Father couldn't curtail his enthusiasm and launched into a description of one of the facts about Kashgar that he hoped would arouse our approval.

"One of the distinctive things about Kashgar is that it only rains once every year or so. And they hardly get any snow in the winter. The whole city relies on an irrigation system that comes from the river. As we get closer you'll notice big ditches on either side of the road. They are part of a unique system of water distribution. Everyone knows when the water will be coming to their area. When the water arrives in a village on the outskirts of town there is a lot of activity because the water has to be directed to the different gardens, water storage pools, and fields. You can identify the pools because they're usually surrounded by willow trees. They're quite deep and will supply water to a community for several weeks at a time.

"It gets cold for about three months, but the summers are warm and pleasant. The soil is fertile and with the elaborate irrigation system the people easily manage to grow an abundance of food. There must be at least fifteen varieties of melon. They grow wheat, barley and maize and there are several fruits and vegetables to be had in season. They raise sheep, goats, cattle, pigs, chickens and ducks. All in all, we won't starve. I think you'll find it quite comfortable living here, Ada."

It was obvious to me that this lecture was intended to impress Mother and soften her up before we arrived in Kashgar.

"Are there any European women for me to visit or talk to?" Mother asked.

"Not really," Father replied ruefully, his eyes downcast. "There's a Russian consulate, but the people working there keep to themselves and don't speak English. Some years ago there was a Swedish consulate but they closed for some reason. I don't know the details. Mr. Gillet, our Consul General, is the only other British person here and he's a bachelor. There are some Indian clerks and a pharmacist who speak Hindi. And they speak the English they learned in school. Mr. Chu, the Chinese-English interpreter, from central China, translates for us when we need to communicate with the civil servants in the Chinese government offices. He and his family live next to us and they speak English fairly well."

Mother shot a knowing glance at Marjory and me, then turned to Father.

"What you're saying puts me in mind of the Falkland Islands. When we lived there we were the only people for miles. We didn't often get together with our neighbours because of the distances. I hope this posting will prove to be different, but it does sound like another form of isolation."

I could tell Mother was discouraged. Although she was a strong-willed, independent woman, she liked to have company and friends nearby.

Trying to cheer her up, Father said, "The house is a lot nicer and there's a large garden. You've always enjoyed gardening, Ada. Once we're settled in I'm sure you'll find plenty to do."

I glanced at Mother and could tell she was not convinced. Gardening was no substitute for afternoon tea with friends.

As we neared Kashgar, I could see the outer wall that Father had mentioned. It was made of mud and stood thirty feet high. It was turreted and had the same outline as old medieval castles built in Europe centuries ago. On closer inspection I could see that the wall was very thick. Later I learned that there was enough room to ride a horse along the top. There were Chinese guards with rifles on sentry duty at the enormous wooden gates. I could see shops and buildings inside as we drove past the gate. These were also made of mud with flat roofs. The shops, stalls and streets bustled with people shopping for fruits, vegetables, meats, spices, earthen ware, carpets, tools, clothes, scarves, leather goods, kites and other toys, shoes and boots, tobacco, pastries and sweets. There were donkeys everywhere, some carrying goods and others carrying riders.

"Where's the Consulate?" I asked.

"It's just outside the east gate. We'll be there in about ten minutes," Father said.

"Do they close the city gates at night?"

"Yes, from sunset to dawn. I haven't been in the city very often. Most of our business is done on the Consulate grounds. We've been advised by the Chinese administration not to go into the city except on official business. The servants regularly do the shopping.

"The only times I've been inside the wall have been when I went to the Chinese Government offices on official business. These are in the centre of town, on a square surrounded by trees.

"The Chinese and the Kashgar residents do not like each other. Fights are common. There was a time, in the not-too-distant past, when this area was a separate kingdom from China and there were some fierce battles when the status changed. Because we are so far away from Peking [as the city of Beijing was then known in English] this is not a very popular posting for Chinese government administrators and they try to get back to China as soon as they can. Many are here as a punishment by the ruling party in China and they come and go frequently. The loss of continuity and the unhappiness of the administrators doesn't help the local situation.

"Here's the Consulate," said Father.

"It looks rather magnificent," said Mother. "We've never lived in a castle before."

"I'm sorry to disappoint you, Ada, but that is the Consul General's house. Ours is much smaller, over there to the right. We will be invited to his house tomorrow for a meal. I think you'll like him. I found him to be very helpful when I first got here."

The truck turned left off the main road and travelled down a short, narrow lane with poplars on each side. At the end of the lane there was a large gate set in an archway. The entire Consulate complex was surrounded by a wall about twelve feet high and three feet wide. The large front gate was guarded by a Hunza man, dressed like Suggi in a red and gold uniform.

"Salaam, Dr. Binns. I see you found your family. I hope you had a good journey," he said, struggling to open the wooden gates to allow the truck through.

At the time, the British Consulate in Kashgar was a large compound that included several buildings. The Consular General's house was surrounded by its own wall with its own guarded gate inside the main walls. The place was a fortress.

As we entered the complex we sped up a circular driveway that went around a garden of shrubs and decorative hedges. There were large shade trees at one end of the garden and, Father said, dug into the ground below them was an ice house. To the left of this garden, close to the main entrance, was a tennis court.

The Vice-Consul's house was the second-largest house inside the walls. It was made of bricks painted red and white. There were two small rectangular gardens on either side of the front door.

"Here we are at last," said Father as we climbed out of the old Ford. "Suggi will get us some tea in a few minutes. Meanwhile, I'll give you a tour."

The house was a bungalow with a study and living room at the front, behind which there was a dining room and a second study with only a skylight for light. On the left three bedrooms opened off a long corridor which ended in the bathroom. The kitchen was at the back of the house, with a door that opened into a small courtyard.

When he found out that Father had children the Consul General separated off an area from his garden for us to use. We could get to this small garden from the kitchen. Mulberry, apricot, plum, and cherry trees grew there and provided fruit for us to eat in season. There were also some beautiful roses that had to be covered with straw in winter because of the cold and a couple of flower beds for annuals. There was no need for a vegetable garden. The Consul General's garden was massive and provided vegetables for everyone living in the compound.

Because there was no electricity in Kashgar, we used various sizes of Aladdin lamps for light. These were fuelled by kerosene. We also had one Primus pressure lamp and several hurricane lamps. All the large rooms in the house relied on open fireplaces to provide heat in winter. And because there was no running water a huge earthenware *chutty*, filled with cold water, stood in the bathroom—similar to the ones we had in India. The lavatory was a "short drop" hole that was emptied every two or three days and relined with fresh straw. Hot water for bathing was brought by the houseboy from the kitchen, through the courtyard and veranda at the back of the house. Free-range chickens roamed this area; during the night they were housed in a small building at the end of the courtyard.

The walls of the house and outbuildings were all about eight feet high. Secondary walls of the same height served as barriers between areas. One of these mud walls separated the servant houses from our house. The servants went back and forth through a heavy wooden door that was wide enough to accommodate a laden donkey and the *Pockshee* man who came around to the back of the house to clean out our "short drop" lavatory. Formerly, the "long drop" lavatories had been dug behind the wall. They were now used by the servants. The depth of the hole of the "long drop" lavatory had been calculated by the Indian army to successfully allow the waste to compost safely over time.

Beyond the servants' quarters was the stable where we kept the pony I had ridden up from Gilgit, as well as the horse Father rode if he had to go out of the complex. There was also room to keep a milk cow and a sheep or goat for fattening and slaughtering later in the year.

The Consul General's house was two storeys high while the rest of the houses in the complex were only one storey. The roofs of these houses were flat and were made from mud and straw, like the walls. They were supported by wooden beams with a very slight camber. As Father had explained, it seldom rained in Kashgar, but when it did the locals all ran outside to watch water fall from the sky. This was treated as a moment of magic. The water for daily living was provided by the irrigation system Father had described and was regulated by the government of Kashgar.

Within our house there wasn't much space in which to play and playing in the garden was frowned upon because we trampled the flowers, so Marjory and I spent a lot of time playing on top of the roofs. We played tag and other childhood games with Mr. Chu's son and daughter who were around the same age as us. It was possible to go from one house to another at roof level once we overcame our fear of walking along the tops of the connecting walls. The tops of the walls were either rounded or an inverted wedge shape. Sometimes broken glass was stuck into the mud. Marjory and I walked the walls all the time and I only fell off once while playing tag. On that occasion I injured my left hip and had a limp for several weeks, but I would not admit to my parents how I had done it for fear of being banned from the roofs. Later on Mother told me that she and Father were well aware of our habit of playing on the roofs and walking on the walls but they thought this was better than annoying the Consul General.

I did not find out what the specific functions of the Consulate were until many years later, but Father walked to the office in the mornings and spent most of the day there. His other duty was to run the dispensary and keep track of the medications and medical supplies that were used. Father was the only western-trained doctor in the area and he saw patients from the city of Kashgar as well as from the Consulate.

Shortly after we arrived in Kashgar Father decreed I needed to be taught the rudiments of reading, writing and arithmetic. I was now ten. Since the Consul General and our family were the only English people in Kashgar, my parents decided that Father would teach me mathematics and Mother would teach Marjory and me how to read and write. Each morning Father would sit down with me before he left for work and teach me some basic maths for about twenty minutes. Then he would assign me some work to do for the rest of the day.

I wasn't allowed outside until I had completed it. Mother was much easier on both of us with the result that as soon as I had completed my maths, Marjory and I would head out to play.

During the next three years my sister and I spent a lot of time with the local children and their families. The most common language spoken in the compound was Turki, the language of the local Kashgarie, followed by Urdu, the first language of the Indian staff. English was a distant third. Marjory and I became fluent in Turki within a few months and we started to speak this language as a first choice to each other. This became such a habit that Father finally insisted that we speak English inside the house and when we were with either Mother or him outside the house. He was worried we would lose our English. This was a valid concern. We were totally immersed in the Kashgar culture and language.

From a child's perspective, I could not understand what the fuss was about. At the time I was verbally fluent in three languages and enjoying the test-free life of a home-schooled program. Neither of my parents realized the implications of our not being able to read or write English and it proved to be a serious problem later on for both my sister and me when we returned to England.

From the rooftops Marjory and I could see pigeons being flown by our neighbours and people who lived within the city. The multi-coloured pigeons flew in flocks of up to twenty. In each flock there would be up to four that were tumblers. These special birds would periodically fly to the front of the flock, rise up, and then throw themselves into tumbling spirals before joining the rest of the flock from behind. I became quite fascinated by them. One morning I went down from the roof and asked Ali, one of the Kashgarie servants, to tell me about the pigeons.

"Quite a lot of people fly them. There are many different kinds of birds and they cost a lot of money," he answered.

"Which are the most expensive?"

"The pure whites and the pure brown ones are the most expensive. The tumblers are also expensive, but they are usually of mixed colours and have a crest on the back of their heads. There are some fantail pigeons, but they are not good flyers and most people only keep one or two of them for show. The owners play games with the birds. They try to catch each others' birds by encouraging the flocks to merge and then calling them down to their home. Sometimes a bird will go to the wrong home. If the owner can catch the bird he gets to keep it or sell it. This is not easy because the bird is often frightened when it is on a strange roof."

"What sort of houses do they make for the pigeons?"

"Their houses are kept on the roofs and made from mud bricks. Inside the house there are perches for the birds to sleep on and some holes for them to nest in. Attached to this brick house is a wooden cage, about six feet long by three feet high and wide. There is a full-width door at the front. The door can be opened and closed from behind the house using a long stick. You position yourself so that the birds cannot see you and catch them when they come into the cage."

"How do you get them to come into the cage?"

"You give them some food, usually a mixture of wheat, millet and corn."

I thought that owning pigeons seemed pretty easy and wanted to try it. "Will you show me how to make a pigeon house? Then we can have our own birds."

"I think you should ask your mother before we start building anything on the roof," Ali answered.

Armed with this information I went to Mother and explained what I wanted to do and how I had talked to the Kashgarie servants who said they would help if I had her permission.

"I'm not sure this is a good idea at all. Looking after pets is time consuming and you cannot expect the servants to do it for you, Bernard," piped in my father, who had been listening to my request.

"I promise to look after them myself and I won't want anyone else helping me, once I've got the pigeon house built and some birds to look after." I was certain that I was responsible enough to look after pigeons.

"I think it would be very nice for Bernard to have some pigeons. He doesn't have many friends to play with here and it'll give him something to do," said Mother in my defence. She smiled, but in a stern way, an expression I had seen her use before with Father.

I continued to plead my case. "Please, Daddy, I promise to look after them all the time. Promise."

Father relented, as I suspected he would. "All right, but I'll have to ask Mr. Gillet what he thinks of the idea. If he gives his permission you can build the pigeon house."

Mr. Gillet granted me permission the next day. He thought it was a splendid idea. It would keep me and Marjory occupied. He did say that the pigeon house would be the only one in the Consulate and stipulated that the task of looking after the pigeons had to be done properly.

Suggi and I built the pigeon house against one of the four foot walls that surrounded the outside edge of our house's roof. It took about a week to build. After it had been inspected by Mother and Father I was allowed to go into the city with Suggi and Ali, the Kashgarie house boy, to buy some birds. I hadn't been in the city before and I got my first chance to see a Kashgarie bazaar.

Once through the Consular gate, we were soon on the main thoroughfare into the city, which was wide enough to accommodate three or four laden horses travelling side-by-side. Merchants attending their stalls lined the road. Everyone wanted to sell me something. Each had a different spiel; all were persistent, almost pushy. The first stalls were piled high with food and fruit. It was obviously the melon season because there were many different varieties of melon displayed. If I showed an interest in a melon, the vendor would quickly cut out a small triangular piece for me to taste. Other stalls had different vegetables, meats, milk and cheeses. Most of these stalls were run by local farmers who didn't have access to the main bazaar in the city.

As we walked through the main gate it became noticeably cooler. The sides of the entrance were like finely polished furniture where thousands of people, over centuries, had rubbed their shoulders as they passed through the gate. Once inside the city the streets were narrow and the houses were mainly one-storey buildings with walls around them. In a few cases, doors into these compounds were open and I could peek in, like a thief planning his next caper. One house had a square compound with a small garden in the middle, surrounding a miniature but deep-looking pool of water, possibly a well. Overhanging this was a single willow tree. On the other side of the garden was the main entrance to the house which had rooms on either side with open windows. I could see an Asian carpet in the hallway and some sandals carefully placed by the door.

"That's a nice looking house," I said to Ali.

"Yes, it belongs to a very rich man who is away at the moment in Urumchi, the capital of Xinjiang province. One of his wives has stayed behind to look after the house and his children."

A hundred yards further on we turned left into a narrow alley between two walls that were fifteen feet high. On either side of the ally trickled a smelly open drain.

"The houses are close together here," I said.

"Yes. There is not much room in the city. The wall around the city hasn't grown but the population gets bigger all the time. It is a very old city. Some of the buildings have been here for hundreds of years."

We turned a corner into a small open square which was home to the crowded pigeon bazaar. Wooden cages of all sizes littered the ground and were attended by the owners. Inside the cages I could see all sorts of different coloured pigeons. Many of the men wandering around carried birds in their hands.

"Look carefully at how the men hold the birds," said Ali. "If you do not hold them like that they will break away and fly off and be lost. If you hold them properly they cannot open their wings and they stay still. It is easy once you learn how to hold them. I will show you how when we decide which ones to buy."

"You will have to show me as well," said Suggi, who was carrying the money to purchase the pigeons. "I, too, have not looked after pigeons."

I could see that the men held the birds in one hand with the bird's feet between their middle fingers. The wings and tail end of the birds were surrounded by their thumb and forefinger. Constrained in this hold the birds were docile. We looked at different birds. I was determined to have at least two tumblers because they looked so acrobatic and fearless when they flew. We bought a small cage to put the birds in so we could get them back to the Consulate. After much bargaining, we bought eight pigeons and headed home. With my purchases I felt much older and definitely more mature.

We had been told by the expert at the market that we must keep the birds locked up for five days and to be sure we fed them well during this time. After five days the pigeons could be let out onto the roof to feed in the mornings and evenings when they were hungry. They were not to be encouraged to fly. At any sign of their wanting to fly I was to throw the grain mixture, which Ali had prepared, at the pigeons to lead them back into the pen. Once they were inside I was to close the door behind them. We were to do this for a further four days, each day extending the time they could be let out of the house. Once they were comfortable and wandered in and out of the pen freely, they were to be encouraged to fly for a short time. Again they needed to be hungry so that they would come back when they saw any grain being tossed onto the roof.

I followed the instructions carefully and only one of my first birds took off and never came back.

Later I was told that there were some pigeons that would always go back to their original homes no matter how diligent the new owner was. The experienced dealers recognized these birds and wouldn't buy them.

I quickly became completely engrossed with looking after my pigeons and spent every free moment up on the roof with them. I gave them all names, proud that I had managed to keep them alive and healthy. One morning, as I climbed the ladder up to the roof, I thought it was strangely quiet. I couldn't hear the cooing of the birds.

When I opened the door between the pigeon house and pen, none of the birds came out as usual. I crawled into the pen and put my hand into the house to see if I could catch one of them. The first thing I felt were some feathers. Then I found one of the birds. It was cold and stiff.

I pulled it through into the light to see what had happened. It was the one I'd named Sally and she was dead. There were some scratch marks on her neck and it looked as though her neck was broken. Carefully I lay her down. I pushed my hand in again and found another bird. This was John, and he was also dead with a broken neck.

Something terrible had happened to the birds, but I hoped that some were still alive. With great difficulty I managed to get my head through the door into the pigeon house. In the dim light I could see that all my pigeons were dead and that feathers were strewn all over the place. Nothing made sense. I sat in the pen and cried my heart out. Finally, Ali came up to see what had happened.

"What's the trouble?" he asked.

"It's the pigeons. They're all dead. I don't know why or how," I sobbed.

"Come out and I will have a look."

I crawled out and Ali squeezed in and had a look around. He reached into the house, grabbed two birds and examined them carefully.

"It must be a cat," he said. "Was the door open when you came up this morning?"

"No. I shut it very carefully last night when I put them to bed," I said and started to cry again. Never before had I felt so gutted.

Ali clambered out of the pen and inspected the top of the house where the vent was.

"Ah! One of the sticks across the hole has come loose and been pushed aside. The cat must have got in this way."

"Why did the cat kill them all?" I asked, becoming more resigned to the slaughter.

"I don't know but they do this when they get into a pen of birds. Maybe they just play with the birds until they stop moving and then go to another until they are all dead. It is very sad and I am sorry for you. Maybe your mother and father will let you get some more. If you like, I will clean up the mess in the pen."

"Thank you," I said, still blubbering. "I need to tell Mother and Father what's happened."

It was early in the morning and my parents were still in bed when I got back into the house. I crept into their bedroom trying to think what I was going to tell them. Although I was now twelve and liked to think I was grown up, the death of the pigeons had devastated me. I had no idea how I was going to replace them. Immediately I started to cry again, which woke my mother.

"What's the trouble darling?" she asked, putting her arm round me.

"It's the pigeons. They're all dead," I sobbed.

"What happened to them?" Father asked sleepily from the far side of the bed.

"Ali says a cat must have got in. They've all been scratched and bitten round their necks. What am I going to do, Mummy? I loved them so much."

"I'm not sure. What do you think Pat, could Bernard get some more?"

"I suppose so," Father replied, "but you'd better make sure the pen is cat-proof this time."

Upon hearing this news I began to cheer up a bit and went back to bed until breakfast time. At breakfast the family decided we should build a new pen—the smell of a cat would probably frighten any new birds. We moved the pen to an outside corner and put the vent through one of the outside walls making it impossible for a cat to get in that way. When the second house was completed it was much sturdier and was better located.

My second lot of pigeons survived for the rest of our stay in Kashgar. I lost the odd one to some of the other bird keepers, but, from time to time, I managed to compensate for my losses by catching some of theirs.

One day while flying my pigeons I heard a whistling sound in the sky over the city. Eventually I recognised that the source of the sound was a kite being flown from somewhere in the maze of streets in the distance. I asked Ali about this. He told me that kite season had arrived and that in the next few days hundreds of kites would take flight. Some of the kites would have whistles attached to them.

These kites were different from the ones I had seen and flown in Abbottabad. They were rectangular with a narrow edge that pointed skywards. The kites could also be made to drop vertically for quite a long time before returning to their high point again. Compared to the Indian fighting kites these were bigger and did not dart about the sky in the same fashion. I asked Ali to get one for me and he taught me how to fly it. My kite was made out of paper and split-dried bulrush stems. Faces or patterns were painted on the surfaces. Later on, Ali taught me how to make my own kites. They were quite expensive to buy and we had all the materials needed to make them in the Consulate. The kite flying season lasted for a couple of months, just before winter started.

I remember the winters being cold and dry. We had a sprinkling of snow one winter but there was not enough to make snowballs. One morning, when I went up to feed and fly the pigeons, the brass lock on the cage stuck to my hand when I grasped it. I was surprised and not sure what to do. The lock and my hand stuck together so firmly that I couldn't pull them apart. In a few moments the lock warmed up enough from the heat of my hand for me to separate the two, but the episode frightened me while it lasted. Father explained the phenomenon but I didn't really understand why the rapid transfer of heat from one surface to another should cause them to stick together.

In the autumn of our second year in Kashgar, Father came home and announced that a British visitor had come and that we would be expected to entertain him during his stay. My first encounter with this visitor took place one morning when I was taking my pony out for a ride. I took him for a ride two or three times a week to keep him fit. The visitor was mounted on a big Kashgarie horse with a high Asian saddle. At the time I rode bareback. I found putting the saddle on the pony too much trouble.

"Hello, you must be Bernard. I'm Bill McLean. Your father said you often went out riding at this time of the morning. Would you like to show me around?"

"I'd be happy to," I said. "I usually go for about an hour and return for breakfast. It'll be nice to have company."

"I gather you've learned to speak Kashgarie since you arrived."

"Yes. I can speak Urdu as well. I have no problems talking to the servants or the locals." Immediately I felt boastful and embarrassed, and felt my cheeks flush. Why had I said this? Also my English was poor.

"You lead the way," he said.

"Let's go down to the river," I replied, feeling a sense of relief. Either he hadn't noticed my boast or, more likely, was ignoring it. "It's a nicer ride than along the wall round the city."

I led him out of the back entrance. The gate opened up onto a road that went to the right, down a hill to the river. The road was bordered by a mixture of Berlin poplars and willows, which lined the sides of the irrigation canals. Past these we could see the fields that contained various vegetable, melon and grain crops. All the farms had donkeys, the main form of transport in Kashgar. Some of the wealthier farms had horses, and a few had a cow. At this time of day there were very few people about and we were able to canter down to the river, a mile and a half away. Here the river widened and got shallower and was used as a ford by farmers who lived farther away on the other side. There were also some deep pools where I often went swimming in the summer months with the local boys.

To rest the animals, Mr. McLean and I paused at the ford. "How long have you been here?" he asked.

"Just over a year. We came up towards the end of summer last year when the rivers were at their lowest. It was a long journey. Six weeks. How long did it take you?"

"We did double marches with the Hunza couriers. It took us three weeks. It's a tough trip for a family to make."

"How long do you plan to stay?" I asked.

"That depends. Officially I'm on sick leave, but there are some other things I've been asked to do before I go back. I should be here for a few weeks. Since I'm told you can speak the local languages so well, I was wondering if you'd like to come along on some of the trips

I'll be making. I've asked your father and he's given his permission, as long as you're willing to come. You would only accompany me on day trips. We don't want to keep you away from home at night. What do you think of the idea?"

"I'd like to very much. What sort of trips will they be?" What he suggested sounded mysterious. I was also flattered and wondered what sort of adventures lay in store.

"I thought of hunting pheasants and rabbits to start with. I gather the locals catch those using falcons. Have you ever done that?"

"No, but I've heard about tame falcons and I've watched wild ones take some of my pigeons out of the sky. I've even heard that large eagles are used to catch deer in the foothills to the south."

A few days after this Father told me that Mr. McLean had arranged a hunting party for later in the week and that I could go with him if I wanted. I was to act as interpreter. He said we would be using falcons.

To get to the hunting site we drove in the Consular truck for an hour. We arrived at a small village at about 7 a.m. Then we transferred to horses. For the first time I saw peregrine falcons at close quarters. The men looking after the birds wore heavy leather gloves on which the birds perched. The falcons were a light greyish blue in colour with some darker blue streaks. Their long, powerful wings were dark grey or black. They were beautiful, proud-looking birds, with yellow feet and sharp black talons that gripped the falconers' gloves like a vice. Little leather hoods covered their eyes keeping them placid. In total there were five hunting birds. Two were smaller than the others. I was told these were young birds and that we had to be careful with them. They might fly away.

To get to the pheasants we would have to ride for about half-an-hour.

Fields gradually gave way to scrub land composed of stunted willows, dogwood, long grasses and occasional clumps of bulrushes. In the waning autumn sun, the willow leaves were turning yellow. The dogwood bark was a vibrant red against the pale brown of the grasses. Some of the bulrush catkins had already burst and their fine cotton-like seeds wafted on the wind.

Arriving in a stand of trees, the leader of the party and the head hunter reined in his horse. "This is where the pheasants are," he said.

"Ask him what we have to do now," Mr. McLean instructed me.

"We will leave the horses here and then walk through the bush in that direction," the leader said, pointing away from the fields we had just come across. "When a pheasant flies up we will stop and let one of the falcons go. We only release one falcon at a time because falcons will fight each other for their prey and they can kill each other."

We dismounted and spread out along the edge of the field with about fifty yards separating us. When we were all in position we started to walk into the bush. At first there was no sign of any birds let alone pheasants. I was beginning to think that nothing was going to happen when suddenly there was a whirring of wings and a squawk as a male pheasant broke cover about ten yards in front of me. The falconer on my left released his bird into the air shouting, "Fetch!" The bird flew up into the air above the pheasant and then dropped like a stone onto its prey. There was another squawk and a puff of feathers as the two birds hit in mid-air. They fell to the ground about a hundred yards in front of us. The falconer ran toward the birds. When he reached them he put the hood on his falcon and then separated the two. This was not an easy job. The falcon had already started to make a meal of his catch. Once the birds had been separated the pheasant was killed according to proper Islamic Halal ritual. One of the men cut the pheasant's throat as he recited the appropriate words.

"This is a good, big bird," the leader said with a broad grin on his face.

By this time we were all grouped together around the catch.

"Why did he cut the pheasant's throat like that instead of just wringing it?" Mr. McLean asked, turning to me.

"It's an Islamic practice. All animals that Muslims eat have to be 'Halal' or permissible. They must be slaughtered in a specific way and certain words spoken or they are not clean and can't be eaten," I replied.

During the rest of the morning we managed to scare up several more birds and the falcons caught over half of them. The ones that got away were the ones that didn't have to fly far for cover. They skittered into the bushes before the falcon could strike.

"Are you enjoying the hunt, Bernard?" asked Mr. McLean.

"I'm not sure I like killing the pheasants. They're such beautiful birds, and I don't think we really need to eat them."

"Hunting is something some people do for sport. They get hooked on the dangers of hunting big game. The thrill it gives them. Guides in India and Africa can make a good living from conducting hunting safaris, but a lot of animals are shot needlessly. I've tried it. Now I only hunt for food. I like the taste of wild fowl and meat, but hunting for trophies no longer appeals to me," he said, pausing to take a sip of his tea. "Ask the men if the falcons can catch anything else."

In response to my question, one of the men said that their falcons could catch rabbits and hares, but that they didn't use the birds for this purpose very often. Rabbits were not part of their regular diet.

"Well, I like them," said Mr. McLean after I had interpreted this for him, "and I think your parents would like some for a dinner. Ask the leader if there are any rabbits round here we could hunt."

"He says there are usually some hares about a mile away from here. If you like, we can go there after lunch."

"Excellent idea," replied Mr. McLean.

After lunch we moved to an area of grasses and dry bush land. The technique used for hunting hares was much the same as for the pheasants, but the falcons would strike a hare on the ground before it reached thick cover. We managed to catch three that afternoon.

On the way back to the village where we had left the truck, Mr. McLean directed me to ask the men if they had ever seen any aeroplanes. They said they had spotted them occasionally in the distance, but, as far as they knew, there were not many. He asked if they ever landed near Kashgar and I was told they occasionally landed on the other side of the city. The men added that the place where the planes landed had been levelled a couple of years ago.

Mr. McLean wanted to know about the size of the airplanes and how many engines they had; I got the impression he was interested in going to see where they landed. My suspicion was confirmed when he asked how the pheasant and hare hunting was near the new runway. Straightaway he made arrangements with the men to show him the area the next day. Unfortunately, I was not invited along on the trip. Mr. McLean turned out to be an excellent linguist and learned to handle his own communications quickly.

I went on several of his other 'hunting trips' and noticed that he spent a lot of time asking about army activities and the roads in and out of the area. At the time I never imagined his interest was anything more than casual.

Mr. McLean stayed at the Consulate for several weeks and then went back to India via the Hunza caravan route. Three weeks after he left we heard that some bandits from Russia had raided some caravans on that route and we feared that Mr. McLean might have been killed. A short time later, the caravan route to Hunza was closed and didn't reopen until we left. I never met Mr. McLean again, but many years later I heard that he had made it through the pass before the bandits started to loot the caravans. Father then told me he suspected that Bill McLean had actually been sent on a spy mission by the British government and that his interest in hunting was his cover. Such a possibility had never occurred to me, perhaps because I was too young and knew little of the world beyond compounds.

I was aware there was a world war going on because Father used to give Mother the news that came over the Consular shortwave radio. Although we were told of the progress the Germans were making and then later, of the progress the English, Americans and Russians made, it didn't mean much to me, and I certainly was not aware of the significance of the war. I could see that Mother was concerned and upset about the welfare of our relatives back in England. And I would listen to Father try to reassure her that the war would not affect them because they lived in the country and were not near any major targets.

The Consular radio ran off a battery that had to be charged regularly and there were only two places in Kashgar where that could be done. One was at the Chinese army base, the other at the Russian

Consulate. The Chinese either wouldn't cooperate or were not asked. Consequently every other week, the battery was sent over to the Russians for charging and I was invited to go along to use their swimming pool. On occasion, Mother and Marjory would accompany us. We would spend most of the day at the pool—the battery took that long to charge—but Mother found the excursion a bit strained as the Russians could not speak English and they weren't hospitable. While there were a few women about the place, there were no children.

My only other contact with the Russians living in Kashgar was when we were invited to official parties at the Consulate for the celebration of various holidays. On these occasions we would all have to sit at a long, formally presented table, usually in the Consul General's garden, and a meal was served. This meant that Marjory and I had to learn our table manners and how to behave properly during public events. It turned out that I was quite useful at these functions. There were two Russians who could speak Turki and I could translate what they said directly into English. Otherwise conversations had to go from three original sources through two interpreters (Russian to the Russian/Chinese speaker then Chinese to the Chinese/English speaker then English and back again—a five-handed exchange). This conversion was time-consuming and often confusing. Ideas got changed in the interpretation. Father and Mother also went on some official events to the Chinese embassy in Kashgar, but these did not include family members. Marjory and I stayed home and flew pigeons. For reasons I was never able to understand, the Chinese administrative staff were a bit aloof and suspicious of our Consular staff.

Mr. Gillet, who was the Consul General when we arrived, left shortly after Mr. McLean did. His appointment had ended. Unfortunately, he had to travel back to England the long way, through Urumqi and Peking because of the bandits looting the Hunza caravan route. I didn't really get to know the new Consul General, Mr. Etherington-Smith—I only met him a few times—and he did not use the tennis court as Mr. Gillet had. Besides, I got the impression he was not fond of children.

A lot of the social life at the Consulate revolved around the tennis court; that's where I learned the basic rules of the game and how to hit a tennis ball. Tennis was played in the evenings after work when the temperature cooled down. There would be tea, cold drinks and sandwiches laid out by the house boys. In the first year the players were Mr. Gillet, my parents, Mr. Chu, two of the Indian clerks, and the driver who had been in Kashgar for a long time, although he had originally come from India. The Indian staff would often bring their children so there was usually someone for Marjory and me to play with.

Next to the tennis court there was a walled-off area that was longer and wider than the tennis court. This was the Hunza polo ground, which was not used. Polo had been banned by the Consul General immediately after a player had been killed during a game. Hunza polo was a rough game and deaths were not uncommon. Small, rugged ponies were used and the "polo mallets" were made from a straight stick with a wicked-looking solid wooden knot at the end. The ball was like a cricket ball, but a little larger. There were seven players a side, which left little room for the horses. No one seemed to know the rules and the game was more of a free-for-all than an organised game with rules. Horses and players were often injured. Suggi told me 'the game' was extremely popular in Hunza.

On holidays and to celebrate world events, such as the end of the war, the Consul General's staff organized large parties. People from both inside and outside the Consulate were invited. There could be up to two hundred people in attendance. These parties were held in the polo ground and local entertainers performed. All the foreigners living in Kashgar welcomed these events. A stage was erected at one end of the polo ground and an outdoor kitchen at the other end. The food was cooked in large cauldrons. I was fascinated by the way the cooks could prepare various chopped-up meats, onions, vegetables and rice all together without burning or spoiling a thing. The meats were partially cooked first. Then the vegetables and finally the rice and water were added. This mixture would then be cooked gradually for an hour or so until ready. Towards the end spices, especially saffron, would be stirred into the mixture. The result was a tasty *pilau* which was distributed to the guests. It was accompanied by assorted side dishes consisting of local foods, some of which were very hot and spicy.

One popular Consulate speciality was ice cream made in its ice-cream churns and its large ice-pit lined with bulrushes that preserved ice blocks brought down from the mountains throughout the winter. The entertainment usually consisted of local dancing girls, comedians, acrobats and conjurers. My job was to translate for my parents and the Consul General. After the meal and entertainment the Consul General would make a speech and the younger members of the audience would be sent home to bed, something I was beginning to resent. I felt I was now old enough to stay up later; my role as translator had earned me the right.

By now I was well into my thirteenth year and had been playing with boys who were as old as fourteen. Some of these boys had reached puberty. Through their stories I became aware of sex and some of its consequences, such as pregnancy or disease. In part, I learned about reproduction from keeping pigeons. The rest I gleaned from the local children, Suggi and Izatu. My parents never told me about sexual matters and I don't recall the topic ever being discussed at home. Suggi and Izatu had come to Kashgar without their wives and they routinely talked about sex and prostitutes. They must have felt that I might be at some risk, because they told me that I should be very careful about what I did and that I should not get involved with any of the older girls in the group that I played with. If I did so, they warned, I could get sick. Exactly how was a mystery.

One day, while playing with a group of the older boys, they took me to one of the farms outside the Consulate. At this farm I witnessed a few of the boys having sex with a donkey. Another boy, who was also watching, masturbated and produced an ejaculate. As this had never happened to me, I asked him about it. He told me that it would happen to me soon and then went on to explain that having sex with the donkey was okay, but it was much better to do it with girls. He added that finding girls who would have sex was very difficult because normally they were not allowed to have sex until they got married. He told me he knew two girls who would do it for money and that he could arrange for me to meet them if I wanted to. Then he admitted I was not really old enough yet. The boys also told me about homosexual activities and warned me about some of the young men in the Consulate who were known to prefer boys.

Shortly after this conversation I was invited to one of the houses in the Consulate where I had my first encounter with some young men who tried to seduce me. Fortunately I knew enough to recognize what was going on and had enough knowledge about rank and status within the compound to rebuff their advances and avoid being raped. I simply threatened to tell my father what they wanted me to do. This was an extremely unpleasant experience, one that has remained with me ever since. I never told my parents. However, I was pleased the older boys had warned me about this type of activity and relieved that I was savvy enough to get out of trouble on my own.

Although World War II had ended in 1945, Kashgar was still cut off from the rest of the world. My father's two-year appointment to the Foreign Service in Kashgar had finished but there was no safe route for us to leave the city. The route to India was blocked by bandits in the mountains to the south and travel through Russia was not possible due to visa issues. The only way out of Chinese Turkestan was through China. This route entailed a long and difficult road journey round the northern side of the Gobi desert to the capital, Urumqi, and then by train to Shanghai. As with Mr. Gillet the year before, the British government had tried to arrange this exit for us. Unfortunately they were told that it was too dangerous and uncertain. China was in the early stages of a revolution and the overthrow of the Chiang Kai-shek regime by the Communists. Father was advised by the Foreign Service to stay put until the southern route to India was open again.

The political unrest and the closure of the passes meant that we didn't get much mail for eighteen months. Luckily there was a telegraph service through China for official messages to the Consulate, but the mail from India and England took many months to travel across the land route from Shanghai. I still have a letter that Mr. Gillet sent out by the first registered mail from Kashgar to England in 1944. It took five months to get to its destination and was then returned to Kashgar because the person to whom it was addressed had died. The return journey from England to Kashgar took just as long.

The isolation and uncertainty of living in Kashgar was starting to upset my mother. By this time, our family had been overseas for over seven years in total, and she wanted to get back to England.

One day in the autumn of 1946 Father came home for lunch—all smiles. "Ada, I've some good news. The old caravan route through Leh and Ladakh (Little Tibet) is open and we're going back to India. The Indian Office sent a telegram today saying that Mr. Etherington-Smith and I will be replaced by a Mr. Eric Shipton, and his wife, Diana, and a Dr. A. Marsh. They'll be accompanied by a new head clerk and a dispenser, along with their wives and two children. We'll meet them in Leh to give them advice about the route. Mr. Etherington-Smith will stay on here until Mr. Shipton arrives. We'll be leaving in three weeks' time."

"Thank God! I was beginning to think we were going to have to stay here for the rest of our lives. How long will it take to get to India?" asked Mother.

"About six weeks, once we get started. It's a longer trip than the one over the Mintaka Pass, and we'll encounter very few people on the way. We'll have to be completely self-sufficient and live in tents for four to five weeks. There's little grazing for the animals so the caravan has to take food for them as well. This means the caravan will be much larger."

"Then I'd better get started planning the packing. I don't think we'll need any more cases. We still have the ones we came up with." Mother's enthusiasm was contagious. As happy as I was for her, I was going to be sad to leave my friends, my pigeons, my freedom. Kashgar was my home; England an enigma.

"What will I do with my pigeons?" I asked, desperately searching for an excuse that might postpone or avert our departure.

"You can sell them or give them away to one of the servants," said Father, an edge of regret in his voice.

"I'll start arranging the packing this afternoon," Mother said. "There must be quite a bit we can give away. Mind you, we've bought quite a lot over the past three years. I don't want to leave it all behind, especially the carpets, which are quite bulky."

At that moment an excited Suggi came in to announce that lunch was ready.

"Sahib, we are going back to India soon," he announced.

"How do you know?" Father asked. "I only found out this morning and I've not told anyone until now."

"Oh, everybody in the Consulate knows about it today. Some caravan men came this morning asking if they could be hired to take you back," he said grinning.

"It's amazing how fast news travels around here. I haven't told a soul and everyone knows about it before I get home for lunch!"

The next day, over a cup of tea, Mother and Father talked about the upcoming trip. I got the impression that it was not going to be as easy as the trip up. To start with it was several years since the route had been used and there was only one old guide in Kashgar who knew the route. It was over ten years since he had made the journey, but he was confident that he could find the way. Father was worried about his age, whether he would be fit enough, and how good his memory was. He was also concerned that, although the Chinese said the route was safe, no one had been as far as the Indian border since the reported presence of bandits, a year previously. Winter would arrive in two months and there was a chance that we could get stuck in blizzards on the other side of the Karakoram Pass. It was imperative we get started as soon as possible.

The alternative was to wait until spring. Waiting would mean that the Shipton party would also have to wait in India or Leh for several months. Father suspected we were being sent down to test the route, but felt we didn't have any choice. He didn't want to leave us in Kashgar for four to five months and do the trip by himself; nor did Mother like that idea. Between them they decided that we should all go as soon as possible and hope for the best.

The next two weeks were busy ones for my parents. My pony and

Father's horse were sent ahead with Izatu to the town of Khokie, at the start of the trail. My pigeons were given to the house boy, Ali. The house was packed up and letters and telegrams were written to my grandparents and aunts and uncles to tell them we were on our way. Everyone was excited although I was still sad if not reluctant to be leaving. Few others had been so lucky as to spend the war, happy and carefree, in such an exotic land.

We left Kashgar in the Consulate truck and drove through Yarkand, then from Karghalik to Khokie. The truck ride took a whole day. Khokie turned out to be a small village in the foothills of the mountains south of the desert. Here we said goodbye to the driver and our Kashgarie servants who returned to the Vice-Consul house to get it ready for the new family.

We spent the next day sorting out the luggage and deciding where things were going to be placed within the caravan. There were several people waiting in Khokie who wanted to tag along with our larger caravan. They felt that the Vice-Consul would provide them with better protection from bandits. This amused Father—we had no guns or armed escort—but it was also a concern because it meant that the locals were not convinced that the bandits had left the area. Eventually we set off, the caravan consisting of twenty-one camels, sixteen horses and a few donkeys. There were eleven caravan men, the four of us, Suggi and Izatu. We carried two medium sized army tents and a smaller tent for the kitchen and Suggi and Izatu. The caravan men had their own tents, consisting of pieces of canvas that they casually draped over some stacked loads.

Once we left the village, the trail set off across the desert towards the mountains that hovered like a mirage in the far distance. After a hot and dusty day we arrived at the last oasis that we would see in Chinese Turkestan (Xinjiang). At this spot there was a Chinese army post and customs office and we spent the rest of the day getting our paperwork sorted out and being assured that there were no bandits around. We departed early the next day. The trail continued through the desert towards the foothills in the distance. We reached a small, slow-moving river that evening and made camp.

During the next six days the trail wound its way slowly up a valley that gradually rose in elevation. When we left the valley we were greeted by a panorama of snow-covered mountains to the south. Right away we knew we would have to go through them to reach the Karakoram Pass. The guide told me this would take us another ten days. Initially the trail was quite well marked, but when we got up onto the high plateau it seemed to vanish. Father was concerned that we would not find the right route into the mountains. He talked to the guide each day with me acting as interpreter and I could sense that Father doubted our guide's knowledge of the terrain. On the other hand, the guide had complete confidence in his ability to find the route.

One problem he did have was estimating the length of each day's trek on the high plateau. Father was uneasy because he knew that camping out on the plateau could be dangerous. We were all at risk of suffering from high-altitude sickness. Years later he told me that he was worried that our guide, who was a very old man, might die if we camped on the plateau, leaving us stranded.

On our second day, as we came over a hill, I noticed a white clump of rocks on the top of the next rise. To me they looked out of place. As we got nearer I saw that they were not rocks but bleached bones.

"How did those bones get here?" I asked the guide

"Those are from a horse that died. You will see a lot of bones in the next few weeks. This trail has been used for several thousand years and many animals have died along the way. Because it is so high and cold here there are very few vultures or other animals to eat them and the bones just lie where the animal died. As we get nearer the mountains you will see dry powdery skin and flesh still on them. If you look down into some of the valleys we pass, you might see human bones. These belong to men who have fallen. It is not always possible to go down to bury them, so they are just left where they lie. I will point them out to you in a day or so, if I can remember where they are."

"When do we get to the mountains?" I asked him.

"In three or four days. Then we will start the climb up a long valley to the Karakoram Pass. When we have crossed the pass, we will be in India. But we will still have to travel ten days before we get to Leh, which is where you will join another caravan to take you on to Srinagar. The mountains on this side of the pass are not as steep as those on the other side. The route from Karakoram to Leh can be very dangerous. It follows a fast river with steep walls. Then we have to cross the Sasser Pass. This pass is always covered with glacial ice. The path there can be difficult to find so it may take some extra days."

Three days later we left the high plains and started to follow a broad river with craggy, precipitous mountains on either side. The landscape was grimly barren. There was little vegetation and hardly any evidence of animal life. One evening, after supper, I was looking up at a steep cliff above our campsite and heard some rocks falling. I looked in the direction of the sound and saw a rock fall, leaving a trail of dust in the still air. Wondering what had caused the rockslide, I looked higher up and spotted some mountain sheep.

The next morning, we approached the junction of two valleys. In the distance, I could see what first appeared to be a herd of animals. As we moved closer, I realized the herd was another caravan going in the opposite direction. It was several weeks since we had seen anyone. I was anxious to discover who these people might be. Suddenly there was a puff of dirt ten feet in front of my horse, followed by a high whine and a sharp crack—a rifle shot. I stopped my pony and jumped off on the wrong side to shield myself from more bullets.

"Over there," shouted Father. "Behind those boulders." We all ran to where he pointed and hid at the entrance to a gully.

"My God, Pat. Who do you think they are?" asked Mother.

"I can't tell at this distance. They could be the bandits who were reported to be in this area last year."

"What are we going to do?"

"First, we'll wait for them to stop shooting. Then we'll try to find out who they are and what they want from us. To be honest, it doesn't look good. I don't think they'll kill us or leave us to die. We're British subjects and the Indian government would take a dim view of that," said Father, trying to be reassuring. I doubt if Mother found his words comforting and I was too wide-eyed at the time to comprehend how lame his explanation was. Why would bandits care if we were British subjects?

The bullets continued to whine over our heads and some hit the rocks we were hiding behind. Father and Suggi put a white shirt on a stick to wave at the bandits, but this didn't make any difference. After about half-an-hour I saw one of our caravan men cantering across to the other side of the valley with a white flag. Father said later he must have been very courageous, had better eyesight than us, or was just plain stupid. Luckily the bandits did not shoot him and once he got to them they stopped shooting.

"That's encouraging," Father said. "They've stopped using us for target practice. I think we'll wait here, though, for them to come over to us in case they change their minds. Keep the flag up, Suggi."

A few minutes later our caravan man and three armed men crossed back over to our side of the valley. As they got closer we could see that the armed men were wearing uniforms. "They're soldiers, Pat," said Mother.

"Let's hope so. It's probably safe now to come out from behind the rocks."

To our surprise, the men approaching us were led by an officer. They were all wearing Chinese army uniforms.

"We're in luck," Father said as he stood up to greet them.

The next problem was that they couldn't speak English or Urdu and their Turki was poor. But through a combination of sign language and Turki we managed to convince them that we were not bandits or armed and that we were from the British Consulate in Kashgar. Father was asked to go with them to talk to their captain and we were told to stay put.

Father was gone for about an hour. In spite of her misgivings, Mother did her best to convince us that everything would be all right. By this time the rest of our caravan had caught up with us and I ex- plained to them what was going on. When Father got back he said,

"It's a Chinese patrol. They had a skirmish with some bandits a few miles from here last week, but they claim the bandits have all gone east. They thought we might be some stragglers. That's why they shot at us. They say that we can go on, but that we should not waste any time. They cannot guarantee our safety. I asked them if they could spare a few men to accompany us to the border, but they said they have to get back to Khotan as soon as possible. They're low on food. I asked if they thought we should turn back and they said we would be safe once we crossed the Indian border, a two days' march from here. I agreed that we would be better going on. It would take us three weeks to get back to Yarkand. Besides, that may be the way the bandits went. They concurred. We'll continue on course for the rest of the day. Please explain that to the caravan men, Bernard."

When I passed on Father's explanation, the men were relieved that we would go on to India and not turn back. The episode had a sobering effect on everyone. We all started to whisper and the men silenced the bells that hung round the camel's necks by stuffing hair into them. They were also noticeably quicker at getting the animals moving and we travelled farther than normal that day.

It was dark when we made camp. We had a light meal and went to bed as soon as the tents were up.

I was woken by what sounded like a rifle shot.

"What's that, Pat!" I heard my Mother whisper. I'd never seen her so jumpy—not surprising after the day we'd had.

"It's all right, Ada. It's just Suggi knocking the snow off the tents so they won't be as wet when they take them down."

"Thank God for that. I thought it was more shooting."

"I think we'd better get going as soon as possible. We're camped too close to where the Chinese encountered the bandits yesterday. There are some shallow graves just over the stream there. I've told Suggi not to bother with breakfast. We'll have a snack in an hour or so."

We got underway quickly. Once I was mounted I could see some low mounds on the other side of the stream and some clothes and a hand poking out of one of the graves. For the rest of that day we were all sombre and tense, as if our caravan had transformed into a funeral procession.

As we climbed up towards the Karakoram Pass, it got colder, and in spite of having a thick woollen vest, shirt, fur-lined coat, padded long trousers, thick woollen socks, knee-length fur-lined boots, and a fur hat that could be brought down over my neck, I could still feel the biting cold wind. I tried to walk for a while to get warm, but became short of breath very quickly—we were approaching 18,000 feet. Although Karakoram was the highest pass we had to cross it was not the steepest or the most difficult. I remember it for the cold wind and the threat of bandits.

Later that afternoon, when we reached the top, the caravan men let out a cheer and began to sing. They removed the hair from the camel bells and everyone congratulated each other for getting to India safely. It did not seem to occur to anyone that the danger from the bandits was probably the same five miles on either side of the pass. The nearest Indian army post was still ten days' fast march away, at Panamik, a town known for its curative hot springs. That night our camp returned to its usual routine. We had lost one camel and a horse. They died on the pass from heart failure caused by the altitude. The death of pack animals was a common occurrence and it didn't concern the caravan men. They had quickly redistributed the luggage and continued on, leaving the carcasses behind on the side of the trail.

The topography after the Karakoram Pass became much more rugged and was similar to the trip up through Hunza. As predicted by our ancient guide at the beginning of the trip, the Sessar Pass did have thick ice and snow at the top. It crossed between the mountains at the junction of two glaciers and was extremely difficult for the animals to navigate; even the camels, which were surprisingly sure-footed, had to be coaxed across the ice by their handlers. There was a steep ascent to the top and then the route descended precipitously into a roaring river gorge. It was the only pass that gave me a headache. Mother, who I thought had the constitution of one of our pack animals and seldom complained, also felt ill at the top. Father said my headache was due to mountain sickness caused by our rapid climb to the top.

One of the men told me this range of mountains was nicknamed the "headache mountains" by the locals in Ladakh, a region in the Kashmir, which was our immediate destination. The people living in the area had come originally from Tibet so it was sometimes referred to as "Little Tibet." The city of Panamik was still one pass and five days away.

We spent hours weaving around narrow gorges. Torrents of water roared past us. At one point some hot springs flowed straight out of the rock face. Hot steaming water ran across our trail and into the river. I was fascinated by the idea that hot water could come directly from the earth. Two days later we climbed out of a gorge and up the last of the passes before entering Ladakh. The last pass, the Khardung, followed a steep narrow trail, but there was no ice or snow at the top. When we descended the other side we met our first Ladakhies. We were more than happy to return their friendly smiles. Other than the Chinese military patrol, they were the first people we had seen in over a month.

That night we camped near a small village and were able to buy some fresh food to cook for dinner—a welcome change from the pre-served food we had eaten for the past six weeks. The next day we reached Panamik and were greeted with the news that Mr. Shipton and his party would arrive the next day. A man from their caravan had been sent ahead to look for us. The Shiptons had decided to come up from Leh where we were supposed to meet them. Leh was still five days away and they had decided to get a head start. They were becoming increasingly worried about the time required to travel the passes before winter set in. They were also worried for our safety—they had heard rumours about the bandits.

We set up camp in an orchard and waited for the Shiptons to arrive. When their caravan turned up, it was obvious they were relieved to see us. After initial greetings and dinner, Father, Mr. Shipton, Dr. March, our caravan guide, and some of Mr. Shipton's caravan men met to discuss the rest of their trip. I had joined Marjory, Mother and Mrs. Shipton, when Suggi came over to us.

"Sahib wants you to help with the translation and interpretation," he said to me. "There are too many different languages for easy discussion."

"Bernard, do you think you can manage?" Mother asked. "They'll be talking about all sorts of difficult problems on the trail and specific details of the route."

"I should be able to manage. There's only one way to find out and that's to try. I can speak and understand Turki and Urdu so it should cut out some of the confusion. I'll also know what the caravan men are saying to each other which should keep them honest."

A major concern of the Shiptons' caravan men was that it had been over a year since they had travelled the route. They wanted to know the details of any major changes the frequent rock slides might have caused. They were also worried about the state of the ice in Sasser Pass. The size of their caravan and how many extra people would be allowed to join up with them was debated. As it was getting late in the year, Mr. Shipton didn't want to lead too large an expedition—this would slow them down, which could be a problem if the weather turned nasty. Payments and bonus money were the final topics I helped clarify. Bartering was expected and was quite fierce; Mr. Shipton was an experienced barterer, perhaps because of his previous mountaineering expeditions, and he delighted in the exchange. Eventually everything was settled and the group broke up.

We spent the next day in Panamik and went to the hot springs for the first bath we had had in about a month. A small house had been built over the springs which made the baths deliciously comfortable. Since it was the last bath the Shiptons were to have for the next month, everyone made the most of the warm, flowing water.

I found out later that Eric Shipton (1907–1977) was renowned in the western world for his mountaineering explorations and mapping which he completed with H.W. Tilman. He was an accomplished climber who had travelled through the Nanda Devi (India) and the Karakoram glacial regions between 1934 and 1939. He was also a key member of four attempts on Mount Everest which paved the way for Edmund Hillary's successful ascent in 1953. What is not well known is that during the war Eric Shipton served as a diplomat for the English government in Persia, Hungary and China. He was headed for his final Consul-General post in Kashgar when we all met in Panamik. After the war he returned to climbing and mapping specific mountains in the Himalayas as well as in South America. His wife, Diana, whom we also spent time with, later wrote a book called *The Antique Land* about her experiences during the two years she spent in Kashgar. In her book, which focused on her domestic life and diplomatic activities, she mentions meeting my family in Leh and my role as interpreter for her husband.

As usual my family and I were a spectacle for the local population. The villagers crowded at the edge of our campsite trying to get a glimpse of Mrs. Shipton, Mother, Marjory and me. I think we were the only white women and children to have visited that part of Ladakh in living memory. The next day we said our farewells and parted company. The Shiptons were looking at four weeks of rugged mountain passes with winter fast approaching and we hoped to get to Srinagar in three weeks.

The route down to Leh was easy compared to the craggy and rutted terrain of the paths we'd followed the previous month. Most evenings we enjoyed the luxury of baths and fresh food in government rest houses similar to the ones we had stayed in en route to Kashgar. The caravan trail ran along the Shyok River, which we forded many times and which grew larger and faster each day. Buddhist prayer wheels, flags, writings and small shrines had been planted at frequent intervals along the side of the trail, perhaps sending us a message of assurance. Occasionally we passed Tibetan Buddhist Lamas in their distinctive red, heavy woollen garments and their characteristic hats. The number of villages we passed increased. Each had small fields nearby in which the villagers grew rice and other vegetables. At this altitude we descended into lush forests where we delighted once again in the songs of birds. For me this was a significant sign that we were returning to a familiar world.

On the last day, before reaching the town of Leh, we had one final high mountain pass to cross. Although steep, the pass had a well-used path which posed no problems after our experiences with the Mintaka, Sasser and Karakoram Passes. My first glimpse of Leh in the distance revealed a large city encircled by a wall. A palace rose from its centre. Behind the city a majestic monastery perched on top of a mountain. I wondered how it could have been built and how the monks could live up there. Later I learned that food, water and other essentials had to be laboriously transported up the mountain by the Lamas and their disciples. The structure had been built over many lifetimes, perhaps centuries and I marvelled at the devotion it would have taken to build such a holy site.

The people who lived in Ladakh were closely related to the Tibetans and shared their religion, language, customs and ethnic origins. A generous and affable people, the Ladakhis offered us small gifts of flowers and fruits as we passed by their homes. The clothes they wore were very different from the Kashgaries; they were much more decorative with many pieces of jewellery. The women wore colourful hats with large ear-like attachments. On these they had sewn all sorts of trinkets and their favourite turquoise stone. From the top of the hat dangled a tail that draped down their backs and had even more ornaments attached. These hats must have been extremely heavy, but they were worn with ease and pride. The women were also adorned with gold and silver bangles and an astonishing variety of necklaces.

The men wore long quilted garments that hung down like skirts. These were all brought together by a long cloth wound around their waists. In pockets, formed by the belted garment, the men kept various valuables, such as small bowls for making tea, knives, whips, and tobacco. They tied their hair in pigtails and also wore elaborate headgear. I was in awe of their dress, which seemed distinctive and ceremonial, yet commonplace.

We spent three days in Leh organizing a smaller caravan to take us to Srinagar, a journey of about two weeks. Because our new caravan used only pack horses, the caravan men spent much time redistributing our luggage. These men were from northwest India (now Pakistan). While our journey involved crossing several passes, the mountain trails were well maintained. Travelling became more comfortable and we were increasingly excited to be reaching the end of our trek and commencing our travels back to England.

On one of our descents, the trail narrowed, bounded by a two-thousand-foot drop into a ravine on one side and a sheer rock face disappearing into the clouds above on the other. In order to get a good view of the valley below I walked close to the edge, despite my parents' warnings. My foot caught on a rock and I pitched forward and found myself hanging over the edge, staring down into the ravine. I started slipping and thought I was going to fall all the way to the bottom when I felt someone grab me by the ankles.

"Stay still, Sahib!" said Suggi as he gradually pulled me back onto the trail. "That was very close, Sahib. You should not go so close to the edge. People die every year on these trails because they stumble like you did."

The experience terrified me and reminded me of my childhood episode in the sea when I'd nearly drowned. I felt the same helplessness and sense of foreboding. Again I didn't tell my parents, for fear of what Father would say and the punishment I would receive for disobeying him.

My final memory of the trip was of a pungent smell of India. I was walking, following a trail that made a gradual descent along a mountainside, when I noticed a clear, fresh smell that I recognized but couldn't name. We had just come down below the tree line and there were silver birch trees just ahead of us, but I knew the smell was not coming from them. I was puzzled. Soon the trail came to a turn and as I approached it the smell became stronger. When I rounded the bend I beheld a long valley that stretched out to my right. The valley was covered with magnificent, tall Himalayan pine trees for as far as I could see. Pine trees! It was their smell I had noticed. It had been three years since I had last seen or smelled them.

Our small caravan eventually came to the end of the trail and my family and all our possessions were transferred into an army lorry which drove us into the city of Srinagar and the army hotel. My father was still a captain in the Indian Medical Service and he was eligible for a year's leave with pay. Given his isolated postings, he had not taken any leave from service since 1938. It was now 1946. Our upcoming trip to England was his well-deserved leave. Since he was a captain he was assigned a "batman" or personal aide. Now there was no need for us to retain Suggi or Izatu. Father released them from our service and they were happy to return to their wives in the Hunza. I was saddened to part with such devoted companions. Suggi had been my confidante, mentor and friend. He had even saved my life. I found leaving my pony equally difficult. Not only had he faithfully carried me to and from Kashgar, we had been a part of each other's daily lives for three years. I was relieved to learn he was going back to the Hunza, back to the familiar, with Suggi and Izatu.

We stayed in the Srinagar Hotel for a few days before being transported by truck to the railhead at Rawalpindi. There we boarded a train to Bombay. The journey took two days. On arrival we learned we would have to wait another two weeks before getting berths on a troop carrier bound for England. True to its name, the Green Sea Hotel was within easy walking distance to the ocean. Here I spent most of my free time watching the fishermen perform a century's-old ritual on the wharf. Adjust rod, bait hook, pull line, cast.

After two weeks at the hotel, Father learned our ship, a Dutch ocean liner, was finally ready to sail. The ship had been retrofitted as a troop carrier for the war, which meant that the men were separated from the women in dormitories. Father and I were in a cabin with six other men. Normally the cabin would have had only two berths. Due to the increased number of passengers, meals were served in three sittings and the passengers were allocated tables according to cabin locations. This meant that Father and I were separated from Marjory and Mother at meal times. We were only able to see them on the promenade decks at prearranged times every day.

Our route back to England took us through the recently reopened Suez Canal. What made a lasting impact on me was the sight of all the derelict ships that had been purposely sunk by the Germans to block the canal during the war. Literally hundreds of ships were beached in the channel that ran between two deserts. Most were rusty, resting half in and out of the water. The scale of the wreckage was shocking and mindless. I couldn't understand why all this destruction had been ordered.

On the way to England, our ship stopped at Aden, Suez, Port Said, Naples and Gibraltar. In all these ports I saw Italian prisoners of war and British soldiers embarking and disembarking from troop ships. Later I realized I was witnessing a prisoner exchange program. This massive re-organization and relocation of human casualties, this sorting of human flesh, went on for years after the war. Many prisoners had nothing to go back to and opted to remain in the communities in which they had been captured.

In Suez I saw skirmishes between Arab boat traders who pulled up alongside the ship and competed to hock their wares to the passengers and crew. The air was hot, even in the shade, and filled with suggestions, offers, feigned anger, accusations, laughter. This boisterous haggling reminded me of the bazaar in Kashgar. Minus the pigeons. Cigarettes in particular were at a premium.

As the boat made its way into the port of Naples, I saw red flames and fire spewing out of the top of a mountain. My first active volcano. I'm not sure if it was Stromboli or Mount Etna. How unlike the snowy skyscapes of the Himalayas.

During the last week of the voyage Marjory fell ill and was admitted to the sick bay. Father was strangely quiet about her condition. I was not allowed to visit her for fear she might be infectious. I did not see her again until we disembarked at Southampton. When I did see her I noticed she was very yellow and Father explained that it was because of the medicines she had been given. Years later he would tell me he thought Marjory had had yellow fever. If this had been diagnosed, the whole ship would have been put under quarantine for ten days. No one wanted to be delayed getting home so close to Christmas. Certainly none of the doctors on board suggested this diagnosis to anyone in authority.

On the last morning of the trip, as we approached the Southampton docks, I went up early onto the deck. We were sailing upstream on a dull foggy morning and I could just make out the banks of the river through the fog. The occasional house was visible close to the shore with big willows, elms and horse chestnut trees close by. Then I heard a cock crowing followed by a dog barking, but I didn't see any people about. Church bells rang and I recognised their distinctive peal, even though I hadn't heard that sound since leaving England eight years before.

My first impressions of England, as I looked over the rail, made me wonder what the future would bring. Most of what I knew was what I had been told. My life was going to be very different. My parents had stressed that there would be no servants. Overseas, I had been in a unique position as a member of the "white" minority ruling class. For the first time I would have to start doing chores around the house. Help with the shopping. Work in the garden. There would be no Suggi or Izatu to do my work for me.

I was also aware I would have to go to a proper school. My previous experiences of formal schooling had not been positive and I was apprehensive. It was likely my new classmates would know more than I did.

"What do you think of England?" Father asked, as he came up beside me.

"I can't see much of it yet and I'm awfully cold. Perhaps it's the fog. I think I'll have a lot of new things to learn, but I'm happy to be returning home."

"Yes," Father said in a hushed voice, "I'm afraid all of us will have much to learn."

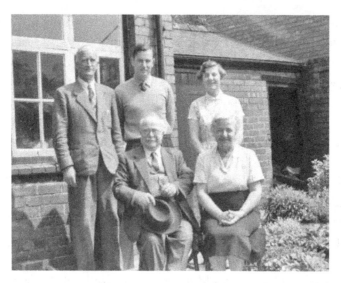

Top row: My father Pat, Uncle George and Aunt Ethel
(standing); Granddad and my mother Ada (seated).

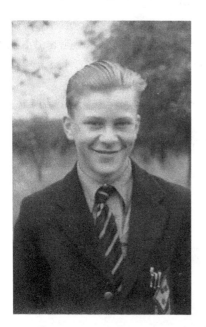

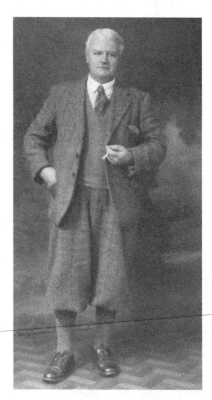

Above: Bernard in 1948.
Right: Bernard's grandfather
Ottwell Binns, vicar and au-
thor, who died in 1935.

Chapter 4
Post-War England and School

All the passengers appeared on deck, looking over the side, as the ship was slowly nudged into the key by three tugs. In the fog it was difficult to make out who was on the dock, waiting.

"Look, Pat. There's Ethel and Father. Father appears to have lost a lot of weight. They've not spotted us yet."

"Where are they, Mummy?" I asked.

"Over there, by the crane, towards the front of the ship. Your aunt Ethel has on a dark blue raincoat and a hat. Do you see her? Your grandfather is the man next to her in the light tan raincoat, glasses, smoking a pipe and wearing a brown hat. The young man next to Ethel must be George Douglas. They got married recently."

I spotted them and waved enthusiastically, like everyone else around us was doing. All at once Ethel started to point at us, and then she started to wave.

"They've seen us," said Father, waving back.

"How long will it take us to get off the ship?" asked Mother.

"At least an hour. Then we'll have to make our way through customs. It may be a while before we actually get to meet up with them. In the meantime, I better go and see how Marjory's getting on. I'll take Bernard down to the cabin to check that we haven't left anything behind. He can meet you back here in twenty minutes or so."

By the time I got back to the upper deck there was a lot of activity on the ship and dock. The two aft holds had had their covers taken off and two dock cranes on tracks were being used to unload them. The dock workers employed enormous rope nets to heft the trunks and baggage. Sometimes the cargo landed on the dock with a crash.

"I hope they're more careful with our boxes," said Mother as we watched one of the nets come open ten feet above the dock, spilling the boxes with a disconcerting thud. "Attention please; we will be disembarking in twenty minutes. Would all passengers please proceed to Deck Two and prepare to disembark from one of two gangways. Please check to see that you have all your personal belongings with you. This will be your last chance to check your cabins before leaving the ship," advised the voice over the loudspeaker.

"You better stay with me," said Mother. "Your father is going to carry Marjory down the gangway. We'll wait for them on the dock."

Eventually it was our turn to walk down the long swaying gangway with its canvas sides. It felt strange to be standing on the dock. It had been nearly four weeks since we had boarded ship in Bombay and I had lost my land legs. I could feel myself swaying to the rhythms of the sea.

We stood to one side and waited for Father and Marjory. They arrived a few minutes later, Father carrying Marjory piggyback. I could see that she looked very yellow; otherwise she seemed normal to me.

Father put Marjory down and she ran to embrace us. "Mummy, Bernard, isn't it a relief to get off the ship?"

"We saw Granddad and Aunt Ethel and her new husband, Uncle George, from the deck. They've come to meet us," I said excitedly.

"Well, I haven't seen anyone yet," Marjory complained, pouting and looking around.

"Let's find the Customs shed and our luggage. We need to catch the boat train for London," Father said. "It's supposed to leave at ten o'clock."

We spent the next hour searching for our trunks and waiting for a customs officer to check them. Father described the contents of each piece of luggage and when the man was satisfied he put a chalk mark on the case. We were lucky. We only had to open one of the trunks. Finally we were allowed out to meet Ethel, George and Granddad, who had been waiting patiently in the fog.

"Home at last!" said Mother as we emerged from the shed.

"Hello, Ada! How wonderful to see you again—after all these years," said Ethel, as they hugged each other. "It's been far too long."

Then the two women stood at arm's length and looked each other up and down. It was as if they were looking back in time and trying to locate an old image of each other in the present.

Then Mother turned and looked at Granddad.

"Hello Pop," she said, and she reached out and hugged him. "You're looking well."

Father said "hello" to Granddad and Ethel and shook hands with them. Unlike Mother, I couldn't tell if he was happy or not. All this time, George had been standing to one side while Marjory and I had stood behind Mother and Father.

"Oh, George, I am sorry. I forgot to introduce you," Ethel apologized. "This is Ada, my sister; Pat, her husband; Marjory and Bernard." We all shook hands.

George seemed to be a lot younger than Ethel. He had sharp features with pale blue eyes and was smartly dressed in a suit and unbuttoned raincoat. He wore a grey hat. Grandfather was shorter than Mother and Ethel and looked very old to me. He wore glasses, had a ruddy complexion, and a pleasant smile. His clothes were not as neat as George's and I noticed that his tweed jacket had spots of different coloured paint on it. I was intrigued by the curved pipe he held clenched between his teeth. Ethel was younger than Mother. She wore a navy blue cardigan and matching pleated skirt. She seemed to be strongly built and strode out when she walked. She also had blue eyes like mine and her hair was cut short and fairly straight.

"The train leaves from over there," said George, pointing to a platform about a hundred yards away to his right. "It will be leaving in about half-an-hour according to the conductor. You have seats booked in first class and we have found space in the next coach. I think it's going to be rather crowded but we'll be able to get together once the train starts. There should be a buffet car available for you, but the meal choices will probably be limited because of the rationing. In fact, you'll be lucky if there's anything more than a few sandwiches, tea or coffee. We've also brought a few biscuits."

We walked over to the train and a porter showed us to our seats. Soon all the seats were taken. Some passengers had to stand in the space between the seats with their luggage tucked between their feet.

The carriage got so full that we were trapped and nobody could get to the buffet car or the bathroom. Everyone smoked and, because all the windows were closed against the cold, the coach soon filled with smoke and became almost unbearable. "I don't think much of this, Pat," Mother said. "We'll probably suffocate before we get to Victoria Station."

Four hours later, as we approached Victoria Station, George managed to force his way to us. "Train's right crowded, isn't it?" he said with a slight Yorkshire accent. "When we get to the station I think we should all meet at the ticket collector's barrier. It's going to be very crowded when we get off and we don't want to get separated. We'll need two taxis to get us to King's Cross, but we should have plenty of time to catch the Retford train. We might even get a snack if we're lucky."

George pushed his way back between the other passengers to help Granddad and Ethel disembark. The train came into the station slowly, its wheels squealing, metal on metal, as the brakes were applied. Then the train jerked forwards and backwards before it came to a sudden stop. Everyone now tried to get off at once and the stampede turned into a jam at the doors.

"We might as well wait until everybody's off," Father suggested.

Once the madness had ended a porter came to help us move our bags and luggage to the barrier where George and the others were waiting.

"The taxis are over there," said George pointing towards the main entrance. When I looked around the station I was reminded of the one in Bombay. This station also had a high curved roof over the platforms and a central portion of glass, much of which was broken and very dirty. The entrance had wide arches of stone, through which I could see double-decker buses, cars and taxis moving around. The number of people in the station astonished me. Many of them were soldiers in uniforms accompanied by cheerful young women. The rest of the passengers were like us, family groups, excited to be going somewhere for Christmas. Bewildered by the commotion and afraid of getting lost, I stayed close to my parents.

We got to the taxi rank. The car was a typical London cab with lots of room inside and extra pull down seats.

"'Ow many of you are there, guv?"

"Five adults and two children," my father informed him.

"Do you have many bags?"

"Just these," said George, pointing to the pile of suitcases we had brought from the boat.

"Oh we can manage that lot," the cabbie said confidently. "Come on. Let's get the passengers in. Women and children first."

So Ethel, Mother, Marjory and I climbed in. "Bernard, you sit on the pull-down seat over there. Marjory, you can sit on my lap. That way I think there will be enough room for the others."

Granddad, Father and George then got in and we were all surprised that we managed to fit, though George had to sit on the edges of the two pull-down seats.

"Sorry, we'll have to put one of the bags inside with you and the piano can go on the top!" joked the cheerful Cockney driver as we all squeezed in. He closed the door, got into the driver's seat and asked, "Where to, guv?"

"King's Cross Station, please," said Father.

"Did you just come in off the Boat Train?"

"Yes."

"You must be back from India then. It's a bit colder here, ain't it? Where are you heading for today?" he asked, deftly steering the taxi out into the traffic.

"Worksop in Nottinghamshire," George answered.

"Never been there," the driver said.

We drove through narrow streets, filled with traffic, travelling much faster and closer to other cars than I was used to. Any second I was afraid there would be a crash. As we came into a brightly lit circus with a statue of what looked like a boy standing in the middle, the driver told us this was Piccadilly and that Eros had survived the war. He also said that London was recovering, that the theatre and night clubs were open and that there were a few things to buy in the shops. He went on to tell us that many of the streets were still impassable because of holes left by the bombing; and that there were a lot of houses still empty because they hadn't been repaired yet. He said it had been a terrible time.

"Here we are, King's Cross Station," said the taxi driver. "I'll take you around to the front where the porters are." He made a big left-handed sweep, through on-coming traffic, into the front of the station. We piled out of the taxi and retrieved our luggage from the top of the car. A porter came with his trolley and the taxi driver bid us farewell.

The porter quickly found the right platform and some seats in a carriage that had a corridor down one side of a row of compartments. Each compartment had eight seats. We settled into one of them and George went with Father to see if they could find some sandwiches and tea. The rest of us were left to guard the seats. The porter had told us that ours would be a very crowded train and that we were lucky to have arrived so early. Father and George returned with some thin, stale sandwiches, which we immediately gobbled up. The train soon filled, but because we had our own compartment we were quite comfortable. The only smoke was from Granddad's pipe and my parents' cigarettes. Eventually I heard the guard's whistle blow and the train started to move.

By now it was getting dark and I was tired. I looked out the train window but all I could see was my own reflection.

I woke up when Mother started shaking me. "Wake up, Bernard. We've arrived at Retford and have to get off the train. You've been asleep for the past three hours."

We packed our bags into two taxis and drove to Worksop, ten miles away on a curvy, hedge-lined road. As we left Retford I noticed some strange, small lights in the middle of the road.

"What are those?" I asked.

"Cat's eyes. They're made out of glass and set in the road so that you can see the middle of the road at night and in fog, like tonight. They were a Godsend in the blackouts when it was cloudy. We weren't allowed to use bright lights then, but the cat's eyes do not need much light to show up," explained our taxi driver. "Fortunately there weren't many cars on the roads because of petrol rationing. People only got enough to go a few miles a month, unless they were doctors or nurses. And even then, they could only use their cars for work. Most folks got about by walking, using the bus, trains or a bicycle."

"Did Worksop get bombed in the war?" I asked.

"No. We were lucky," said George. "The bombers were after Sheffield, which is sixteen miles further on. When we heard them coming, we ran for the air raid shelters, but they never hit us. Sheffield was hit badly for two or three nights. The Germans were after the ball-bearing works, but fortunately they missed the factory. It could've made a big difference to the war if they had hit it because it was the only factory making ball bearings for Spitfire engines.

"One bomb landed in a potato patch on a farm just outside of Worksop, to the south. They think the pilot got frightened and dumped his bomb trying to get away. The other excitement was one of those V1 bombs that came down just past Worksop and landed near another farm. They had to get the bomb disposal unit in to blow it up. It hadn't gone off. Those bombs were funny things. We could hear them coming because they made a different noise from the planes. We knew we were safe as long as we could hear them. When the noise stopped we would run for shelter."

"The V2s never got this far, but they were a different story. They hit the ground before you heard them coming. Your Aunt Alice was in London and said they were very frightening," Granddad added.

"We had no idea what was going on in England while we were in Kashgar," Mother said. "It must have been terrible."

"The blackouts were difficult," Ethel said. "You didn't go out at night unless you had to, and the rationing, which is still bad, made life hellish. We've not had oranges, bananas or fresh fruit in the shops for a long time now. One egg a week is not much if you want to bake. The one ounce of bacon allotted does not go far. Added to that, the sugar rationing means that you can have sugar on your corn flakes or in your tea, but not both. Meat is terribly scarce, but there is some fish. I think we have all lost some weight. Your Granddad has lost a lot but he always fancied sweet things. Even though we have coupons there are no sweets or chocolates in the shops. Without sugar it's difficult to make cakes and nice puddings. Clothes and shoes have also been rationed and they're in short supply up here and will be for a while.

"Coal for heating the house is hard to buy even now and even though we live right next door to two coal pits. There are some things that you just can't get. Other things, like cigarettes and tobacco, you have to queue up for when they come in. Fortunately your Granddad has a few friends that keep him supplied. George and I don't smoke so we're not bothered. They keep saying that things are going to get better, but we haven't noticed any change. The children get extra milk at school and can get school lunches. That helps a bit although a lot of them complain the food is awful. When I'm on school lunch duty I notice that most of the food is eaten. The children don't look too bad," Ethel informed us.

"England's had a hard time of it," said Father. "It sounds as if we were better off in Kashgar."

The taxi stopped on a corner outside a three-storey, red brick, semi-detached Victorian house. Along the front of the house ran a low wall with the remains of a wrought iron fence sticking out. On the other side of the wall was a narrow patch of grass with two empty flower beds. Overhanging these was a bay window covered by curtains. Up six steps, the entrance was set back into the house. Granddad opened the heavy front door and we all went in. A small narrow hallway led past a door on the left. Beyond this I could see a straight stairway going up to the first landing.

A short, plump lady with a reddish face and dark hair bustled along the corridor from the back of the house. "Merry Christmas to you all! I was beginning to wonder if you'd get back tonight with all the fog about."

"Miss Knowles, do you remember Bernard and Marjory?" said Mother, nudging us forward to meet her.

"You have grown a lot, haven't you, Bernard. Of course, Marjory was just a baby when you went out to India. I've got some supper for you in the back."

Miss Knowles led the way to a large cosy kitchen. A coal fire glowed in an old-fashioned farmers' stove. A square table was laid out with a plate of sandwiches, homemade cakes and cheese. In one corner, a tall grandfather clock stood beside a well-worn settee. Some wooden chairs were set around the table. To the left of the fireplace a door led out to a scullery and the backyard. An old roll-top writing desk with a wireless and several pieces of paper on top nestled next to a small window. Beside the wireless, propped up against the wall, was a six-by-eight-inch rectangle of thin, silver-plated metal.

"I'm afraid there's not much butter on the bread and we're a bit short of sugar, because of the rationing—and with Christmas coming tomorrow," she said.

"Don't worry about it, Miss Knowles. A good cup of tea will go down nicely," said Granddad.

Surprisingly, there were Christmas stockings at the end of our beds in the morning and presents for us to open. After three years in Kashgar, where there were only local products, the toys we got that Christmas were numerous and novel, imaginative and colour-ful. Thanks to these presents I became aware of some of my other relatives in England. There was an Aunt Alice, Ethel's twin sister, in Birmingham, who worked as a district nurse. George had a brother, Ron, and sister, Betty. I got a present from an Aunt Marjorie and a Grandmother in Derry Hill, and discovered I had an aunt and uncle who lived in Rochdale. We learned about an aunt and uncle who had sent us gifts from Jamaica. Another aunt and uncle lived in Wash-ington, D.C. And finally, there was an Uncle Max, who, for whatever reason, remained a mystery.

Marjory and I spent the morning playing with our new toys. At lunch time Ron, Betty and Alice arrived to spend Christmas with us. That evening I had my first proper Christmas dinner. A feast, in spite of rationing. Marjory and I had never eaten a meal like it, with so many people gathered around a large dining table in the front room with an open coal fire to keep us warm. There was ham and turkey with all the condiments. Christmas pudding and custard, which was new to us, topped off the meal.

During the next couple of weeks Granddad showed me around

Worksop. I learned that he owned and ran a painting and decorating business out of the house and that the shop was in the back yard at 80 Carlton Road. He had worked there most of his life but his parents had come from Scotland. He was a gifted artist but only painted in his spare time. The silver-plated rectangle I had noticed in the kitchen on Christmas Day was a coffin plate. I was enthralled by the way he did them, completely free hand, and he always added decorative touches to make them more attractive. Each one took him about ten minutes.

Granddad also took me to my first church service. Aunt Ethel warned me that he tended to fall asleep and snore in church and that it was my job to keep him awake by elbowing him when this happened. I was not sure what to make of church services, but I felt religion was something about which I needed to learn. My parents never went to church and did not discuss religion with Marjory and me until we were much older. This always surprised me as Father had been brought up in a strict Church of England family. His father, Grandfather Ottwell Binns, had been a parson who, towards the end of his life, had become disillusioned with the church. Perhaps this explained Father's misgivings. And silence.

Worksop was a typical North Midlands coal mining town of approximately 50,000 people. Located on a small river canal, it had several schools, a public library, four cinemas, a small park, a railway station, many public houses, churches and a busy shopping street. The only large store was the Co-op, which had five storeys. Everything was within walking distance of 80 Carlton Road. Two coal mines were located just outside of town. We were only aware of the tip smoke when there was a south wind. The prevailing wind was from the east. In the winter of 1947 there was a lot of fog, made worse by the pits and the use of open coal and coke fires for heating houses. Those first Worksop weeks were cold, damp and foggy. My discomfort was compounded by the fact that I had to wear clothes brought from India, which were very different from those worn locally. I looked out of place and felt embarrassed when other children laughed at me.

Fortunately, because of the holiday, I didn't have to worry about school when we arrived in Worksop. It was not until Aunt Alice had gone back to Birmingham, and the other visitors had left after Christmas, that Father broached the subject. At breakfast, in early January, he said, "I've been down to the local school and talked to the Headmaster. He says you are too old to take the 11 Plus exam. Therefore you'll have to go to the Secondary Modern school here. I had hoped you'd be able to attend the Grammar school in Retford, but you have to pass the 11 Plus exam to be admitted there. Anyway, I have arranged for you to go down to the school on Monday. I've asked your Aunt Ethel if she can take you."

"Do I have to go to school, Daddy?" I asked. The prospect of facing other children who already found me peculiar was daunting.

"Yes, it's the law. Besides, a proper education is important. I've told the Headmaster that for the most part you've been home-schooled. The Headmaster said he would put you into one of the classes with younger boys to see how you get on. I think you'll be all right, but don't be afraid to ask the teachers if you don't understand something."

"I'm not sure I'm going to like school here. The other day, some boys in the street laughed at me. They all have school uniforms, shorts, long socks and special pullovers or jackets. All I have to wear are long trousers and a brown jacket," I said.

"We can't do anything about that at the moment. Your ration book has not arrived yet. You'll just have to explain to them why you're dressed differently."

Worksop Central School, a Secondary Modern School, catered to pupils aged eleven to sixteen. It was a single-storey building with two tarmac playing areas. The whole school was surrounded by a six-foot wrought iron fence. There were several hundred boys and girls enrolled and the individual classes had up to thirty-five children in them. Most of the students came from mining homes. They spoke with a broad Nottinghamshire accent that I found difficult to understand.

My humiliation and isolation intensified when it became apparent in class that I couldn't read. This was also a surprise to the teacher who decided that learning to read was my first priority. I soon found myself at the back of the class trying to learn this skill while the rest of the class did other lessons. My teacher designated two of the better pupils to help me. I was also given special work to take home. After a few weeks my reading did improve but my writing was another story. The script I had been taught in my brief lessons in Indian schools was different and was considered unacceptable. I hadn't been taught how to wield a pen. I repeatedly tried to write things out for the teacher and was told that my penmanship was terrible. Nothing but chicken scratch.

I was so embarrassed about my reading and writing problems that I didn't tell my parents. Consequently, they remained ignorant of my deficiencies until the half-term reports came out. My report card stated that my English teacher thought I was illiterate. The proposed solution was that I should be sent to a special school. Worksop Central did not have the time or the staff to give me the special tutoring I needed. This came as a terrible shock to Father, but not to Mother. She was confident that I would learn fairly quickly once I got over the initial steps. Father was not so convinced. He was worried about what he should do with me. He wrote to the headmaster at his old school, Nottingham High, which was a public day school (one of two in England at the time) asking for advice. In response, he was invited to take me to the school for an interview.

A few days later, Father and I travelled to Nottingham by train, changing stations at Mansfield. Nottingham High School was perched on the top of a hill overlooking an Arboretum and the city of Nottingham to the south. A public park area called the Forest was located to the north. The grounds were surrounded by an intimidating nine-foot grey stone wall. The school, also built out of grey stone, looked a bit like a medieval castle. The building was five storeys high with four turrets which, I was to discover later, housed the prefects' rooms. At that time there were five to six hundred boys attending the school.

The main entrance was up a set of stairs and through a Gothic arch inset with nine-foot double doors. When Father and I stepped through the heavy wooden doors into the front foyer, the first thing I noticed was the high walls and ceilings. Light flooded the space from towering windows. Down three steps to the right there was a long hardwood corridor. Straight ahead, up five steps, was another wider, more modern corridor with windows on the right and doors off to the left. One of these was a big wooden door with 'Library' printed on it. Just behind us was a door marked 'Secretary' and on the other side of the entrance was a door marked 'Headmaster'. Father went over to the secretary's door and knocked.

"Come in," a female voice called. A slim middle-aged woman got up from behind her desk. "You must be Dr. Binns and son. The Headmaster is expecting you. I'm Miss Morley, Mr. Reynolds's Secretary."

"Wonderful," Father said, "Mr. Reynolds was the Headmaster when I was here as a boy, twenty-odd years ago."

"Yes, the Headmaster has been here for a very long time. He's free now. I'll go and tell Mr. Hardwick that you've arrived. He wants to talk to Bernard after you've introduced him to the Headmaster."

We left the office and Father tapped on the Headmaster's door.

"Come in," called a deep voice. Father opened the door and I saw a tall, gaunt man with a prominent hooked nose standing behind a large wooden desk. He wore a black academic gown over a dark suit. There were a few books, papers, and a mortarboard on the desk in front of him.

"I remember you, Binns! You went off to London to do medicine. Whatever happened to you after that?" he asked.

"It's a long story," my father said. "After I qualified in medicine I got married and went to the Falkland Islands for two years. Then I joined the I.M.S. after a short stay in England. During the war I spent two years in the Middle East and then ended up in Chinese Turkestan in the British Foreign Service. Unfortunately there were no schools there and Bernard didn't get any formal schooling. I'm hoping that you will be able to help out."

"How do you do, Bernard? What do you think of England? Were you born in India?" He came round the edge of the desk and loomed over me. He had striking blue eyes behind his spectacles.

"I was born in the Falkland Islands, sir. I've found England to be very different from India and China. I haven't made any friends yet so I can't say much more about it."

Just then there was a knock at the door and a short man wearing a black gown with a mortarboard on his head entered with a flourish.

"Ah, Mr. Hardwick, this is the boy I talked to you about at lunch. Could you take him while I talk to his father?"

As worried as I was about what might lie in store for me at this school, I was determined to please Father.

"Hello, Bernard," said Mr. Hardwick, motioning his head toward the door, "would you come this way? I want to talk to you. I also need you to take a little test." He led the way out of the office, turned right, and we walked down the corridor I had noticed earlier. We went past three closed doors behind which I could hear voices. The fourth door was open and Mr. Hardwick led the way into a small classroom with about twenty desks in it.

"Take a seat at that desk in the front there. How old are you?"

"I'll be thirteen next month. My birthday is on the second of April," I answered.

"Have you ever been to school?"

"Yes. When I was six or seven I went to Ooty in India for two terms, but spent most of the time in the sick bay. I've been going to the local school in Worksop for the past two months, but they don't think I can manage there."

"What's the problem?"

"I can't read what the teacher writes on the blackboard and the other boys and girls make fun of me. I don't like it, especially because I try hard."

"Do you think you can read and write?"

"Not very well, but I'm good at maths. I know a lot more than the boys in the Worksop school."

"That's a good start. Is there anything else that you can do that they cannot?"

"I can speak Urdu, Hindi and Turki. But I can't write in those languages either."

"Let's just see what you can do, shall we? Here's a paragraph from a book by a man named Bernard Shaw. What I want you to do is to read the paragraph and then in your own words write down on this piece of paper what you think the paragraph means. Write your name and address on the piece of paper first. I will be back in about half an hour."

He swept out of the room, closing the door behind him.

A lot depended on how I got on in the next half hour, so I started by trying to read the paragraph out loud to myself. It was headed by a quotation and included a lot of words I had never come across before. Some I could not identify because I had been taught to read phonetically. When I tried to pronounce them they did not sound like words I had heard before. However, after twenty minutes I had come to the conclusion that this man Bernard Shaw was commenting on how the poor lived in England and how hard it was for them. Having established this I proceeded to start writing my name and address at the head of the piece of paper. I got as far as *Bernard Binns, 80 Carlton Road.*

When Mr. Hardwick returned he looked at what I had written. "You don't seem to have gotten very far, do you?"

"Sir, I've read the piece and can tell you what it says. But I've not had time to write anything down."

"Tell me what it says, then. We'll forget about the writing part for now."

So I told him what I thought the paragraph meant and asked him who Bernard Shaw was. Mr. Hardwick told me that he was a very famous writer and that I should have known about him. Then he said, "You seem to have some idea what the writing was about, Bernard, that's very encouraging. Now let me see you write the rest of your address out."

I did as he asked, but I noticed that he was getting a bit agitated as I puzzled over each letter. Finally he said, "That's enough; you can't write properly yet, can you? I'm not sure what we'll do with you if it's decided to admit you here. Tell me, have you been taught any geography, history, English literature, French, German, Latin or science subjects?"

"No sir, but I have been taught a lot of maths, with algebra and geometry."

"I suppose that's better than nothing. Let's go back to the Headmaster's office to see what he has to say." Later I discovered that Mr. Hardwick was the senior English teacher and did not think much of the sciences or maths.

When we got back to the Secretary's office Mr. Hardwick asked me to stay with her while he went and spoke to my father and the Headmaster. Ten minutes passed before I was asked to go into the Headmaster's office again.

"Bernard, you seem to have a problem with your reading and writing. I have talked it over with Mr. Hardwick and your father. I think you'll be able to attend here, but you will have to work very hard to catch up on all the things you've missed. Your father has suggested some private lessons after school hours. I think this is a good idea. You will be starting after the Easter break, in form Three Red. You will be a little older than the other boys, but don't let that worry you. What do you think of the idea? Do you want to come to school here?"

I knew this was a great opportunity and that Father wanted it. "Thank you, sir. I would like to come here very much. I will try hard to catch up with the other boys."

I could see Father relax and I knew he was pleased. As we were about to leave the room, he stopped and turned back to the Headmaster: "Could I ask you one more favour? Do you know of anyone who could help find a place for Bernard to stay while he attends school?"

"I don't know of anyone off hand, but I'll make some enquires and let you know. There are a few weeks left before Bernard starts so there should be no problem finding him a place to live. On the way out, ask my secretary to give you the details about uniforms and other information that you'll need," said Mr. Reynolds.

"Thank you again. You don't know what a relief it is for me to be able to give Bernard an opportunity like this," said Father, shaking hands with the Headmaster.

"We have a lot of things to do when we get back to Worksop," Father said as we settled into our seats on the train for the return journey. "Most important is to find you somewhere to stay in Nottingham before the term starts. I hope you'll do all right at this new school. Mr. Reynolds said you have one year to prove yourself. The main thing he's interested in is your willingness to learn. If you don't put in an effort then you'll be back at Worksop Central Secondary, learning a trade. It's not what I had hoped for you, but it's still an option. However, if you manage to do well at Nottingham then you should be able to go to University. We will have to buy a house in Worksop and I have to find some work soon. With everyone coming back from the war there aren't many jobs available in England at the moment. It may take me some time to find a suitable position. Anyway, I'm sure things will work out in the end. Do remember, it's your own effort that will be important at Nottingham." The idea of going back to Worksop Central was distasteful, so I decided, then and there, I would do my best to stay at Nottingham. Luckily my Aunt Ethel was a teacher and my parents arranged for her to come over in the evenings to help me with my reading and writing skills. Surprisingly, understanding Aunt Ethel's lessons was challenging, for reasons I did not yet understand.

Grandfather had a radio and I was allowed to listen to *Dick Barton, Special Agent*, every evening at quarter to seven, just before the news. He also had a half-size billiard table in the front room and taught me how to play billiards and snooker. On the weekends he showed me round the paint shop at the back of the house and took me for walks with Mitzie, his dog, who was not very bright. She used to get lost and could not find her way back to the house even if she was just around the corner. Everyone in the neighbourhood knew Mitzie and they would bring her back to the yard when she got out.

Grandfather took me to work with him a few times so I learned a bit about painting and decorating. More importantly, he took pride in showing me how to paint people and scenery and I discovered how difficult it was to create a picture that had proportion and perspective.

During the Easter holidays, my father and mother bought a house.

It was located on a quiet street close to the centre of town. Built of red brick, it was two storeys tall, set behind a three foot high wall. A small gate on the main road opened into a pretty garden split into two by a path that led to the front door. On either side of the front door were windows that looked into the front rooms. Inside the front door, stairs rose up to the four bedrooms and bathroom.

The main living area extended across the back of the house. A window on the right looked into the yard and onto our neighbours' brick wall. A short flight of stairs led to a small damp cellar. On one side of the room stood an old built-in, wood-burning cook stove that brightened up the room when lit. To the right of the stove was another door that went through to the kitchen which had a draining area with a hand-action water pump. Recently hot and cold water taps had been added over the sink, and a new gas cooking stove had been installed. A door opened into the backyard. Most of the yard had been paved with tarmac, except for a small area of garden, a coal shed, an outside toilet and two horse stables, one of which had been converted into a garage.

We had nothing for the house, so over the next two weeks the whole family went on a shopping spree for furniture, cutlery, crockery, kitchen items, linen, and other essentials. For me visiting the shops became an expedition of discovery. Not only did I meet new people, some of them like the characters Mother had read about in stories during homeschooling, but I learned something of the history and gossip of Worksop.

One evening, during the holiday, Father announced that the next day we would be going to Nottingham to see a Mrs. Jackson. "She's offered you a place to stay while attending school in Nottingham. The minister at the local church says it's most suitable. We'll take the bus from here; that way you'll know the route, where to get on and where to get off. You don't have to change buses anywhere. That makes it simple."

Mother, who was folding linen, interrupted Father: "I gather Mrs. Jackson has two children, a boy, Philip, who is a year younger than you and a girl, Katherine, who is four years younger. Mrs. Jackson's husband did not return from the war and is presumed killed, so don't ask about him when you meet them."

The next day our entire family took a double-decker bus to Nottingham. We went to the upper deck so my parents could smoke. I sat next to a window. It seemed a long drop down to the road and I was a bit frightened, especially when the bus went fast and leaned over, as if it were going to roll, when going around corners. Father said there was no danger because of the bus's low centre of gravity. I soon got used to this swaying motion, as I had riding a horse, and began watching the scenery pass by.

The road out of Worksop started with a climb up a steep hill. As the bus struggled towards the top the driver kept changing gears and, at one point, almost lurched to a stop. I thought we might have to get out and push as we had done on one occasion in India.

Outside Worksop the countryside became rolling farmland dotted with farm houses and the occasional clumps of massive oak and beech trees. There were cows and sheep, but most of the fields had been recently ploughed and planted. I saw a few crows and two magpies fly off the road as the bus accelerated towards them.

"Look, Pat. Two magpies. Isn't that supposed to be lucky?" asked Mother.

"Yes, but it's a silly superstition, Ada," Father replied. "I don't believe in that sort of thing." Father had an abiding faith in science.

"The country we're going through now used to be all oak forests," Father said. "Legend says this is where Robin Hood lived with his band of outlaws. We pass two towns that were famous in his time. Ollerton is the first and the other is Edwinstowe, about seven miles further up the road. There is a famous oak tree standing near Edwinstowe known as Robin Hood's larder. Robin Hood used to store food in its hollow interior. Unfortunately there is very little of the old forest still standing. The remaining trees are all on private land."

"How far is it from Worksop to Nottingham?" I asked.

"It's twenty-seven miles as the crow flies, but the bus route takes some twists and turns, so it takes an hour-and-a-half to get there when the weather is good. Fog, which is frequent through the fall and winter months, can slow the bus down to a crawl. I have no doubt you'll have some long trips during the next few years. In the summer it's a very pretty trip, but in the winter it can be dreary."

The bus continued through the rolling countryside and eventually crept up a long hill. When we got to the top I could see the city of Nottingham spread out below us. It was a beautiful cloudless, sunny day. I could see a big stone castle in the distance.

"What's that place over there?" I asked.

"That's the famous Nottingham Castle, where the Sheriff used to live," explained Mother.

As we came down the hill we entered a heavily built-up area. The main streets were wide and the gardens large, some with old, well-established trees. My first impression of the city was that it would be a nice place to live.

"The Odeon, Sherwood!" bellowed the conductor and I heard the stop-bell ring for the driver.

"This is our stop," said Father.

The walk to Mrs. Jackson's was three to four hundred yards along a short road. Number 27 was at the top of a slight grade and overlooked a valley where I could see open countryside and family farms.

Mrs. Jackson was a small, vivacious lady with a round face and dark tightly-curled hair. I liked her right from the start and ended up staying with her family for the next six years.

After a tour of the house my parents decided that the accommodation was more than adequate for my needs. I would arrive in a week's time, when I started at Nottingham High. After leaving Mrs. Jackson's we went into Nottingham city to buy my school uniform—a grey suit, school tie, shirts, socks and two pairs of black shoes. Since I was entering the third form in the upper school, I was allowed to wear long trousers. Rationing was still in place so Mother had to use up a lot of the family clothing coupons for the purchases.

Nottingham was the first big-city shopping area I had explored, but to my surprise the shops were less busy than the market stalls in Kashgar. And instead of horses, camels and donkeys, quiet trolley buses glided along the streets. At first I was startled by the overhead wiring that crackled and threw out blue sparks when the trailing arms went through junctions in the wires. So much was completely foreign—at times I felt speechless.

My school routine proved simple. I would board the bus at Worksop at 7 p.m. on Sunday evenings and arrive at Mrs. Jackson's at about eight-thirty. I would have a cup of tea and a snack and go to bed. Mrs. Jackson woke us up at quarter to eight in the morning. I had to be out the front door by eight-thirty, down to the end of the road, to catch a bus into Nottingham. After reaching my stop, it took me another ten minutes to walk to the school.

Within six months of my starting school at Nottingham High, Father took a job with the Colonial Office in Northern Nigeria. Once again he had been hooked by the allure of adventure.

He started his first tour in October 1947. Consequently the next six years of my life were sometimes a bit muddled and lonely. My parents' absence left me feeling adrift. Yet even as a school boy I could see why Father was attracted to working for the Colonial Service. He liked travelling, changing environments, challenging work, meeting a mix of people, and the job security. On the other hand, he and Mother both disliked being away from Marjory and me and the rest of their family.

During the ten years they were in Nigeria, between 1948 and 1958, my parents were stationed in six different cities. While I was in school, they came back to England for a total of fifteen months, on leave, plus nine months when Father did his Diploma of Public Health course in London. Any friendships they made during tours were short-term—people moved so often it was impossible to keep in contact.

Perhaps the greatest concern for people who went overseas was the physical risk, especially when most of the assignments were to tropical countries. Tropical diseases were common and colonial staff were frequently shipped home or reassigned. Alcoholism was also rampant amongst the colonial expatriate 'club'. Drinking excessively all too often came with the lifestyle. Added to this, marriages suffered from multiple moves and separation from children and spouses.

Initially Father was posted to a hospital station in Minna, Northern Nigeria. With my sister and me both enrolled in good schools, my parents thought it was better for us to stay at school in England. To facilitate this, Ethel and George moved into our house to look after Marjory and me when we were not in school. I would be in Worksop every weekend and every school holiday, while Marjory, who was enrolled in a girl's boarding school in Rutland and later Skegness, would return to Worksop for Christmas, Easter and the summer holiday. A typical 'tour' lasted for twenty-two to twenty-six months. Between tours my parents would take a two- to three-month holiday and return to England and our house in Worksop. The whole family had to adapt to this 'colonial' lifestyle. As strange as it might seem, I rarely thought there was anything unusual about having two 'homes' and absent parents. And yet I don't recollect meeting any other boys at Nottingham High School who lived similar parentless lives. Nottingham was a day school, not a boarding school, so all the students lived close by and their parents had jobs in the city. On the other hand, Marjory had several school friends whose parents lived overseas like ours.

Because home-schooling had left such deep gaps in my knowledge, my academic performance during the first two years at Nottingham was poor—the work gruelling. I was placed in a class of boys who were all at least a year younger than I was, but who all knew more than I did. All were much better at reading and writing. Although the masters were aware of my educational history, I did not get any special treatment and my classmates and I were all assessed using the same tests and exams. The subjects that required reading and writing skills were a total disaster for me. I had not been taught the basics needed to do well in geography, history, French, general science, English language or literature—essentially the entire curriculum.

To fill in the gaps in my knowledge, I stayed on after school once a week for special tuition in French and English Language. The tutorials continued for my first two years. Luckily most of the boys in my class were sympathetic and for the most part didn't tease me, but there were times when they couldn't resist taking the Mickey out of me. Fortunately there was one area where I could hold my own and that was in mathematics. I was soon put into the upper-stream class in this subject.

As I struggled with the sheer amount of work I needed to do to be successful, I became well organised and disciplined. Until I'd finished my homework, I was a prisoner. I was slow and methodical and at first homework took up most of my free time. I would get back from school at about 5 p.m., have an early high tea with the Jackson family, then go up to my room and do school work until 8:30 p.m. At 9 p.m. we would sit down and have a sandwich and cup of cocoa before bed. Often I would read one of the library books I had borrowed until ten. Then Mrs. Jackson would call "lights out."

I continued to read library books. I even read on the bus back and forth to Worksop. Eventually I came to appreciate new and alternative visions of the world, some rash, some clumsy, some beautifully conceived. It was a pleasant way to pass the time. Initially I would only get through a book every two to three weeks, but towards the end of my high school days I would check out two novels a week.

I found adventure stories the easiest and the most interesting to read, but I also read quite a lot of non-fiction, mainly in the sciences and travel. One book, by Julian Huxley, started me thinking about astronomy. He explained how vast the universe was by suggesting that if each known star were represented by a grain of sand, there would be enough sand to cover the entire British Isles with six inches. This concept was awe-inspiring, suggesting to me that the world was a very insignificant place. And that humans were even more so.

To improve my sadly neglected knowledge of English literature I tried to read the English classics. Some authors, like Sir Walter Scott, Jane Austen, and Charles Dickens, I found difficult, while others, like Aldous Huxley and Joseph Conrad, told a good story and shared ideas and images that stimulated my imagination. They had something to say about how I should live my life. At school we covered the usual Shakespeare—*Macbeth*, *A Midsummer Night's Dream*, *Othello*—as well as a Goldsworthy play and a Shaw play. Mr. Hardwick enthusiastically explained what these plays were all about, but I was never interested enough to read more of their works on my own.

Ultimately, it was the sciences that captured my interest. Initially we took a general course which covered basic concepts in all the sciences. But as the years progressed the subjects became specialized into physics, chemistry, and biology. Like my father, I found the sciences suited my temperament and aptitude. In these areas I could hold my own with the other boys and eventually I even managed to rise to the top of the class.

The fact that I was mildly dyslexic was not recognized until years later.

Throughout my school years I don't remember spending a weekend or any vacation time in Nottingham. Consequently, I never got to know any of my schoolmates very well. Nor, to my surprise, do I remember spending any 'free' time with the Jackson children. Most of my discretionary time was spent with my aunt and uncle.

In 1947, on what was to be the last family outing before my parents went off to Nigeria, the entire family went to Skegness on the east coast of England for a week's holiday. There were eight in the party and we all stayed in a boarding house two streets from the sea. Our party included my parents, Marjory, Uncle George and Aunt Ethel, Aunt Alice, Granddad Grant and me. There wasn't much room in the house and we had to share bedrooms. I ended up sharing a double bed, which had a bolster down the middle, with my grandfather. George muttered something about Granddad's snoring, but I hadn't a clue what he was talking about. In the middle of the first night I was wakened by a horrendous noise. As I crawled out of my slumber I thought it must be the sea, and then I realized we were too far away from it for it to be the source. Finally it dawned on me—the noise was coming from Granddad. I had no idea how to escape his snoring, nor did I think it was my place to complain, so I spent a sleepless week.

It was a hot summer and the sea at Skegness was reputed to be warm, at least by East Coast standards, so we were all expected to go swimming. In fact, the water was frigid and I concocted every excuse I could imagine to avoid going in. I spent a lot of time walking up and down the promenade and going out onto the pier.

My Aunt Alice loved the slot machines. She spent hours at them and I used to watch her and the other players, beguiled by the promise of great wealth. I was only allowed to put in six pence a day and soon found that I did not get much in return; but the attraction of winning held me and I have since liked to have 'flutters' on the pools in England and lotteries in Canada. The strict rule about only putting in a set amount of money was a good education for me and has probably stopped me from becoming an ardent gambler.

Ethel, Alice's twin sister, had no interest in the slot machines. My mother enjoyed them but was not as addicted to them as Alice. Father, George and Granddad were not at all interested in the slots and insisted they were just a waste of money. One evening we all went to one of the vaudeville shows, which was a review and a bit bawdy. I wasn't old enough to understand most of the jokes.

But it's the crowds of people and people-watching that I remember most—they were everywhere—walking on the promenade, sitting on the beaches tanning, playing games, queuing up for food at the shops along the front, queuing up to get into the public toilets. Gaudily dressed in stripes, polka dots and bright colours, most of them had strong Yorkshire accents. Between laughing, drinking, partying, dancing, and gambling, the occasional argument would erupt or a child would scream. Street photographers roamed the promenades, picking out likely subjects and pointing a camera at them, then asking them if they wanted to buy a photo. Sometimes they took the picture before asking you if you wanted one taken; other times they asked you to pose, as if you were a celebrity. I could never figure out what determined which approach they would take. What surprises me now is why crowds of people would cast such a spell on a boy who had spent his formative years in India.

* * *

One Saturday afternoon when I was fifteen, my parents' house in Worksop was invaded by a troop of girls. My Aunt Ethel had invited the school netball team over for tea. I was in the front room listening to the radio when she came in.

"Bernard, would you like to join us?"

I was rather shy about the idea of meeting new people, but it was teatime so I went into the kitchen where there were seven girls. This was the first time since my weeks at Worksop Central that I had met girls my own age. After the initial introduction most of them ignored me. They were excited about how their team was doing in the inter-school competitions. One of the girls was quieter than the rest. She came over to me and introduced herself as Shirley. She told me she liked to go for walks on Sunday afternoons and asked if I would be interested in joining her. Embarrassed to explain to my aunt and uncle that I was meeting a girl, I used walking their dog, Jimmy, as an excuse for our rendezvous.

Shirley came from a mining family about whom she was reluctant to speak and of whom I sensed she was ashamed. I was never invited to her house. Walking along the canal and through an abandoned RAF airfield, we grew closer and intimate, each of us transfixed with discovery and experiment—with our first encounter with the opposite sex.

One evening at supper my aunt asked: "Bernard, would you like to go Youth Hostelling over the Easter holidays? I have to book the hostels this weekend. We have a group of five netball players from the school and I need to even out the numbers. Marjory's not coming back from Rutland for the holidays."

"What's Youth Hostelling?" I asked, a little apprehensive.

"It's an organization that runs hostels for young people who are interested in touring. They provide dormitories with blankets and bunk beds, some meals or cooking facilities, at very modest costs.

They run hostels all over the country and Europe so that you can see different places cheaply. Our plan this time is to walk in the Yorkshire Dales, which is gorgeous walking country. We will be away for four or five days."

"Will Uncle George be with us?" I asked.

"No, unfortunately I have to work that weekend and can't come," said Uncle George. "But you'll enjoy the trip, Bernard. It'll be better than staying home alone with me."

I hesitated, worried about being the only male in the group. What would we talk about? What did we have in common? What would they think of me, the only boy on their outing?

But I had been trapped. I'd been caught by my own indecision. I needed to be quicker.

A week later, Aunt Ethel gave me the booklet that came with my membership to the Youth Hostel Association. The organization was for people who wanted to walk, cycle, canoe, or kayak. Cars were not allowed and hitchhiking was discouraged.

Three weeks later I met my fellow hostellers at the Worksop railway station. We took the train to Northalerton where we transferred to the train to Castle Bolton, in Wensleydale. Aunt Ethel had found an old rucksack for me and had told me what to pack: a sheet sleeping bag, towel, change of clothes, rain gear, soap, toothbrush and paste, plus several other odds and ends.

During the next four days we walked an average of twelve miles a day over hilly terrain. Under a cloudless sky, we hiked up one dale, found a path over the top into another, and then returned to Castle Bolton. Ethel had an Ordinance Survey map, which showed official walks, streams, rivers, farms, forested areas and height contours. She showed us how to read maps and use a compass. The only thing I got was a nasty blister on my right heel. I think Aunt Ethel had been expecting the problem because she made sure I packed a good supply of Elastoplasts and antiseptic solution. At day's end, I was also surprised by how sore my muscles felt.

At each hostel we were given tasks to do during our stay. We were not allowed to leave until the warden had inspected our work. Some wardens were strict, others more tolerant and forgiving. The porridge pan after breakfast was one job I avoided, if possible. I met people from all over the country and several hikers and cyclists from the continent. There were people from all age groups. Some of them must have been in their sixties, which surprised me, but most of them were young adults. Ours was the only school group. Many of the languages and accents were new to me. To my embarrassment there was a group of cyclists from North Birmingham that I couldn't understand, mistaking their thick accents for a foreign language. They thought this was a great joke.

During that same summer Ethel and George took Marjory and me on a cycling trip into Lincolnshire. We also went on a walking trip to the Lake District with some of the netball team. This walk was long and the terrain rocky and rugged. I came to love Youth Hostelling and I looked forward to these treks. While out on the land, I was free from the pressures of school and I could feel the possibilities in my life grow larger.

In the years that Marjory and I were in India and Chinese Turkestan various relatives had put birthday and Christmas present money into post office accounts for us to use on our return. I had about sixteen pounds and decided that I would like to spend it on a good road-racing bike. George was supportive, but Ethel was not too sure about the idea; she was worried about my safety on the roads. But I was determined to get a good bicycle and for my sixteenth birthday I asked everyone to give me money for the cause. I ended up with eighteen pounds, which was just enough to get the bike I wanted—a turquoise Carlton three-speed road-racer. I showed it to my Aunt Ethel in the shop and she finally let me buy it, but she was not very keen on my taking off on long trips on my own. I had to prove that I was a responsible rider first by surviving a couple of short, one-day trips on the weekends before she relented. I purchased a rear-seat pannier to put my gear into and was ready to begin my cycling adventures.

When the weather was good, I cycled the twenty-seven miles to Nottingham. By doing this I was able to save the bus fares, which supplemented my pocket money with half a crown a week. I soon found that I was fast enough on the bike to beat the bus from Worksop to Nottingham.

Soon I was cycling around the English countryside—Lincolnshire, Nottinghamshire, Shropshire and Derbyshire. Through Youth Hostelling I made friends with a couple of boys who were members of the Worksop cycling club. I used to cycle with them on weekends and I went to some of their meetings. Usually I planned on riding sixty to eighty miles a day, which I managed comfortably. One cycle trip I remember with great fondness was a day's outing from Worksop to Skegness and back. The round trip was 120 miles, which was the farthest I ever rode in one day. On one memorable weekend I watched world champion and Olympic medalist, Reg Harris, racing.

My father's sister, Aunt Marjorie, lived in Derry Hill, near Chippenham, Wiltshire. My sister Marjory and I visited her on a few occasions during our holidays. Grandfather Binns, who had been the vicar in Derry Hill and with whom Aunt Marjorie had lived, died in 1935. Aunt Marjorie was a teacher at the local church school and she and Grandmother Binns were allowed to stay on at the vicarage cottage after Grandfather died. To keep us entertained Aunt Marjorie toured us around the area in her old Austin Seven for which she managed to find some petrol. She took us to Devizes, Stone Henge, Salisbury Cathedral, Melksham and Marlborough.

Grandfather Ottwell Binns had also written adventure books. There was a small library at the house which he had used as a writing room. He wrote a total of seventy-five books which were published in the twenties and thirties, some under the pseudonym Ben Bolt. My father later told me that these books had paid for the tuition of his two brothers, Max and Bernard, and his sister, Marjorie, all of whom went to Oxford University, and for his own medical school fees in London. Grandfather Binns initially sold the stories to the *News of the World* to print in the entertainment section in instalments. In the 1920s the *News of the World* was a solid news organization with a huge circulation. Later his books were sold to the publishers, Ward Lock and Co.

His novel, *A Mating in the Wild*, was published in the US by Alfred A. Knopf.

Marjory and I learned that there were stringent rules of etiquette to be followed at Derry Hill. Afternoon tea was invariably delicate cucumber sandwiches and cakes which were not to be scoffed down when one was hungry. Table manners were strictly enforced and we soon discovered to be careful how we addressed our Aunt and Grandmother.

Aunt Marjorie was a big, daunting woman with whom I found it difficult to talk. Grandmother was completely different. She was a small, delicate person who liked to hear about India and Kashgar. She was interested to know how I was doing at school and if I liked Worksop. She also insisted that I start writing to her, which resulted in her sending me my grandfather's books to read. I used to get one or two a month which I read and then sent back to her. I continued my correspondence with Grandmother Rose for many years, until her death in 1965.

During the years my family had a house in Worksop, I visited Derry Hill several times on my own as part of my Youth Hostelling trips. It was at Derry Hill that I first met my cousin Anne. She had been sent back to England by her family, who were in Italy. Her father, Sir Bernard Ottwell Binns, had worked for the British Foreign Service before the war in both India and Burma. Anne and her mother were evacuated from Rangoon just before the Japanese invasion, and my uncle was one of a group of evacuees who walked out of the country to India.

After the war he joined the World Food Organization (part of the United Nations). At the time he was a leading expert in rice cultivation and was responsible for the development of certain strains that increased the production of this staple food worldwide. He was knighted for this work.

Anne and I shared a lot in common. We were of a similar age and, like pieces of luggage, had both been dragged around the world after our parents. She had lived and gone to school in Burma, Switzerland, the US, and Italy. Like mine, her schooling had been disrupted. In the summer of 1952 she was completing her secretarial training course in Torquay on the south coast of England and I cycled down there from Worksop to visit her. It was my first experience of a South England holiday resort with its beaches, theatres, theme parks and museums. We chose to spend much of our time rambling about the undulating countryside behind Torquay. Our friendship has lasted to this day, even though the Atlantic and Pacific Oceans have separated us for most of our lives.

Marjory and I also holidayed in Rochdale, Lancashire, where our Great Aunt Lil and her husband, Freddy, lived. They were both retired teachers who had married late in life and didn't have any children. When visiting them we would usually go for picnics on the moors. Freddy had a pair of binoculars through which he used to look for wildlife. One day, when I was fourteen, I noticed movement through the binoculars close to a stone sheep pen. I couldn't figure out what it was. I was about to ask Uncle Freddy to have a look when I realized that what I was watching was a couple having sex. When the woman stood up I saw she had no clothes on. It was the first time I had seen a young woman in the nude. Enthralled, I hung onto the binoculars—until Uncle Freddy became rather insistent.

"Bernard, what are you looking at?"

"Oh," I said, "nothing really. I saw something move over there on the right and thought it was a partridge. But I've lost it now."

Reluctantly I handed over the binoculars, pointing well away from the couple. By the time I got the binoculars back the couple had dressed and were walking across the moors.

After I had settled into the routine in Nottingham, Mrs. Jackson suggested I should take some time off schoolwork and go to the local social club with Philip and Katharine on Fridays from seven to eight. The club was held in an old army Nissen Hut just down the road and was run by the church. I took her advice because it gave me a chance to meet and play table tennis, cards, dominos and board games with other kids.

I also joined a swimming club at Arnold, about two miles away. Six of us from the school walked to the baths on Tuesdays and swam for an hour-and-a-half. Mr. Martin, the organizer and a friend of Mrs. Jackson, had three children who belonged to the club and he taught me how to swim competitively. The club organized events with races for different age groups and it was here that I discovered my passion for competition.

At school we were expected to participate in the Combined Cadet Forces. However, I soon got frustrated with the CCF army section. I didn't like being ordered around on the parade ground by Mr. Bennet, who had been a Sergeant-Major during the war and treated us as if we were soldiers in the regular army. To me there didn't seem to be any point in marching up and down the school yard and I felt that my time could have been spent more productively. As well, there were the boots, brass buttons and gaiters to be cleaned and polished, another job I disliked. But I soon learned that if I didn't keep a shine on my kit I would spend even more time on the parade ground. Marching.

Nonetheless, there were some positive aspects to the CCF. We learned how to look after firearms and how they worked. We were taught marksmanship, both small-bore and .303, whose kicks were tough on thirteen- and fourteen-year-old bodies. We also learned how Bren guns and machine guns worked, and went on field days where we ran amok playing war games.

A couple of times during the year, army trucks picked us up from the school and took us to one of many army camps that were within fifty miles of Nottingham. We were shown manoeuvres and tactical warfare and made to crawl around in fields and were allowed to try the obstacle courses. The leaders of the CCF showed us army equipment like tanks and field guns in action. We saw how British soldiers lived and the discipline they needed in order to do the right thing at the right time. But I was not convinced it was the sort of life I would enjoy.

My experiences with the CCF did prove helpful. One day, towards the end of the school year in 1948, Mr. Bennet called us all together.

"Boys, next year you will have a choice to make. Those of you who like the Army can stay on in the Army which is what I hope most of you would like to do. Some of you might like to try the Air Force or the Navy. The Air Force is run out of this school but the Navy is across the road. They are very small and don't have much in the way of equipment. For those of you who are really interested in the Air Force or Navy please let me know by the end of today and I will put your names down for them."

All the marching and the time spent on spit and polish had not endeared the Army to me. Having heard that the Air Force did less drill work and did not wear boots and gaiters, I was happy to sign up with them.

Once enlisted in the Air Force, I found the training much more to my liking. We had to do some drill work, but mostly we spent time learning the principles of flight, studying piston and jet engines, navigation, meteorology, and aircraft armaments. We went on field days to local Air Force bases and learned about parachutes, how bases were run, what was involved in becoming a pilot, and the functions of the Air Force. When weather conditions permitted we were taken up in trainer planes and allowed to take over the controls for short periods of time. The CCF was a good introduction to National Service, which was expected of us when we finished school.

Slowly I had been gaining confidence in my swimming ability so I went to see Mr. Neville about the swimming options available at Nottingham High. "Now, Binns, how far can you swim and how many different stokes can you do?" he asked.

"I can do fifty lengths of the Arnold pool without any trouble. I can do the breast stroke, crawl, backstroke, side stroke and I have tried that new stoke called the butterfly."

"Hmm, not bad. I'd like to see you in the pool. Can you come to the baths on High Pavement Road next Thursday afternoon? I'll clear it with your form master."

On Thursday afternoon I went to the public baths, which the school rented for the afternoon. The pool was 33⅓ yards long with black tiles marking the pool bottom into lanes. Hollow sounding, the damp, cold building smelled slightly of chlorine. The sides of the pool were grey concrete and the changing rooms grimly Spartan. Wooden benches, strewn with towels and loose clothing, stood beside a few toilets and six open shower heads, each with a single tap that delivered only bitterly cold water.

I found Mr. Neville at the side of the pool with about twenty boys from different levels of the school. Some were in the pool swimming lengths, others talking to him. Mr. Neville wore swimming trunks, which surprised me. He was a short, almost bald man with broad shoulders and his body was almost completely covered with curly black hair.

"Ah, Binns. Go and change and then come back here. We'll see if you are as good as you say.

When I got back he sized me up. "You look a bit skinny. How old are you?"

"Fifteen, sir."

"Can you dive?"

"Yes, sir."

"OK. I want you to dive in at the deep end, then swim the first length using the breast stroke, the second the back stroke, the third the crawl. The first three are to be done slowly. I want to see how good your stroke is. On the fourth length I want you to use the crawl again, but I want you to go as fast as you can. You can use lane two when John gets out. Do you understand?"

"Yes, sir."

As I walked to the deep end I tried to remember what Mr. Martin had taught me about the three basic strokes. I couldn't believe how icy the water felt when I dove in but it became more tolerable after the first few strokes. I swam the first three lengths as carefully as I could, trying to avoid splashing as much as possible. On the fourth length I splashed away trying to go as fast as I could. By the time I got out, I was gasping to catch my breath.

"Not bad, Binns. Your technique is good, but needs some work. You were fairly fast on the third length, but out of control on the last one. In fact, you were slower on the last lap, in spite of trying to go faster. Does that surprise you?" he asked.

"Yes, I thought I was going a lot faster on the last one."

"Would you like to swim for the school if we can improve your time?"

"Yes, sir. I'm not much good at rugby and don't like it. I like swimming. I go to the Arnold baths once a week. I could practice there," I said.

"Good enough. Let's get started. We'll begin with the basics."

I got into the pool and was taken aback when he got in with me. During the next fifteen minutes he showed me how to improve my strokes. He was a strong swimmer and clearly enjoyed being in the water showing me what to do.

"Okay. That's enough to start with. As you can see, there's a lot more to swimming well and even more to going fast. Spend the next half hour trying out what I've just suggested. Then you can join the rest of us for the last half hour."

Thanks to swimming I found my niche in school sports, something that had previously eluded me. After a few weeks of training, I was selected for the school swim team and over the years enjoyed success at freestyle as well as diving.

Mr. Neville taught botany and zoology to the six forms. He accompanied the swim team to the matches that were organized outside of Nottingham. Some locations were a good distance away, and he kept us entertained on these trips with all sorts of stories, discussions and games. His most memorable story was about how he broke his back while on active service in the Middle East. He was a dispatch rider in the army and had to ride a motorcycle between companies delivering messages. While he was on leave in Cairo one weekend, he and some friends were swimming and they dared him to perform a double back flip dive. While attempting the dive he slipped and caught the back of his neck on the diving board. He did not lose consciousness but felt very woozy. During the next few days he suffered some low backache, aggravated by riding his motorcycle. He went to see a doctor who told him that he was malingering. Nothing was wrong with him.

A week later he still had a lot of pain while riding his motorcycle and he returned to the same doctor who reluctantly ordered some x-rays. When the doctor saw the x-rays he said, "Sit in that chair and don't move until I get the ambulance to take you to Cairo."

He had crushed three spinal vertebrae.

He was put in a full-body plaster cast and sent on the upper deck of the ambulance ship that went through the Suez Canal and the Red Sea, eventually arriving at Capetown Hospital. Here they decided to change his full body cast. Unfortunately it had become very hard and a highly offensive odour emanated from it. The medical attendants broke two sets of plaster shears trying to get the cast off. Eventually they resorted to taking him into the carpenter's shop and pushing him onto the circular saw, which did the trick.

At the end of my second year at Nottingham High I excelled in the sciences and math but, despite extra tutoring, continued to have problems with English Literature and French. If I couldn't pass these two subjects in the National Exams I would not be able to go on to University. At the time I didn't see how this could be a problem. I enjoyed my other subjects and rebelled against doing the homework assigned in English and French.

On the last day of the year, my classmates and I were all sitting in class about two hours before breaking up for the summer holidays when the form master, Mr. Beatty, said, "Binns, the Headmaster would like to see you in five minutes. He is in his office. You'd best go and ask the secretary to show you in."

I had no idea what I'd done wrong but I could only think I'd done something terrible. Frightened and apprehensive, I made my way to the Headmaster's office. The secretary told me to knock on the door and wait for him to call me in.

"Come in," he called when I knocked.

"Ah, Binns, come in," he said as I entered timidly. "Sit down," he said pointing to the chair in front of him on the other side of his desk.

"How do you like school?" he asked.

"I like it here, sir."

"Well, you don't seem to be doing too well in all your studies. When you first came we knew that you had problems because of a lack of schooling but it is now two years on and you still seem to be struggling with some subjects. What have you got to say for yourself?"

I was a bit taken aback by this and was not sure how to answer. However, the thought of going back to Worksop Central Secondary still intimidated me so I attempted an explanation, one that made sense to me.

"I know that I've not done well in French or English, but I'm doing well in the sciences and I feel I should spend more time at them. I find French and English very difficult. At least I can read and write now. I thought that would be enough, sir."

"From what I hear from your teachers you're far from good enough in either subject. You cannot get on in this world, Binns, without a basic knowledge of English literature. Added to that, your French marks are terrible. You certainly won't be able to go to university without receiving your School Certificate and you have to pass both French and English language to do that. I admitted you into this school as a favour to your father and I'm now beginning to wonder if I made a mistake. Although you seemed to try in the first year, you have not continued to do so this year. I am rather disappointed in you."

Fearing he was going to tell me that I could not come back to Nottingham next term, I could feel tears coming to my eyes. "Please sir, I know that the School Certificate is not for another year. My Aunt Ethel is a school teacher. She could help me with English during the summer holidays. And if Mr. Whitty could give me some extra work in French to do during the holidays, I'm sure I could catch up."

"I'm not convinced, Binns. Where are your parents at the moment? I'd like to talk to them about this problem."

"They're in Nigeria, sir, and will not return until Christmas, when they come back for three months' leave. You would have to write to them."

This news surprised the Headmaster. Clearly he was not aware that my parents had taken jobs overseas or that my Aunt Ethel and Uncle George lived in their house and looked after Marjory and me when we were home from school.

"Who do you stay with while they're in Nigeria?" he asked.

I explained to him that I spent the week days in Nottingham at the Jacksons and the weekends in Worksop with my aunt and uncle. I then told him I would be with my aunt during the summer holidays.

"Hmm, that makes things a bit difficult. Tell me honestly, do you really think you can improve enough at English and French to pass if I let you stay on?"

"Sir, I don't know if I'm good enough to pass, but I would like to try. I promise to work as hard as I can to get to a level that will get me through. Until now I didn't think these subjects were that important."

The Headmaster thought for a bit. "All right, then, I will let you come back next term but remember, if you do not show an improvement, I will not let you stay on any longer. I will write to your father and let him know what I've decided. Have a good holiday. You may go back to your class now."

"Thank you very much, sir," I said. I got up and left the office, rather shaken.

"What did the Head have to say to you, Binns?" asked Mr. Beatty when I got back to the class.

"He told me that I have not been doing well enough in French and English and if I don't do better next term I'll not be able to stay on at Nottingham."

"I'm pleased you're staying. I thought he was going to give you the boot. You must have said something that made him change his mind."

"Sir, you will be my English teacher next year. Could you give me some extra work to do in the summer holidays and could you ask Mr. Whitty about assigning some extra French?"

"Yes, I think we can manage that. Come and see me after the last bell. You can go and sit down now. Think about some of the things the Headmaster said to you."

On the bus back to Worksop I thought a lot about what had happened that day and wondered if I would be able to cope with the problems facing me next term. I had only a three-month summer holiday and two school terms in which to satisfy the Headmaster. I knew I would get some help from Aunt Ethel with English, but French was going to be a problem.

I was in for a further shock when I got home to Worksop. A letter had arrived from Mother announcing that I was going to Nigeria for the summer holidays.

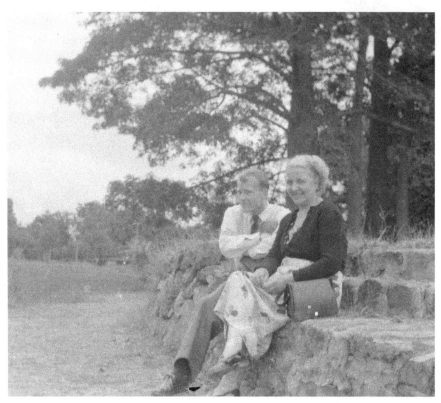

Above: Bernard and his mother in Nigeria, where his parents lived
for about a decade starting in the late 1940s.
Below: Bernard studying anatomy while at medical school.

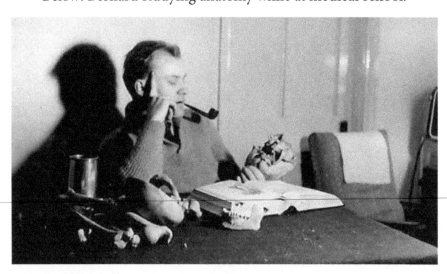

Chapter 5
Nigeria: First Contact with Medicine

At the beginning of the summer of 1950 Uncle George took me by train to London Airport. When we got to the airport we were met by a stewardess named Pam who knew that I was on my own and who explained she would be looking after me during the flight. She told me the trip would take about ten hours with a stop at Tangiers for refuelling. Once I was safely seated on the plane she went off to help other passengers get settled. Luckily the seat next to me remained empty.

The airplane was an old York, a civilian version of the wartime Lancaster bomber. It seated forty-five to fifty people in pairs on each side of an aisle that ran down the centre of the aircraft. I had a window seat from which I could see a wing with its two engines, each having four propeller blades. Just as the chief steward finished giving us his list of safety instructions, I heard a dull explosion from outside my window. The propeller nearest me began to rotate. A cloud of blue smoke blasted out of the spluttering engine. At first, the propeller rotated slowly, gradually picking up speed and wafting the smoke away. Once the inside engines were humming, the outside engines turned over. As each engine fired up, the whole airplane shook noticeably. After idling for a few minutes, the engines revved, producing more noise and shaking. I glanced around. No one but me seemed concerned.

Once all the engines were running smoothly, the airplane taxied out to the runway.

"Would you like a sweet?" asked Pam. "They'll help keep your ears clear until we reach our cruising altitude."

"Thank you," I said, taking one from her basket.

"Take more," she said, "they don't last very long."

When we got to the end of the tarmac the aircraft came to a stop; the pilot announced that we would be taking off shortly. He revved the engines for a couple of minutes with the aircraft stationary. More smoke. Then, with an enormous roar and a lot of shaking, we took off down the pavement, gaining speed. I wondered if we had enough runway when I felt the plane rise into the air. I saw the ground receding and took a deep breath. We were airborne. Soon the airplane levelled off and the noise died down to a low hum.

Out the window I saw the buildings and roads of London; the countryside south of London; the English Channel; several small boats, yachts and even one ferry. The farms in France looked different from those in England, more regular and rectangular in shape. As we flew south, I saw the sun set over what appeared to be a castle surrounded by fields and woods beside a river. I settled back into my seat. I was carrying one of grandfather's books to read on the journey and retrieved it from my bag.

A couple of hours into the trip Pam arrived with dinner on a small tray. She told me that after dinner the cabin lights would be lowered so that those who wanted to sleep could do so. She showed me how to adjust my seat should I want to sleep. Later I woke as I felt the plane start to descend. It was dark, but after rubbing my eyes I could see lights on the ground ahead and below us. The cabin lights came on and the steward announced our approach to Tangiers.

The airport was a ramshackle old place, filled with badly worn furniture. We were scheduled for a stopover of about an hour while the airplane was refuelled, but after half an hour, an announcement was made over the loudspeakers that our flight would be delayed for at least an additional two hours due to a mechanical problem. We were invited to have breakfast while the repairs were being made. The idea that the plane had a mechanical problem worried me. This was not something I had bargained for. Nor was I comforted by my accompanying thoughts. I'd seen too many newsreel clips from the war. When I'd finished breakfast, I decided to go for a short walk outside the terminal to have a look around.

In the 1950s there were only a few commercial airline routes and the idea of security had not yet entered the public imagination. For me to move about at will, the most I was asked to do was show my passport. I walked out the front door of the airport unchallenged. The complex was surrounded by desert and sand dunes. I walked around the terminal building and discovered hangers built with corrugated iron. I could see numerous holes in the walls and slowly it dawned on me that these were bullet holes which must have been made during the war, perhaps by Rommel, the Desert Fox. That memory and the horror it had brought had now become a silent and accepted part of the architecture.

There wasn't much to see outside so I returned to the terminal and waited to board the plane with the other passengers. We took off without any difficulty and headed across the desert toward Kano, Nigeria. Endless sand dunes stretched to the horizon like a rippled sea. Never before had I seen such a desolate and featureless landscape. We were flying fairly high but I could identify animals and human beings in small patches of green daubed on the expanse of sand. Oases. Two camel caravans plodded across the dunes and I wondered how far they had to go before reaching the next oasis. As we got closer to Kano the landscape changed; a few trees, bushes, and the occasional village appeared. Around midday the plane circled Kano, then landed. Pam accompanied me through immigration and customs to where my parents waited anxiously in Arrivals.

"Bernard," Mother said as she rushed up to hug me. "How was your flight? Did they take good care of you? You look well." She turned to Pam, smiled and thanked her.

Before I could say anything, Father stepped forward and shook my hand. He cleared his throat and spoke, as if our reunion required a degree of formality. I was surprised by his awkwardness.

"They told us you had been delayed in Tangiers," he said, "because of mechanical issues. We've got a six-hour drive from here to Minna, so we had better get going soon. Have you had lunch yet?"

"No. Just a snack, but I'm not hungry."

"Excellent. We can start as soon as your bags arrive."

"I made some sandwiches to eat on the way back," Mother said. "Our plan was to drive for an hour or so before stopping for a picnic lunch."

We went out into an oppressive heat and walked to the car, a Vauxhall 14, similar to the one we had had in India. The road to Minna went past the ancient city of Kano surrounded by a high red mud wall. Through the main entrance I saw many mud houses, *duhkas*, and several mosques whose minarets pierced the blue sky. People wearing flowing white robes gathered near the wall's entrance. Coils of variously coloured cloth were wrapped around their heads. Father told me most were Nigerian men. Their full-length costumes surprised me, especially in such stifling heat.

Laden camels and donkeys moved in and out of the gate.

"It's a big city," I said to Father.

"Yes, it's the largest in northern Nigeria and the main centre for trade in this area. Many different tribes come together here to exchange goods. The majority of the local people are Hausa but a number of different people come down here from the Sahara and the Sudan to trade. The goods you find in the city have come from all over North Africa, even from the rest of the world. You can buy items from almost anywhere, but you have to be prepared to bargain for everything."

A short time later we entered the West African bush, a mix of tropical trees and tall grasses, which I had seen from the plane. The rainy season had just ended and everything was lush and green. The bushes came right to the edge of the road, graded red laterite, red because of the high iron content. Because it hadn't rained for a few days, a great cloud of red dust rose up behind us. There wasn't much traffic on the road, but whenever Father saw an approaching car or truck he'd pull over and we'd wind up all the windows to keep out the dust. Passing was impossible.

The journey to Minna was about two hundred miles. We skirted by Kaduna and Zaria, two relatively large cities, but we did pass though several villages of round, mud-walled huts with thatched roofs. A constant parade of donkeys, chickens, dogs, naked children, and brightly dressed women carrying water pots, firewood and other objects on their heads shared the road. When they saw our car approaching, they jumped to the side as fast as possible, sometimes spilling water or dropping a few sticks of firewood. Most of the men, dressed in their familiar white robes, sat near the mud houses, smoking and chatting. We happened on four main crossroads going to Katsina, Gusau, Zaria/Kaduna and Yelwa.

After a few hours of driving we pulled over into a small clearing just off to the side of the road. "I think this is where we stopped on the way down," Mother said, as she glanced around.

We spread a canvas sheet on the ground to help keep the ants away and sat down to a picnic lunch of cold chicken, tomatoes, bread and butter, followed by cake and tea. Time and distance, I thought, can make for strange juxtapositions. In just a short time, I had travelled from one of the largest cities in the world to a remote stopover in the African bush.

"Are there any wild animals here?" I asked. "I was hoping to see a lion or two from the car."

"There are all sorts of wild animals in the bush, but they're shy and usually move away from the road when they hear cars coming. Since we've been here we've seen the odd elephant and giraffe but no lions yet. Sometimes you'll see baboons and chimps crossing the road, and there are a lot of hyenas about, but you only see them at night. When you go walking in the bush you have to be careful where you step. Some very poisonous snakes live in the grass and trees. To see the wildlife, though, you have to go on a safari with a guide. They're all hunting safaris and, as you know, I've no interest in hunting," Father said, "but we can check into it if you like."

"In Minna we live on the top of a hill and can hear leopards, hyenas and baboons," said Mother. "Occasionally we see snakes in the garden, but they usually flee when they hear someone coming. And there are lots of brightly coloured birds around the house."

"Where is the nearest big town?" I asked.

"Zaria. It's about one and a half hours away. We passed the turning at the last village. They have the only petrol station between Minna and Kano. We didn't stop because I get petrol cheap from the government and we have plenty to spare on this trip. There are four gallons in the boot just in case we run out, but usually this car does the whole trip without having to fill up," explained Father.

We were about to get back into the car when I heard some chattering in the trees on the other side of the road.

"What's that noise?" I asked.

"If we wait a minute I think you'll see your first African monkeys."

Soon after, a family of small brown monkeys came skittering across the road towards the car. They were quite brave and went over to where we had been eating our lunch. They nibbled away at crumbs of food that had fallen on the ground when we'd shaken out the ground sheet, and then emboldened, they investigated the outside of the car. After a few minutes, they lost interest and bounded into the trees. Just watching them exhausted me.

During the rest of the journey to Minna, I fell asleep.

"Bernard, we're almost home," Mother said, patting me on the shoulder. "Our house is the second one on the hill over there. We turn off here to the house. The road goes on to the town and hospital, about half a mile away."

I looked out of the window and saw a hill with four houses visible through some trees. I noticed that there were some rocky outcrops below the houses. The houses, which had corrugated iron roofs and stood on stilts to keep them cool, had several flowering trees in their gardens. A mass of bright red bougainvillea grew up onto the roofs.

My parents' circular driveway encompassed a big garden. In front of the house there were two large avocado trees which gave a fair amount of shade. Several smaller flame trees lined the drive. Pink and white oleander bushes, blue jacaranda, and some others that I didn't recognize were interspersed between these. Later on, I found mango, lemon and grapefruit trees in the back garden. There were all sorts of coloured flowers in the beds round the front of the house and in the centre of the circular drive.

"I see you've been working hard in the garden, Mother."

"Not really," she said. "I just tell the garden boy what to do and make sure that he waters things when it gets dry. We get most of our fresh vegetables from the garden patch at the back. And we pick the odd pawpaw [papaya] from a lovely tree growing next to the garden. Much better than the ones the cook gets from the market."

"And probably a lot cleaner!" Father added.

The entrance was impressive. Ten wide steps led up to a shaded veranda. At the top of the stairs a big black man, dressed in a white uniform, stood at attention. He was obviously waiting for us. When we had stopped he came down the steps to help get things out of the car.

"Good afternoon, *Bwana*. Did you have a good drive from Kano?" he asked.

"Yes, thank you," Mother said. "This is our son Bernard, Mbula. Bernard, meet Mbula. He is the head house boy."

"Nice to meet you, Mbula," I said and shook his hand.

We climbed the front steps and entered a colonial-style entrance hall with a high ceiling. There was a sitting room with a view down the hill across the bush and a dining room with a large wood table and wicker-backed chairs. A side board stood against the far wall and the window looked out onto the garden. A wide corridor led to the back of the house where there were three bedrooms and a kitchen. Cooking was done on a wood stove.

From the kitchen a few steps descended to a small clearing, on the other side of which were three two-roomed huts that the servants lived in. Off to the right of the huts there was a small shed that covered the well. There was no running water or electricity, but there was a telephone that linked the hospital to the house but went no further.

A shaded veranda extended round three sides of the house. The floors were red stained concrete. Each room had Indian carpets or copra mats and whitewashed walls. The furniture was mostly heavy wicker-backed wood with large cushions on the easy chairs and settee. Jugs of orange juice covered with bead-edged squares of fine netting, to keep the flies off, stood on several small tables. All the beds had mosquito nets over them, held in place by wood frames. The house was cool and airy. In the sitting room, there were two kerosene Tilly lamps, similar to the ones that we had had in Kashgar. They were placed on small shoulder-high shelves that were fixed onto the walls. The other rooms were lit by Primus lamps that Mbula lit and brought in at dusk.

In Minna I was re-introduced to the colonial life style. Four servants did all the menial tasks in the house and garden. Father would go to the hospital at six in the morning and return for breakfast at 8:30 a.m. by which time Mother and I would be up. Father would leave for the hospital again at 9:30 a.m. and finish at 2 p.m. when he would return for lunch. While Father was at work Mother would organize the meals for the day with the cook, look around the garden and tell the garden boy what to do. We spent some mornings at the *dukhas* buying tinned and non-perishable foods, drinks, cigarettes and anything else that Mother felt we needed. Compared to life at school I felt totally pampered.

On some mornings we went round to the neighbours for morning coffee or tea. During these visits recent events in Nigeria and the UK were discussed in detail. We would always organize our outings to make sure we returned to the house in time for lunch with Father. Twice a week Mother would go to the hospital with Father after breakfast—she helped as a volunteer at the maternity clinic. I used the time to do the school work I had brought with me. When Mother was not at the hospital she would help me with English grammar but she was of no help with French.

After lunch we would sit and talk, read the mail if there was any, and generally take life easy; it was usually far too hot to do anything outside. We had afternoon tea and biscuits at 4 p.m. After tea we strolled around the garden and then returned to the house to read. Sometimes Mother and I would go down to the club where there were usually up to a dozen people. A few children would be there with their mothers.

The club had two tennis courts, a snooker table and bar. I was not allowed into the bar where the snooker table was, which was a pity; Granddad had introduced me to the game and I would have liked to have had a go. I spent time watching the tennis and after a few visits Father explained the rules and showed me the basics. He had been quite a good player as a young man. After a few weeks of practice I was good enough to play with the adults.

After dinner Father and Mother would often play classical music together. Father played the flute and Mother accompanied him on the dulcitone. This instrument was a kind of piano that worked with tuning forks instead of metal strings, which made it a lot easier to keep tuned in places where the temperature and humidity changed rapidly. We also played cards, usually whist, and listened to classical recordings on an old-fashioned gramophone.

One morning, after breakfast, Father invited me to go to the hospital with him to see what he did. For a moment I was dumbstruck. "Yes, yes," I stammered, "I would like to. My teachers at school have often asked me if I've ever thought about becoming a doctor. But I couldn't answer them. I wasn't really sure what a doctor does, even though you are one."

I could see Father was pleased. And I was proud to be included in his world.

That morning Father drove us all down into town. Just before we got to the main street we turned right into a wide drive and pulled up in front of the hospital building. Father parked the car under a large flamboyant tree loaded with brilliant red flowers.

"I'll be in the maternity clinic," Mother said, as she got out of the car.

Father and I climbed three steps to a narrow veranda. Like all the other buildings I'd seen, the hospital had whitewashed walls and open windows. The door we went through led to a corridor with offices on each side.

"My office is over there on the right, opposite the common room. The other rooms are used by the nurses," said Father.

As we entered the common room, two Nigerian nurses stood up from a table that was pushed against the wall. Besides some cups and a teapot, there was a bottle of Camp concentrated coffee and some biscuits on a plate.

"Good morning, Dr. Binns. We're just having coffee before going back to work," said a plump nurse who was dressed in a pale blue uniform with a black belt that had a large buckle at the front. A white starched nurse's cap sat firmly on her head.

"Good morning, Sister. I've brought my son, Bernard, who's here for the summer holidays, to see what we do. Bernard, this is Sister Adjola who looks after the maternity ward."

"How do you do, Sister," I said, and we shook hands.

"And this is Head Nurse Matumbu. He looks after our busy out-patient department."

"It is a pleasure to meet you," Matumbu said as we shook hands. He wore a crisp white uniform and looked like a man accustomed to taking charge. "I hope you'll have a nice stay in our country. Are you going to become a doctor like your father?" he asked. "That would be a good thing. You can always work here. We are always short of doctors."

I could tell Father was pleased by this encouragement.

"I'm not sure yet," I said. "I have a lot of exams to pass first."

As the two nurses left the room, Father and I sat down to a cup of tea. Out of the blue he asked, "How old are you now, Bernard?"

I wasn't surprised by this question. It had been nearly two years since we had last seen each other and such matters were usually trivial to him. "I was sixteen last April," I replied. "Why do you ask?"

"Good, that's good, I think you're old enough to see most of the things here, but we'll take it slowly. Finish your tea. We'll go and see what kind of patients are on the wards."

He got up and led the way out of the lounge, down the corridor to the back of the building where a door opened onto half a dozen steps which dropped down into the hospital compound. In the compound there were eight buildings of various sizes. Across from us, on the other side of a pair of flame trees, was the largest building. It was a single storey with large double doors at one end. Its huge shuttered windows had all been thrown open. Sitting under the trees were several people chatting away. Some were obviously patients. They had plaster casts or bandages on various parts of their bodies or limbs.

"That's the main ward. On the left you will see patient beds for the women while the men's beds are on the right. There are about twenty beds on each side, but we often have many more patients than that in the hospital. When that happens the patients sleep on the floor, between and under the other beds.

"The building over there on the left is the operating theatre where we do all the surgeries, and the one behind it is the maternity wing where the babies and postpartum patients are housed. Sick women who haven't had their babies yet are also kept there. If we have to do caesarean sections or forceps deliveries we take the patients to the theatre. Over on the right is the children's ward. Behind it you can just see the isolation ward where we keep all the TB patients. Sadly, that ward is always full."

As he turned I caught a glimpse of his face and I could have sworn I saw his lips quiver, and I tried to imagine what this otherwise stoic man was feeling.

"Over there, where all those people are milling around, is the outpatient clinic. About a hundred patients are seen there every day by the outpatient nurses. These nurses are specially trained to treat most of the common problems you find here like malaria, dysentery, hookworm, bilhartsia [schistosomiasis], pneumonias, various colds, coughs, and boils. They hold the difficult cases for me to see each afternoon. In amongst those trees, you can see the top of the kitchen and laundry. All in all there's a lot to this place."

"Who looks after all these people?" I asked.

"I'm the only trained doctor for a hundred miles but there are enough nurses to look after the wards. Two of the nurses have finished two extra years of training and can give anaesthetics so we're able to do some surgery and look after emergencies. Midwives look after the maternity wards. There are also some clinics out in the bush that are run by nurses. The midwives go out to them regularly to check sick patients. Some of these clinics are a long way out and the only way of getting there is on foot or by bicycle. In the whole of the northern region there are about sixty doctors to look after several million people, so a lot of the work is done by nurses. And, this might surprise you, by witch doctors. There are two mission hospitals in the region that are not government run; they do a lot of good work, but, regrettably, many people don't get any treatment at all."

"Does that mean many die needlessly?" I asked Father who was clearly upset by what he had just said. I could understand why this knowledge would wear on him.

"Unfortunately, yes! There are too few doctors to provide people with the services they need. And, at the moment, there's not enough money to bring more doctors to Nigeria. Which is a shame. I don't suppose there ever will be," Father added sadly. "Anyway, let's go and see what we can do here today."

Uncharacteristically he put his arm around my shoulders and led the way to the main ward and into a small office with "Sisters Office" painted in white letters on the door.

Sister was waiting for us. "Good morning again, Doctor." And with a nod to me, "Bernard."

"Did anything new come in during the night?" Father inquired.

"Yes. There is a man over in Bed 16 who has been vomiting for the past two days and has a lot of abdominal pain. He came in after midnight and vomited some thin green vomit several times during the night. He looks quite sick. The man with the hernia that you operated on four days ago wants to go home and is eating well. The girl with the miscarriage is ready to go and so is the girl with the boil that you lanced yesterday. The others are much the same. Do you want to go round now or would you like to see the man in Bed 16 first?"

"Let's go to Bed 16 first. If he's as sick as you say, we may have to do something about him later today."

"Nurse Bhula," Sister called out through the door, "please prepare the patient in Bed 16 for the doctor to see."

"Yes Sister," a voice called back.

"While she's preparing the patient would you like to sign the orders that you left yesterday?"

Father moved over to Sister's desk by the window where seven manila charts had been neatly placed in a row. He sat down and started to sign the orders.

"How is the man with dysentery getting on? He should not really be in the ward. He could infect some of the other patients."

"He is a lot better today and his pulse is slowing down. We could send him home. He lives in the town and has a wife who can look after him. We only admitted him because he was very weak and needed some intravenous fluids yesterday."

"Good. I'll sign him out." He paused and took a deep breath. "What about the man with malaria?"

"He died during the night," Sister replied.

I was shocked by how matter-of-fact this conversation between them was. Death, in this instance, obviously required calm, but I despaired that a person's dying could be treated with such ease and routine. And yet Father and Sister carried on as if they were simply filling out requisitions for supplies.

"Let's go and see the man in 16," said Father, standing up.

All the beds in the ward were occupied. Many of the patients, on seeing Father, scurried back to bed and seemed quite cheerful about being in hospital. Others were obviously ill and remained covered up. One of the nurses had put green and white striped curtains around the man in Bed 16. The curtains travelled on wheeled metal frames that could be folded away against the wall at the end of the ward when not in use.

The patient was the first really sick person I remember seeing. He was probably in his forties. He looked ill in a way I'd not seen before. His eyes were dull and sunken and he lay on his side in a foetal position, moaning. He was obviously in pain. A kidney dish at the side of the bed was filled with green vomit and there were green stains on the sheets. I could make out the smell of vomit and sweat, and a scent, I was to learn years later, that was the stench of acidosis. The man's hands were wizened and wrinkled, his lips dry and cracked. He looked up at us with a vacant expression.

My father could not speak Hausa, the common language in that part of Nigeria, so all communication with the sick man had to be done through an interpreter. On this occasion, Sister acted as interpreter, but as Father explained to me later, sometimes the patients, especially the women and children, did not speak Hausa but some other West African language. Then a second or even third person had to be used to retrieve the required history.

"Sister, please ask him how old he is?"

"He says he doesn't know. He looks about forty and from what he says that should be about right."

Following this Father asked a whole series of questions that to me seemed to be a bit pointless. They included questions about the duration of the vomiting and pain, about any previous episodes, change in bowel habits, when he had last had a bowel movement, any urinary problems, fever, pain, type, duration, whether there were any relieving factors or whether any other members of his family were having similar problems. To my surprise, his final question was, "What does he think the problem is?"

"He says that it is not the dysentery because he has had that many times and this is different," replied Sister.

"Interesting," Father said to the patient, "let's take a look, shall we?"

"You better get a glove, Sister."

"I have one ready," she replied.

"I thought you might," said Father with a smile. I found out later that nurses have an uncanny way of predicting what equipment a doctor will need.

Father took the man's hand and looked at his palm. Then he turned the hand over and pinched the skin on the back, raising the skin and releasing it. The skin-fold seemed to take forever to return to its original shape. Following this, Father felt the man's pulse, put a hand on his forehead and looked into his eyes, pulling the lower eyelid down as he did so. He then asked the patient to open his mouth and stick out his tongue. Next he ran his hands over the man's neck and chest. Then Sister lowered the bed sheet to expose the man's abdomen which Father pointed out to me was obviously distended.

"If you watch carefully, Bernard, you may see the bowel moving under the skin. We often see it in thin patients like this when they have an obstruction to the normal bowel function. Sister, can you ask

148

him if there is any point in his abdomen that has been painful in the past week?"

"Yes, he has had some pain down the right side," Sister answered after talking to the man for a moment.

"Can he point to the exact spot?"

After a few more words with Sister the man put his finger on a point just above his right groin.

"Pity, if he had shown us the other side, we could have almost certainly excluded the appendix as the cause of his problems."

Father then proceeded to press down softly on the man's abdomen.

"Bernard, what I'm about to do is called palpating."

This was done in two phases. First Father ran his hand over the patient's whole abdomen very gently to get a feel of what was there and to see if it was soft, rigid, or tender. Then he administered a deeper palpation to the four quadrants of the man's abdomen. I noticed that Father watched the patient's face while doing this. The patient grimaced when Father palpated the right groin area. The last thing Father did was press into the abdomen and then release the pressure quickly. He did this over the four quadrants, again watching the patient's face. There did not seem to be any particular point where this manoeuvre caused the man pain.

"Let's see if he has a hernia."

Sister covered up the man's abdomen with the sheet, exposing his legs and genitals. She said something to him and he drew up his legs and parted them so that Father could examine his scrotum.

"Do you notice anything, Bernard?" asked Father.

"No," I said

"Well, the right side is enlarged and you can see that the enlargement goes up into the right groin. Let's see if it's tender." Gently, he picked up the patient's scrotum in one hand and started to feel its contents. He felt the left side first and this did not seem to cause any pain, but when he felt the right side the man groaned and grabbed Father's hand to pull it away.

"Sorry," Father said apologetically. "Sister, could you explain to him that we need to do a rectal examination. That will be a bit uncomfortable but shouldn't hurt too much."

After Sister's explanation the man turned over onto his left side, manoeuvred his rear onto the edge of the bed and then drew up his knees. Father put on the glove Sister had been holding and applied some petroleum jelly to use as a lubricant. He then gently stuck his finger into the man's anus and felt around inside. I was a bit taken aback by this procedure and, when Father had finished, I asked, "Why did you do that?"

"There are several possible causes for this man's problems. The most common is dysentery or malaria, which can cause a lot of nausea and vomiting. In this man's case, that diagnosis does not seem to apply. Fever hasn't been a problem and he hasn't had much in the way of diarrhea. The other possibilities I have to consider are appendicitis, which can be very difficult to diagnose, or an obstruction of some sort. He does have a tender inguinal hernia, but hernias are very common in this part of the world and they do not get fixed unless they cause a lot of pain or other problems. To answer your question, a rectal examination is done to exclude the presence of any major tumour or other problem in the pelvis that could be causing his problems. If he had had a pelvic appendix, which was inflamed, he would have found the examination extremely painful and we would have had our diagnosis. There is an old saying in medicine, 'If you don't put your finger in it, you will put your foot in it.' There is a lot of truth in this advice because there are many things that can go badly wrong in the pelvis that do not show up unless one feels for them.

"Sister, I think our man has a strangulated hernia. We'll have to operate on him this afternoon. Can you explain this to him and ask him if he has any questions?"

Sister had a long talk with the man. Finally, she told Father that the patient agreed to the operation and did not have any questions. On the other hand, I had a question and a thought: I wondered how much of Father's explanation the patient had understood? And I was astonished by the extraordinary faith the man had in Father's diagnosis.

"I will leave you to organize the theatre and nursing staff, Sister."

Father turned to me. "Bernard, we'd better get on and see the rest of the patients."

We started at the first bed and worked our way round the ward. Many people had injuries of one sort or another. Some were the result of accidents, many from falling off bicycles. A few were from knife, spear or arrow wounds following fights or hunting accidents. One man had been mauled by a warthog and his condition was serious. There were a few post-operative patients, most of whom had had emergency surgery for appendicitis or hernias.

The only cancers that he could do anything about were the ones caught early. Unfortunately, most cancer patients were far too advanced by the time they arrived at the hospital and there was nothing that could be done for them. The only large hospitals to which Father could refer patients were in Lagos and Kaduna, and their facilities were not much better than those in Minna. Although patients had access to general surgeons, there were no radiotherapy units in Nigeria at that time to treat cancers.

Next we toured the female ward and the maternity unit. Fortunately there were no babies being born so I did not have to watch a delivery. Otherwise I might have been put off medicine forever. A lady in early labour showed some distress, but Father said this discomfort would be controlled with some pethidine. We spent the last hour of the morning on the outpatients ward where Father saw and decided what to do with the patients that the special-grade nurses had saved for him.

One of these was a middle-aged man who looked very sick, thin, and miserable. He had been sitting on the floor waiting for us. He could hardly stand, even after the nurse had helped him up.

"What's his problem?"

"He says that he has been feeling ill for over a month and that he is getting weaker all the time," said the nurse.

"He certainly looks poorly. Has he noticed anything else?" asked Father.

I was surprised and impressed by how much a patient's answers formed a part of my Father's assessment. This collaborative approach to diagnosis was to influence my own practice of medicine in future years.

"He says that he does not eat well, has some sweating at night, and thinks he may have a fever sometimes. But not every day."

"Any diarrhea?" asked Father.

"No."

"Any cough?"

"Some, but no blood."

"Any pain?"

"No."

"We better have a look at him, then. Have him sit down in the chair and ask him to take off his shirt," said Father.

By the time the man had staggered over to the chair and was seated, I could see that he was breathing very heavily and that this had caused him to cough a couple of times. Father tapped the front and back of the man's chest, then listened with his stethoscope.

"Bernard, come over and listen to his chest. Then tell me what you can hear."

I put the ends of the stethoscope into my ears and placed it on the man's chest like Father had done.

"First, I want you to listen here," said Father, putting the stethoscope over the left side of the man's chest. "Listen carefully for a few breaths."

At first I could hear very little, but when I concentrated I thought I could hear air going through fine tubing.

"And now listen to this," he said, and moved the stethoscope to an area of the man's back. This time I definitely heard something different. Every time the man took a breath it sounded like air bubbling through water.

"Do you hear the difference?" asked Father.

"Yes, it sounds as though he has some water in his lungs."

"That's not a bad guess, but it's more likely thin puss than water, which sounds a lot finer. I think our man has pneumonia and needs to be treated in hospital with antibiotics for a few days. Can you arrange that?" Father asked the nurse.

"Yes, doctor," the nurse replied.

"It is also possible," he said to me, "that he has tuberculosis. TB is very common here. Most of these patients, though, have a history of coughing up blood which they will readily tell you all about. We don't have an X-ray machine so if he doesn't improve on penicillin in a day or so we'll send him to Kaduna for an X-ray."

Just then another man, around twenty years old, walked in. At first I thought he looked well and I wondered why the nurse had bothered asking Father to see him. He seemed cheerful enough, but he had many spots on his face.

"Ah. This patient's story is completely different," Father said looking at the young man's chart. "He's been sick for a couple of weeks and now has a rash all over his body. We see a lot of this illness here, and there's nothing we can do about it except give the patients calamine lotion for the itchy rash. It looks like chickenpox, but it isn't."

"How do you know? The spots look just like the ones I had when I caught the chickenpox in India. I remember because they itched terribly."

"There are two things different in this case. One is the distribution of the spots, and secondly, these spots come in waves. Show us your hands," Father said to the young man, who understood English.

"If you look carefully and then feel, you'll notice he has some raised reddened areas on the palms of his hands." Father showed me what he meant. I found it easy to feel the little raised areas but the redness was not so obvious because of the young man's natural pigmentation.

"Please show us the soles of your feet as well," asked Father.

"They feel a bit sore but I can't see anything," said the man.

When I looked at the man's feet, I couldn't see anything except soles that were thickened from walking barefoot.

"Bernard, you'll have to feel carefully, but the spots will be there. They'll be a little sore if you press down on them," said Father.

Sure enough when I felt firmly, especially in the softer part of the sole, I could feel the small nodules. The man reluctantly admitted they were sore.

"Bernard. You have now seen your first case of what was once the scourge of Europe and is still a serious but quite common disease in Africa. What do you think he has?"

"I have no idea," I said. I wondered how he could possibly think I would know the answer to his question.

"He has a mild case of smallpox." Father then turned to the patient and said, "Don't worry. You have had it long enough now for it not to become serious. Just take things easy at home, stay away from work for the next four weeks, and we will give you something to put on the spots to stop the itch. Try not to scratch too much and keep the spotty areas clean so that they don't get infected. Or they will scar even worse."

"Thank you, sir. My friends thought I had chickenpox but I thought I had had chickenpox before and I was worried," said the man as he got up to leave.

"That's all we have for you this morning, sir," said the nurse.

"Thank you," said Father. "We'd better wash our hands, Bernard. You may have noticed that I do so after examining every patient."

"By the way," he said as we dried our hands, "I noticed you were concerned when I mentioned smallpox. Don't worry. You've been vaccinated several times. Vaccination is a very effective way of controlling diseases. In Europe they have been using vaccination against smallpox, measles, whooping cough, polio, yellow fever, typhoid, as well as cholera, and they are adding to that list almost yearly. Vaccination and other public health measures probably save a lot more lives globally than the efforts of practicing surgeons and physicians, but many doctors don't find public health a very satisfying occupation."

At this point Father became thoughtful and his eyes wistful. "What did you think of the morning's work?"

"I was impressed seeing what you do, but I'm not sure I could do that every day."

"I don't suppose you've thought much about work or what you're going to do when you leave school. There are many things one can do—ranging from manual labour to being a university professor, from playing a musical instrument to being a composer. Businessmen and traders often start right after school and, if successful, can make a lot of money. I had a choice between playing music and becoming a doctor and decided on the latter because my Father thought it was a good idea. I have never regretted doing medicine. It has taken me all over the world and I've never been without a job, but I doubt if I'll ever be rich compared to some of the other people with whom I went through school.

"Medicine is certainly not for everyone and there are physical risks that one takes on a daily basis, especially if one practices in countries like this. However, if you want to do any of the so-called professional things in life, you'll have to go to university. I gather you may have trouble passing the necessary exams to get you into a university, so you may have to consider working in something that does not need a university education. Your grandfather could probably help you out a bit in that area if you wanted to get into the painting and decorating business.

"Anyway, let's not worry too much about that at the moment. You're here to have a holiday and spend some time with us. We'd better get back to the house for lunch."

A couple of days later Father asked me if I would like to witness an operation. I was a little dubious, wondering if I had the stomach for it. On the other hand, I didn't want to miss out on the opportunity. What a story I'd have to tell back home. So the next morning we went down to the hospital and into the operating room.

"Good morning, Doctor. I see you've brought your son with you again. Is he going to help you with the operation?" asked the scrub nurse.

From the deadpan expression on the nurse's face I couldn't tell if this was a serious question or not.

"No," Father laughed. "He's here to observe what goes on during surgery. I just hope he doesn't pass out. All he needs is a cover gown, mask and cap. If he feels queasy he can go next door to where his mother is doing a clinic."

The nurse showed me how to put on the gown, mask and cap. I was surprised that the gown was put on back to front, but my father explained that this was done so that our clothes were kept away from the patient's sterile drapes during the operation.

"The first thing I have to do is administer an anaesthetic," Father said. "Since the patient has a hernia we can do the operation under a spinal anaesthetic. A local. He will be awake during the operation but will not feel anything below his belly button. We do this by putting a needle into his back. Once the injection is in it only takes a few minutes to take effect."

The patient was already on the table and sitting up with his back to me. I moved around in front of him and smiled, but then realized this wouldn't be of much comfort since I had a mask on. Father was at the sink washing and scrubbing his hands and arms. When he finished he dried them and put on a sterile gown and gloves.

"Whatever you do, don't touch any of the sterile items on that trolley or get too close to me or Abdulla when he's scrubbed," said Father. "The first thing we do is paint the patient's back with iodine to sterilize the skin. Then I cover the area with a drape that has a hole in the middle. Sterilizing the skin prevents bacterial contamination of the needle that I'll be using. He could possibly get meningitis if that happened and the outcome would probably be fatal."

He then turned to Abdulla and asked him to explain the procedure to the patient. There followed a brief conversation in Hausa and then Abdulla said, "He understands what we are going to do and does not have any questions."

"Right, let's get started. Bernard, if you feel weak-kneed just step outside for some fresh air. We don't need two patients to worry about."

Abdulla gave Father a sponge holder with a swab in its jaws and a small metal bowl containing iodine. Father dipped the swab into the iodine and painted the patient's back, starting over the spine and going outwards. He did this twice using a different swab for each painting. Then he put the drape over the man's back and adjusted it so that the hole in the drape was over the man's lower back. Abdulla gave Father an empty syringe which had a small needle attached and a separate needle that was about five inches long. Father then used the syringe to suck up some clear fluid from a vial Abdulla held out to him.

"The needle I use for injecting the anaesthetic into the patient is called a spinal needle and is this one," he said, picking up the long one. "It's thin and bends easily so it has a stylette to stiffen it while I put it into the patient's back. Once I think it's in the right place I'll take the stylette out to see if there is free flow of spinal fluid before injecting any anaesthetic."

Although I couldn't take my eyes off what was going on in front of me, I noticed I was beginning to sweat. Initially I thought it was because of the gown I was wearing. "Now I have to find a space between the vertebrae so that I can get the needle into the spinal column and inject the anaesthetic. I do this by feel, like this." With two fingers of his left hand Father started to palpate the man's back, in the midline, about a quarter of the way up from the tailbone. "The needle has to go in at a level that is below the spinal cord so that no damage is done to it. Ah, this feels like a good spot." He started to push the needle into the man's back at right angles and parallel to the floor. When it had gone in about three inches, Father stopped pushing and removed the stylette from the needle. Clear fluid started to drip out of the needle.

At this point I began to feel quite lightheaded. I turned to Father, "I'm sorry but I think I'd better go out and get some fresh air."

One of the nurses came over and gave me an arm to hang onto, afraid I might faint.

"Don't worry about it," Father said. "Go next door to the office and sit down. Your mother might be there having coffee. I'll finish here and see you later."

I hardly remember getting to the office, but things came back into focus once I was sitting and Mother arrived. "Well, that's a pity, Bernard. But a lot of people feel faint when they see an operation for the first time," Mother said and she gave me a hug.

I was disappointed and explained that it was before the operation even started that I began to feel woozy. "It was seeing Father put the needle in and seeing the spinal fluid come out—I think that's what set me off."

"Don't worry about it. I've finished here for the morning. We can go back to the house. Father should be ready for lunch in about an hour. Do you feel up to walking out to the car?"

"Yes, I think so, but I'm still feeling a bit funny," I said and stood up slowly.

"Walking to the car will probably help," Mother said as we left the office.

When we got to the house and were sitting on the veranda Mother thought of a solution. "Perhaps you could do with a drink. I'll get you a gin and tonic to buck you up."

She returned quickly. "There you are. See if this helps. I didn't put too much gin in it because I don't imagine you've had alcohol before, have you?"

"No. It'll be my first drink," I said, and took a sip. I was not impressed by the taste, but after a couple of mouthfuls I felt better.

Mother continued to reassure me that my reaction to the sight of the spinal needle was not unusual. "A lot of people faint at the sight of needles or blood or babies being born or seeing operations for the first time. Men are more likely to faint than women. It doesn't take long to get used to these things, especially if you're actively involved in the procedure. Watching as a bystander, doing nothing, allows you to think about what's going on and seems to affect people more. We don't know why we faint, but it seems to be some sort of reflex."

I could feel my face flush from embarrassment and said to Mother: "Thanks, except I was thinking that going into medicine could be a possible occupation but feeling faint at the sight of a needle going into a patient's back isn't exactly an exemplary start. Nor a good omen."

"Medicine's not so bad. It is a calling, especially for someone like your father. Not everyone has the disposition to put up with the long hours, dealing with sick people all the time, lack of funding, a lot of stress and endless night calls. Not to mention the disruption to family life. On the other hand, you get to travel, the pay's not bad, you meet lots of people from all walks of life, and you get to heal the sick and save lives. You'd never be bored. Your father has never regretted being a doctor and I have never had any problems as a doctor's wife. I would have liked to have seen more of you and Marjory these past few years, but our choices were limited when we got back from India. Finding a job in the Colonies seemed to be our best solution. There have been times when I've wished we had stayed in England, but after four or five months without finding a job your father felt that going overseas was our only option. We'll be here for another few years then we should be able to retire home."

She stopped talking, to muse, I think, on a life that had been happy but not always to her liking.

During the next three weeks Father took me down to the hospital several more times and on these occasions showed me some of the more unusual cases that came into the hospital. I saw many different tropical diseases, including elephantiasis of the legs and scrotum, Mosey foot, guinea worms which come out at the ankles, blood slides of malaria and filariasis, and several other parasites. He never invited me into the theatre again or the delivery room, which was probably a good thing.

One morning we were on the way to the car to go home for lunch when a group of men carrying a stretcher came through the gate. "I better go and have a look and see what this is all about. Do you want to come along?" asked Father.

"Yes, please," I replied. By this time I enjoyed seeing new cases.

We met the group half way across the hospital compound and Father asked the first man what the problem was.

"There was a train accident and this man has been killed. He was run over by the train."

"I'd better have a look," said Father.

The stretcher bearers parted so that we could get a good look. The muscular young man on the stretcher looked dead to me. He wasn't breathing or moving. His eyes were closed and blood covered his head, the upper part of his body, and his tee shirt. Banana leaves hid the lower part of his body. Father picked up the arm and hand that hung over the side of the stretcher, felt for a pulse, and then said, "I can't feel a pulse but he's still warm. How long ago did this happen?"

"About an hour ago and he has stopped bleeding. There was much blood and we could not do anything to stop it. We came here as fast as we could," replied one of the men.

By this time Father had put his hand on the man's neck. "There's a very faint pulse in the neck so he's still alive. Bring him over to the theatre where we can take a good look. You can come as well, Bernard. I might need your help."

When we got to the theatre the nurses moved the man onto the operating table. A nurse removed all the banana leaves. The man's right leg had been completely mashed below the knee. Bits of bone stuck out through muscle and skin in all directions. His foot lay in a pool of clotted blood at a grotesquely abnormal angle. The condition of his left leg was even more baffling. It did not appear to have been broken but the skin and sole of the foot had been stripped away and were attached by only a few shreds of skin. All the tendons and muscles of the foot and lower third of the leg were exposed. Curiously I was unfazed by this gruesome sight. Perhaps I could be a doctor, after all.

"Come over here, Bernard, and hold this bottle of saline while I try to get an intravenous going," my father instructed. "Nurse, find out if he has any relatives here who can give us blood. If we're to save his life he's going to need some." By this time Father had put a tourniquet around the man's arm, had stretched the arm out and was feeling for a vein. The bottle that I was holding was attached to some red rubber tubing, which had a drip chamber a few inches from the bottle and a metal clip below this that blocked off the tube. At the end there was a simple metal lock to attach a needle to.

"Bernard, see that drip stand over there by the wall? Fetch it here and hang the drip on it. Then open the clip to make sure that the drip chamber and the tubing is full of saline; we don't want to let any air into his vein. I think I've found one. Nurse, give me the widest gauge intravenous needle you can find, please."

I was amazed by the stillness that surrounded us; a mixture of solemnity and calm, as if we were all participants in a mysterious sacred rite.

"Thank you. Now let's see if we can get this drip going." Father inserted the needle into the man's elbow at about a forty-five degree angle and then reduced the angle a little before pushing it in a bit further. The attached syringe started to fill up with blood. "When I detach the syringe I want you to give me that tube, Bernard. Nurse, I will give you the syringe with the blood, so that you can put it into a heparinized tube in case we find some relatives who are willing to give him blood."

Father then proceeded to detach the syringe from the needle and blood flowed freely. By putting pressure on the point where the tip of the needle was in the man's arm, Father stopped the blood flow. With his other hand he took the drip tube from me and attached it to the needle in the man's arm. "You can open the clip now and we'll see if the needle is in the right place."

I opened the clip and saw that the saline was running freely in the drip chamber.

"Good. Now we can see how bad his injuries are. Leave the drip wide open for the time being, nurse."

Father turned the stripped leg over to see how much skin was still attached to the sole. It was fairly broadly attached to the back of the leg and he said there might be enough blood supply to keep it alive once the man's blood pressure normalized. If that occurred he thought we might be able to save the lower limb on that side.

"I'm afraid the other leg will have to come off at the knee or just below it. That will depend on how much damage the knee has sustained. Now let's look at the rest of him. The abdomen is soft and not distended yet. The arms seem to be okay apart from some bruising. There is some bruising over the left side of his chest but I don't think he has any broken ribs. He has a superficial cut on his forehead but his skull seems to be intact." While he talked Father examined the affected areas by running his hands over them. "Nurse, can you roll him over a bit towards you? I'd like to have a look at his back. Be gentle. He's in a state of shock and the less we aggravate the situation the better."

Two nurses then rolled the man on to his side away from Father who was then able to have a good look at the man's back.

"How's his blood pressure doing?" Father asked the nurse.

"I can feel a very faint pulse. It's going very fast, but I have not been able to take his blood pressure," replied the nurse who was at the head of the table.

"Let's lower his head and see if that helps. He'll probably need a couple more bottles of saline before we see much improvement. If he starts to bleed from the broken leg put a tourniquet on, above the knee, but release it every twenty minutes for three minutes. Keep him here for the time being and put a blanket over him once you've got him cleaned up. Has anyone gone looking for relatives?"

"Yes, sir. He's a local man so we should be able to locate someone from his family."

"That's good news. I'm going to take Bernard home. Then I'll be back to see how the patient's doing. I won't be long. Come on, Bernard, perhaps I can get some food. I may end up here for most of the day."

"Do you think the man will survive?" I asked as we made our way to the car.

"Probably, if he doesn't have any internal injuries. He's going to lose one leg and I may have to take both off if there's not enough blood supply to the skin that's been stripped on the other. Fortunately he's a rail worker and will get a pension; otherwise his life expectancy would be pretty poor in this country," Father reflected.

"Thank you for your help, Bernard. I noticed that all the trauma and blood we witnessed today didn't trouble you. That's probably because you were involved with what was going on. You don't see many injuries as bad as that, especially the strip injury to the foot. The train wheel must have just caught the sole. I saw a similar injury during the war when I was in Egypt. On that occasion a man had been caught between two vehicles and was in a real mess. He died in spite of our efforts."

After a very short lunch Father returned to the hospital. I didn't see him again until breakfast the next morning.

"How did that man make out last night?" I asked.

"By the time I got back he had woken up. We found some relatives and were lucky to find two whose blood was compatible for a transfusion. We eventually got him to the theatre and then spent a couple of hours sorting out and rearranging the parts. I had to take one leg off above the knee. Losing the joint is bad because the prosthetic knees available here are cumbersome and not tolerated by many amputee patients. I hope the skin I put back onto the stripped foot will survive, and that he doesn't get a serious infection. Otherwise he'll lose the foot below the knee. It's sad, because he has a wife, two children, as well as his parents who depend on him for food and shelter. I hope the railway is good to him and gives him a decent pension. All I could do was patch him up and make recommendations."

Two weeks later Father came home for lunch and said to Mother, a note of displeasure and annoyance in his voice, "Ada, I have some bad news. I've been transferred to Zaria because the doctor there has had to go back to England on a family emergency."

"Oh dear, not again. When do we have to leave?" asked Mother.

"Next week. They have a replacement for me coming from England in about two weeks, but they want me in Zaria as soon as we can get there. I've written and told them that it will take at least a week for us to relocate," replied Father.

"Why is it always us who have to move in mid-tour? This is the third time and I'm fed up with it."

This was one of the rare occasions when I heard Mother express anger at the way they were treated by the Colonial Service. Mother always felt it was to be expected when Father was in the Army, but when they had gone to Nigeria she had expected to move less. On this occasion they had me to worry about as well. Our precious time together was going to be affected.

"I'll get Mbula and the garden boy organized to do the packing in the morning. It won't take me long. I'm used to it now," she said forming her mouth in a grim line and shaking her head. "All the boxes and packing materials are in the storeroom and I have Bernard to help. It's a pity. He only has three weeks to go before returning to England and I'm enjoying having him here. We certainly won't have time to find our feet in Zaria before he leaves. What terrible timing!"

* * *

Zaria was a larger station than the one in Minna. The colonial-style concrete brick house with high ceilings and airy rooms was bigger. The furniture was similar and the concrete floors were painted the same red. My parents, however, did have the luxury of electricity, running water and a telephone.

Three days after we got to Zaria I woke up in the middle of the night with a severe headache and abdominal cramps. I felt terribly hot and was sweating profusely. I lay in bed for a few minutes wondering what was going on and then was struck with a violent fit of vomiting. I tried to get out of bed but was too weak to do so. I felt so miserable that I was not even worried about the mess I had made and was still lying in. The light was turned on and I could see Mother and Father standing in the doorway looking at me.

"Oh dear, you are in a state. What happened?" asked Mother.

"I woke up feeling awful and then was sick. I tried to get to the bathroom but was too weak to get out of bed. It all happened so fast. Sorry."

Father came over to the bed, put his hand on my forehead, picked up my hand and felt for my pulse.

"Your pulse is fast and you certainly feel as though you have a fever. Ada, can you get the thermometer, I think it's in the bedside table drawer? Now let's have a look at your tummy."

Father sat on the bed next to me, avoiding the vomit as best he could. He pulled the sheet down and looked at my abdomen.

"Does it hurt anywhere?"

"Not really. I woke up with some cramps but they've stopped since I was sick."

"Were you feeling well when you went to bed? Or have you been off color this past day or so?"

"I was fine before bed; I've not noticed anything unusual since we got here."

"Any diarrhea?"

"No."

Then he put his hand on my stomach very gently. I was surprised at how cool and gentle his hand was. He felt around the four quadrants of my abdomen. On the second pass he exerted more pressure, but there was no pain—although I did experience a general feeling of discomfort.

"The good news is that there's nothing out of place or particularly tender. You've not missed any of the anti-malarial pills that you're supposed to take every day have you?"

"I don't think so," I replied after pausing for a moment.

By this time Mother had returned with the thermometer, which she put under my tongue.

"Close your mouth, but don't bite," she instructed.

"The most likely diagnosis is malaria," Father suggested. "We'll take a blood slide and put him on Mepacrin to start with. I think I have some slides and a needle in the bedroom," Father said as he walked out of the room.

By the time he was back the minute was up and Mother was reading the thermometer. "No wonder you're feeling ill. You have a temperature of 101.4 degrees. I'll bring you some juice and clean sheets."

"Now let's get some blood from your finger, Bernard. Give me your left hand."

Father took my finger squeezed it a bit, wiped it with some cotton wool soaked in alcohol, then stuck the needle in and out quickly. I felt a sharp, stabbing pain for a second and blood appeared almost immediately. He squeezed a drop onto the slide, put the cotton wool swab onto the end of my finger and told me to squeeze it where the needle had gone in. He proceeded to get a second slide and spread the drop of blood in a very thin film onto that slide as well.

"That will do for now. Here are four tablets of Mepacrin I want you to take right now. We'll give you some more in the morning, after breakfast. You'll be staying in bed for the next day or so if you've got malaria, which I'm fairly certain you have," said Father.

With a slight feeling of trepidation, I swallowed the pills, which I noticed were very bitter. "Do you often have violent vomiting with malaria?" I asked.

"Quite often with the variety we have here. The malaria that we saw in India did not behave in the same way. This one seems to be much more aggressive and sudden in onset."

I felt much better the next day but Father would not let me out of bed for two days. The slide confirmed that I did indeed have malaria. He said that if I was well without a fever in three days' time we could assume the disease was under control. I was to take Mepacrin three times a day for a week. He warned me that I might turn quite yellow because of the drug. He explained that even though I had been on the recommended dose of prophylactic anti-malarial sometimes the disease would gain a foothold, possibly because of poor absorption of the anti-malarials from the gut. Whatever the reason, I felt as though my brain and gut had been spun round in a butter churn.

Within two weeks of my recovery from malaria it was time for me to return to England. Visiting my parents in Nigeria, seeing them working at the hospital, had been an illuminating experience; for the first time, I felt like a future had been seeded in my thoughts, one rich in possibility and promise. Now I needed to make it happen.

During my holiday in Nigeria I managed to complete most of the work that Mr. Beatty and Mr. Whitty had assigned me to improve my test results. Mother helped a lot and encouraged me to practice my writing. By the time I was due to return to England I had a better understanding of some English grammatical principles, but it was apparent to both Mother and me that spelling was always going to be a problem. I did not seem able to visualize words as a whole. I read and spelt words phonetically and this meant that I would spell the same word in different ways depending on how I pronounced it mentally. Deciphering words was laborious and resulted in my being a slow reader. There was no one in Minna or in Zaria who could help with French, so I concentrated on increasing my vocabulary as much as possible. Pronunciation was a problem. Father never said anything about the letter that Mr. Reynolds was supposed to have sent him and I never asked if he had received it.

* * *

On returning to Nottingham High in the fall of 1950, Mr. Beatty made the following announcement to my class: "Boys, I hope you had a good summer. Now you are going to have to start some real work because the School Certificate is only eighteen months away and it's important that you take these exams seriously. They are National Exams set by a board of teachers from all over the country. In order to go on to the sixth form and then to university you have to pass them. You are lucky in a way because you are the first year to take the General Certificate of Education (GCE) exams which are going to replace the old School Certificate. The major change is that the exams may be individually tougher but if you pass one subject you keep it and don't have to take all the subjects again the next time you try for the certificate." At this point the room erupted in a chorus of groans and mutterings about making things harder for us and questions about why we were being made guinea pigs.

"You were allocated your houses last year and will stay in the same one until you finish school. You are expected to participate in the activities of the Houses," continued Mr. Beatty. "If any of you have problems, I'm always here to help. Any questions?" he asked and paused a moment. "Since there are no questions, let's dip into the first chapter of the English grammar text." And so the term began.

During the first few weeks back at school I had a vague notion that engineering might make a challenging occupation, but this also meant that I needed to be accepted by a university. If I didn't improve in my weaker subjects I could end up pushing a broom on a factory floor. Worrying about my future, I felt quite lost and down in the dumps.

One day on the bus to Nottingham I got into a conversation with a gentleman who was interested in my history. He was a teacher at a borstal school, a youth detention facility, just outside of Nottingham. He told me that his was a rather depressing job because of the low success rate. Sooner or later most of the boys he dealt with ended up in prison. He felt the reason for this was that once his detainees returned home they went back to their old ways and friends, where peer pressure usually trumped ambition. The boys stayed at the borstal school for relatively short periods of time and came from all social backgrounds, but their problems were similar. Many were repeaters and they had all been in trouble with the police.

I met him on the bus several times in the next few months. It was he who suggested that I should divide my homework hours into segments and write out a schedule that I could refer to and maintain. He helped with this schedule and suggested how many hours I should spend on the various subjects. He stressed the importance of adhering to my schedule and over time took an interest in how I was progressing.

With the support of Aunt Ethel and this kind gentleman, I settled into a strict work regime, which in the end paid off. My next two term reports were good and I was encouraged by being told I could stay on at Nottingham until the GCE "O" level examinations. I never felt I was going to be a French or English scholar, but gradually I became confident that I could pass the exams.

I took these exams in July 1951 when I was seventeen. The exams took two to three weeks. Each exam lasted two or three hours, so it was a bit of a marathon. I had to pass General Maths, Physics and Chemistry as well as French and English Language if I were to continue into the Sixth form the following term. Those who did not achieve passing grades could attempt the exam again after completing a revision class during the winter term.

By the time the exams were over I was deeply depressed because I didn't feel I had done well enough to pass the required subjects. In spite of my misgivings, my teachers continued to encourage me, while Mrs. Jackson became almost a surrogate mother. She was always able to give advice that brought a sense of balance into my agitated world.

All I could do was thank her and go back to Worksop and wait for the results. Over the next few weeks my mind was in turmoil. The more I thought about the exams and what I had written the worse I thought I had done. I even thought I might have failed the science subjects. With my parents in Nigeria, I felt lonely; and I definitely didn't feel I could talk about these problems with my aunt and particularly my uncle. I ended up going for long, aimless walks or cycle rides on my own.

One weekend I walked up to the Canns' house, the parents of Shirley who I had met while at Worksop Central. They asked me in for tea even though Shirley was still at school in Ireland. They were kind and observant people who soon realized I was troubled. They asked me about my problems and I unloaded my worries on to them—about the exams, about the fact my parents were in Nigeria, and about how I felt that I had likely failed the exams, which would be a big disappointment to my parents. The Canns listened attentively to my ramblings and dreams and doubts, and although there was nothing specific they could do, my age and experience was never a barrier to their understanding. For me, just being able to talk freely to someone was a huge relief. They treated me as an equal. This was the beginning of a long friendship that continued until they passed away some thirty years later.

Eventually the exam results arrived in the mail one Tuesday morning. It was a brief note:

Dear Bernard A.O.Binns
Exam No. 3632
    I have been instructed to inform you that you were successful in the following subjects at the "O" level of the General Certificate of Education.
- General Mathematics
- Physics
- Chemistry
- English Literature
Yours Sincerely,
Mrs. E. Roberts
Secretary

Aunt Ethel was there when I opened the letter, "How did you do?"
"I only managed to pass four subjects. That's not enough to get

me into the Sixth Form, especially since I missed French and English Language. Now what am I going to do?"

"I seem to recall that they'll let you have another go at the exams you failed. I'll write to the school if you'd like."

"Yes, please," I said, thinking I should be able to pass them on the second try.

Ten days later we received confirmation that I had been accepted back at Nottingham and that I had been added to the revision class in preparation for the next set of examinations. On the first day back to school I went to the assigned classroom. Mr. Rhoe came in and said, "Binns, the Headmaster wants to see you, now."

"Thank you, sir." I had not expected to have to see the Headmaster and I wondered what the problem was. Being told to go to the Headmaster's office nearly always heralded a problem.

When I got to his office he said, "Binns, you better sit down. What sort of a summer did you have? Did you see your parents this year?"

"No, they're still in Nigeria and will not return to England until next year. The holidays were a bit depressing. I was worried about the exam results and the more I thought about them the worse things seemed to get. At one point I thought I had failed the whole lot. My aunt and I did go Youth Hostelling in the Lake District for two weeks and I went to Skegness twice for weekends, Sir." I replied.

"How old are you now?"

"I was seventeen in April, sir."

"Yes, that's why I've called you in. We have a problem with you because you'll be due for National Service next April. The school can get you deferred for one year but you'll need two years in the Sixth before you can take the GCE 'A' levels. This means I'll have to put you in the Sixth Form now or you will have to continue any further education when you get out of the service in two year's time. If you go into the service your only choice once you get out will be Technical College. My problem is that you don't have enough 'O' levels to be admitted to the Sixth. But, if you think you're capable of doing the work necessary to pass the French and English exams, as well as the work required in the first year of Sixth Form, I can think of a plan for you to do both."

I couldn't believe my good fortune. The Headmaster was offering to make an exception for me; using his authority to influence the direction of my life, although at that time I wasn't aware how momentous his offer was.

"Sir, I think I can do the work necessary to pass the exams and I would like to start the Sixth Form, right away, if that's possible."

"What subjects were you thinking of taking?" he asked.

"Civil engineering appeals to me which means taking Physics, Chemistry, Maths and Advanced Maths."

He considered my answer for a moment or two. "That wouldn't work. The Advanced Maths course takes three years and you don't have the time. Have you any other ideas, Binns?"

I thought for a moment. "I could do Physics, Chemistry and Biology with a view to doing biological sciences at University. Can that be done in two years? My second choice is a career in Medicine."

Mr. Reynolds looked relieved. "I was hoping you might suggest that. I think it's the best alternative. Don't get me wrong; what I'm proposing you do is going to be very difficult for the first year." He paused and then continued. "You can go now, and good luck. Mr. Neville is in charge of the Biological section of the Sixth Form and is expecting you. He tells me that you're quite a good swimmer."

I quickly settled into the Sixth Form routine. I was already familiar with Physics and Chemistry, but I had never done any Biology, a new and mysterious discipline, although my time assisting Father helped me appreciate its subtleties. I took the English and French exams in November, passed the English and French oral but had to wait until the summer exams before I finally passed French Grammar.

Toward the end of the first year in the Sixth Form, the students were advised to send out applications to the universities they were interested in. I was encouraged to apply to Birmingham University to enter their medical program.

At the time, Father and Mother were back in England for a holiday. Since Father had trained at Guy's Hospital in London he suggested I apply to them as well. Applications included an interview with the admissions department. Father accompanied me to London for the interview, but before it was scheduled we took in a theatre show and did some sightseeing—Hyde Park, Oxford Street, Piccadilly Circus, the British Museum and the Science Museum. The show was a London revue at the Palace Theatre. I was spellbound and tickled by its antics, acrobatics, jokes, songs, dance and music.

London was a new bustling world to me.

On the day of the interview, Father and I climbed out of the Underground at London Bridge. It was a bright spring morning. The first thing I noticed as we came up the damp, concrete steps was the smell of vegetables. I wondered where it was coming from. As we rounded a corner I could see a street market with several barrows piled high with vegetables. We turned and walked down to Burgh High Street. On the right I could see the start of London Bridge. We took the next turn into a narrow street with old red-brick three-storey buildings on each side. The street opened into a large courtyard with a wide wrought-iron gate at its entrance. In the centre of the courtyard there was a bronze statue of Thomas Guy. Immediately ahead was the main entrance to the Hospital by way of a colonnade.

Several cars were parked in the courtyard and most of them were Rolls Royces, Bentleys or Daimlers.

"The consultants park here," Father said, clucking his tongue. He seemed to be enjoying a private joke.

Entering the hospital, we were met by a distinguished looking man who stood outside the porter's office. As we approached, he turned to Father and said, "Good morning, Dr. Binns."

Father was rather taken aback by this. "Good Lord, how did you remember my name? It must be twenty-five years since I was here last."

"Happily, I have a long memory for names. What brings you here today?"

"I've brought my son for an interview. I presume it will be in the Medical School building?"

"Yes sir, the interviews are being held in the board room. The office is in the same place. Mr. Cook is still there and he will be interested to see you again. Good luck with the interview, sir," he called after me as Father and I walked down the colonnade to the small park that lay at the centre of the Hospital's Medical, Dental, and Nursing Schools.

After waiting for half an hour with three well-dressed boys who said nothing, I was called into the board room, a large room with a highly polished oak floor. There were three large windows down one side with drawn, heavy, dark red curtains. At the far end of the room was a long table. Five gentlemen sat on the other side of the table. The man seated in the centre had a black patch over his left eye. On my side of the table there was a single hard-backed chair. As I closed the door behind me the gentleman in the middle said, "You must be Mr. Binns. Please take a seat. We won't keep you too long."

Once seated I noticed how remote and stern-looking my interviewers seemed. I felt totally out of place and wondered what I was doing there. The ambience was quite different from the colonial hospitals I had experienced through Father in the middle of Western Africa or northern India.

"Let me introduce the panel. On the far right is Mr. Blackburn. Next to him is Mr. Grant-Massie. They are consultant surgeons. On the far left is Dr. Mann, and next to him is Dr. Houston, the Assistant Dean. They are consultant physicians. I am Dr. Boland, another physician and Dean of the Medical School."

"I don't know why there are always more physicians than surgeons on these panels," commented Mr. Blackburn in a jocular tone. "I don't think there are more of them in the profession, Mr. Binns. They just have more time on their hands."

"That's a lot of rubbish. We have time to think and are not cooped up in operating theatres all the time," said Dr. Houston, bantering back.

"Mr. Binns, when did you come down to London and what have you been doing here?" Dr. Boland asked.

"My father and I came to London two days ago and we've spent a good portion of our time looking at the cultural highlights. It's my first extended visit to London, sir, and I'm surprised by the variety of things to see and do."

"From your application form I see you have only been at school in Nottingham for the past four to five years. What happened before that?" asked Dr. Houston.

"It's quite a long story, sir. During the war our family was in India and then Kashgar in Chinese Turkestan. There weren't any schools there. So the only schooling I got was from my parents."

"How did you get to Kashgar?" asked Mr. Blackburn.

"On horses. It took us six weeks of trekking through the Himalayas."

"How old were you when you made the trip?" asked Dr. Mann.

"I was ten when we went up and thirteen when we came back by the old silk route through Leh, in Little Tibet."

"How fascinating. What do you think of England?" asked Mr. Grant–Massie.

"It's a lot different from India and Kashgar. The weather's colder but the summers are pleasant enough. Here there are a lot more people and cars. School at Nottingham was a bit tough for the first three years. I was so far behind the other boys. Overall I like it here."

"Are you involved in rugby or cricket at school?" asked Dr. Boland.

"Not really. I swim for the school in the spring and summer terms and do some cross-country running in the autumn. I'm also on the reserve list for the tennis team. I have played both cricket and rugby but not well enough to get onto the teams," I replied.

"Pity. We could do with some good players for the hospital teams. Was your father a Guy's man?"

"Yes, sir. After he finished here he joined the Colonial Service and went to the Falkland Islands for two years. That's where I was born. Then after a short spell here he joined the Indian Medical Service and spent ten years there. He saw active service in the Middle East during the War. He is now in the Colonial Service working in Nigeria."

"I remember your father. He was a year behind me. He was a good tennis player. Why do you want to become a doctor?" asked Dr. Mann.

I had been warned about this question by my father who told me not to say "for the benefit of suffering humanity."

"Because I like the sciences. I think being a doctor would be a fascinating job where I could meet a lot of different people and travel like my father has," I replied.

Dr. Boland removed the patch from over his left eye. He did not have an artificial eye and I was a little shocked. I had never seen an empty eye socket before. I tried not to stare, but his eyeless socket was distracting.

"How do you think you will do in the GCE 'A' exams?" he asked.

"I hope to pass, sir. At least I seem to be doing better at school now than I was a couple of years ago, and my teachers seem to be quite pleased with my progress."

"Thank you, Mr. Binns. I think that will do for now. Give our regards to your father. We can't tell you now if you'll be offered a place at Guy's, but we'll write to you soon. Of course, you realize that any offer will be dependent on your obtaining the minimal requirements for entry to London University and Guy's Hospital. Good luck. You can go now," said Dr. Boland.

And just like that, the interview was over. Feeling like I had been dismissed rather perfunctorily, I left not knowing what to think. Father, who was talking to Mr. Cook, was waiting for me in the Medical School office.

"Ah, there you are. How did it go?" he asked.

"I really don't know. It was an unusual experience," I replied. "I'm not sure what they know about me now that they didn't know before I went in. Apart from a little personal history."

Two weeks later I received a letter from the university offering me a place in first year at Guy's and outlining the provisions as they had been stated in the interview. This meant that I had to pass Physics and Chemistry at the Advanced level, something I was confident I could manage.

My last year at Nottingham High was the only one that I truly enjoyed. I was doing work that interested me and I was well up in the class academically. I felt that I had a good chance of passing all my exams. I was still running the swimming club, which I enjoyed, and my social life in Worksop flourished, perhaps because the number of people I knew multiplied. Life became less stressful and frantic as my confidence grew.

During the last week at school I ran into Mr. Hardwick in one of the corridors.

"Ah, Binns, how are you doing? This is your last week at school, isn't it?"

"Yes, sir. I have a place at Guy's Hospital, University of London. I hope to do medicine, like my father" I replied.

"Congratulations. When we first met I didn't think you would manage to make the progress you have. I'm sure your English reading skills and spelling will always plague you, but remember, there are a lot of people out there who can help you out when you need documents and communications corrected."

"Thank you, sir, for the advice and for all that you've done for me during the past six years."

"As a teacher it gives me a great deal of satisfaction to see a pupil with problems get over them. And progress. I have no doubt that you will become a doctor and that you'll enjoy your chosen profession. Best of luck in the future," he said and shook my hand. At that moment he exuded a sense of happiness, of genuine pleasure, that has stayed with me all these years. I knew right away we shared a feeling of accomplishment.

I passed physics, chemistry and biology at advanced and scholarship levels. That summer I went on another visit to Nigeria. By this time Father was in a full administrative job so I was unable to see any more of his practical work in medicine. In a way that was a relief. Just spending time with my parents laughing, telling stories, hearing about their adventures, exchanging small talk over meals, reading, listening to them make music, made up in a small way for all the time we had been apart. Perhaps I was reassured I had not been forgotten. When I got back to England I spent ten days with my Grandfather, Ethel and George in Worksop before heading down to London to start my medical training.

Chapter 6
London: Medical School

Sunday, the fifth of September, 1953. Aunt Ethel, Uncle George, Granddad and I were waiting on a cold damp morning for the train to London. I was to start medical school at Guy's Hospital the next day. My parents were still in Nigeria so Ethel, George, and Granddad had come to see me off on this important day. They seemed to be more excited about the event than I was. The trip itself didn't worry me as I had now been down to London by train a few times and I had clear instructions on how to get to Mrs. Perry's house where I would be staying.

"Have you got everything?" asked Ethel.

"Yes, I think so," I replied, looking at my two suitcases on the platform. They contained most of the clothes I owned and the usual toiletries. They also contained a few books and writing materials I thought would be useful. I had twenty-five pounds in my wallet, the first of my monthly allowances from Father.

Granddad gave me a last minute pep talk: "You are about to start on a big adventure, Bernard. I have spent all my life here in Worksop and have only been to London four times. I've never been across the channel to Europe or anywhere else for that matter. Fortunately, you have already seen a lot of the world and now you are about to start learning for a serious career. It's going to take a lot of hard work and dedication. I hope you enjoy it."

"Don't forget we're still here. You can always contact us if you have any problems. Remember, Granddad now has a telephone. Use it, even if you just want to chat," said Aunt Ethel. She was fussing but I appreciated her concern.

Then George added a final bit of wisdom. "Bernard, remember, there are a lot of places in London that you'll have plenty of time to explore. You'll meet many people from all walks of life, some will become friends for life, and others will annoy you, some you will never understand. Try to be both tolerant and understanding. This is particularly important, as you get closer to becoming a doctor. The trick at university, as far as I understand, is to be self-disciplined."

His comment surprised me. It was not the sort of observation I had come to expect from George, who had always seemed to me rustic and on the quiet side. As he shifted from foot to foot, he seemed nervous and a bit awkward.

Ethel dug into her handbag and brought out some wrapped sandwiches. "Don't forget to change trains at Retford, and ask the conductor on the London train where the buffet car is. You can get yourself a cup of tea."

When the train came to a stop, George walked over to a coach door, opened it and ushered me up the stairs, all with great ceremony. He then passed up my two suitcases, closed the door, and gave it an extra nudge with his shoulder. "Have a good trip. We'll see you at Christmas."

"Remember to write," called Aunt Ethel who was on the verge of tears.

Just then the whistle sounded and the train started to move out slowly. I stood at the window and waved until they were out of sight, then I picked up my cases and stowed them away for the short trip to Retford station.

I spent the ride to London thinking about what might lie ahead. I was leaving the familiar behind, the comfort and security it brought. London was a long way from Worksop. I had no idea what my digs in London were going to be like and Mrs. Perry was a complete unknown.

When arranging to stay at Mrs. Perry's, the Medical School secretary had told me that I would get breakfast and an evening meal during the week, plus lunches at the weekends. She also assured me that many of the horror stories I'd heard about student accommodation in universities were exaggerated, but I still wondered. The Medical School office had set up the accommodation so I was pretty confident that all would be as advertised. The other important thing was that

Mrs Perry would look after my laundry. For all this I would have to pay her four guineas a week, which had to come out of my monthly allowance of twenty-five pounds. There wouldn't be much left for books, lunches and transport within London. Father had told me, just before he and Mother had returned to Nigeria, that he had made enquiries about expenses and had been assured that my allowance would be enough, providing I was careful. He had opened an account for me at his branch of Lloyds Bank on the Embankment, near the Houses of Parliament.

Idly I watched the countryside speed by. The morning had started in a dreary fog but by the time we got through Peterborough it was a beautiful sunny day. We passed by farm fields recently harvested, cows and horses, trees turning red and yellow, and small villages. After Stevenage we entered a more urban area with a number of factories. The houses were close together, many terraced with small gardens at the rear. Most had outhouses in the gardens. Perhaps because it was Sunday and it was the only day women had off, rows and rows of washing hung on lines were strung out to dry. All of the houses were grey from a thin covering of soot, which I assumed came from the trains that passed frequently. Set back from the tracks only forty to fifty yards, these houses must have been very noisy and shaky to live in.

As we got into the outskirts of London the buildings got bigger and grubbier. There were old car dumps, broken windows, and empty buildings that looked as though they might collapse at any moment. Finally the train slowed down and entered the tunnel leading into King's Cross station.

To get to Mrs. Perry's I had to make my way to the Westcombe Park metro station, which was located past Greenwich and north of Blackheath. I could see Guy's Hospital from the right side of the train just after London Bridge station.

Mrs. Perry's house, an old two-storey Victorian residence with a small garden surrounded by a privet hedge, was on Beaconsfield Road. A wrought iron gate opened to a short path that led to a covered front door. As I knocked, the door was opened by a fairly large, middle-aged woman with reddish hair. "I'm Bernard Binns," I said. I'm not sure why I felt so self-conscious. "I think you're expecting me."

Mrs. Perry appeared to be quite jovial and bustled around the entrance as I carried in my luggage.

"Welcome," she said warmly, "the other Guy's student arrived a couple of hours ago. His name is Morton Wilson and he's in the same year as you." She led me into the hallway. "Yours is the first room on the right." She opened the door and showed me into a small room with a single bed against one wall and a small desk and chair under a window that looked out into the front garden.

"Your evening meals and lunches at the weekends will be served in your room. Breakfast is at ten past eight in the dining room which is the room on the left as you came in. The bathroom is across from your room, and the kitchen is down the hall. Morton's room is next to yours. Come, I'll introduce you. You can unpack later. Supper won't be ready for a couple of hours yet. And don't forget to give me your ration books." She led the way out of the room, knocked on Morton's door, and introduced us.

"Thank you Mrs. Perry," Morton said with a politeness I felt was exaggerated and with an accent I didn't recognize. "Come in," he said closing the door behind me, "have a seat on the bed." His room was a little larger than mine but similarly Spartan.

We spent the next hour talking about where we had come from and a little about what we expected from Medical School. Morton, like me, had come directly from a public school into first-year medicine. He was two years younger than me and had not seen much of England. Nor had he been aboard. He had been brought up in the West Country and came from a small town. His hopes were like mine, to take the medical course and become a general practitioner somewhere in England. Other than this, neither of us really knew much about the profession we hoped to embark on. However, we were both optimistic and looked forward to our first day at Guy's.

He told me the trip to the Hospital took twenty minutes and that there were trains every few minutes in the mornings. Mrs. Perry had given him instructions about which train to catch. Morton also mentioned there were two female medical students in the house, upstairs. One was Mrs. Perry's daughter, Gill, and the other was Elaine Parker. They were both starting their second year and were taking courses given by the Royal Free Hospital program. Because it took them longer to get to their classes they had their breakfast scheduled a little earlier than ours.

The next morning I woke up early and became bored sitting in my room. At eight o'clock I wandered out of my room and into the kitchen where Mrs. Perry was busy preparing breakfast.

"Good morning, Bernard. You're a bit early, I have to get the girls their breakfast first. You can wait in the dining room if you'd like."

I wandered down to the dining room, which had an oak sideboard against one wall, a drinks cabinet, a few spare chairs and a big round oak table in the centre with four matching chairs set around it. A large oriental rug covered the floor. I took a seat at the table, and looked out the window into the garden, wondering what the day would bring, when I heard someone hurrying down the stairs.

"Your breakfast is ready, Elaine," I heard Mrs. Perry call out from the kitchen.

"Thank you, Mrs. Perry."

An attractive young woman came into the dining room with eggs and bacon on a plate and sat down opposite me. She was of average height, athletic looking and had dark brown hair that came down to her shoulders. Her skin was an attractive bronze colour and she was not wearing any make-up. She wore a skirt and no stockings. I thought her face striking, although perhaps a little too angular to fit the cinematic definition of beautiful. And yet I found her looks appealing, especially her brown-flecked greenish eyes. They were intense and lively, accompanied by an inquisitive and spirited smile that was filled with impish delight. As if she knew something I didn't.

"Hello, who are you? I'm Elaine Parker, one of the students here."

"I'm Bernard Binns, a medical student starting at Guy's today."

"I heard from Mrs. Perry that there would be two of you."

"Morton's the other one. We both arrived yesterday. Morton tells me you're studying at the Royal Free Hospital."

"Yes, that's right, and, as usual, I'm late. Must rush off. I'll see you again soon, I expect. Oh, if you want a seat on the train, go to the back, there's often more room there."

After breakfast Morton and I walked down to the station. Everyone else was in a hurry, some actually running. This was my first introduction to the tempo of the London commuter who always seemed to be trying to get somewhere fast. At the front of the platform a crowd had gathered, two to three deep. Remembering Elaine's advice I pulled Morton towards the far end of the platform through the crowd that was behaving like a rugby scrum.

As we walked down the platform the crowd thinned out, just as Elaine had predicted. We still had a few minutes to wait before the train arrived. The station had been carved out of a hillside that was covered with some untidy grass and a few bushes. Above these there were some trees that lined the road that came into the station. Two concrete platforms, separated by tracks, were connected by an old, wooden, covered footbridge at the London end. There were toilets, a small waiting room, and a guard's room—all made of grey stone. A dull green wooden roof overhung most of the platform.

We stopped at three stations before reaching London Bridge. The twenty minutes passed quickly. Most of the passengers were men dressed in pinstriped suits and dull ties. The majority wore bowler hats and carried rolled umbrellas, as if they had stepped out of a scene assembled that morning by René Magritte. Although there was the odd empty seat, most of the passengers preferred to stand and read the morning newspapers. Some filled in the daily crosswords. In the crowded areas, where people stood elbow to elbow, they folded the papers carefully, lengthwise, so they didn't interfere with the person standing next to them. Those that didn't have papers craned their necks and read other passengers' papers. The choreography was meticulous and over the months would be repeated daily, coming and going. There was minimal conversation, which made the ride remarkably quiet.

Morton and I walked the rest of the way to Guy's Hospital. The first thing on our agenda when we got to the Medical School was to register at the office with Mr. Griffin and Mr. Cook. They gave us keys to our lockers, which were located in the basement under the Office, timetables for the rest of the term, and told us how to get to the "Spit," the student cafeteria. Obviously this was the hub of the student universe. We were also expected to attend an introductory lecture by the assistant dean, Dr. Houston, at ten-thirty. Our initiation, a hodgepodge of rites, was all a bit confusing, but Mr. Cook reassured us there was always someone in the office to help us out.

While Morton went off in search of his locker, I found mine at the very back of the locker-room, in the darkest corner. I put my raincoat and some books I'd not need that day in the locker and decided to go exploring. I discovered the library directly above the locker rooms. Opposite the library was a large lecture theatre, which could accommodate up to two hundred students at a time. Behind the theatre I found the physics, chemistry, biology and biochemistry laboratories. I avoided rooms on the second floor because the arrow pointing up the stairs said "Anatomy Department" and I was wary of what I might find there.

The School had two other lecture theatres. In the basement were the men's toilets and a long corridor that went out the back of the School to Nuffield House, a private psychiatric ward. The Medical School gym, which had a boxing ring and two squash courts, was at the end of this corridor. A few days later I located a swimming pool in the nurses' home that medical students were allowed to use during restricted hours.

Even with all this exploring, I still had more time to spend before the Assistant Dean's lecture and decided to go in search of the infamous "Spit," which was situated in the basement of the residents' quarters on the other side of the hospital park. As I walked across the park I was struck by its tranquillity in spite of being smack dab in the centre of London. A few nurses and people in white coats with stethoscopes sauntered to various hospital destinations. None showed any sense of urgency, as if they were out for an evening stroll; as if their rushing might disturb a long, hard-won moment of peace.

Nobody noticed me as I entered the "Spit" with some trepidation.

I was the lowest of the low in the university ranks and I was not even sure I should be there. I lined up with a few other people, purchased a cup of tea for tuppence, and took it over to an empty table in a corner of the lower level. Seated, I felt brave, a man about to make his mark on history, while at the same time I was conscious of trying to remain as inconspicuous as possible. A mouse of a man. Looking around I could see that there were two main groups of people, those wearing long white coats and those wearing suits. There were very few women. I later discovered Guy's had only just started to admit female students.

When I'd finished my tea I hastily returned to the Medical School for the lecture. I took a seat about halfway up from the front and sat down next to a tall man about my age who had longish dark hair and deep-set eyes. I wondered if he was as relaxed as he looked. Or as apprehensive as I was.

As the clock over the blackboard approached ten-thirty, the theatre filled. A hush came over the room when a stern-looking man in a dark pinstriped suit entered through the door at the front of the theatre. He looked up at the clock as he walked behind the podium that was next to a plain desk, the only other piece of furniture in front of the large blackboard. At precisely ten-thirty he started.

"Good morning ladies and gentlemen. First, I would like to introduce myself. I am Dr. Houston and I am the Assistant Dean. It is my privilege to give you this introductory lecture but I am never sure how I should set about trying to give you an idea of what you have let yourselves in for. Five and a half years is a long time and that is the minimum that it will take you to qualify in medicine. And that is just the beginning. It is often said that your troubles really start when you get through your finals. There is a lot of truth in this. However, that is not your worry at the moment. About a third of you in this room are going to do dentistry, but most of what I am about to say applies to you as well.

"Your first year will be concerned with Physics, Chemistry and Biology. Although many of you have already done these subjects at school there will be a bias towards the medical sciences and you will find that there is a lot of new material to learn. Some of you will be exempted from taking the first MB exams in some of these subjects, but we expect to see you at the classes."

Dr. Houston's last comment provoked laughter and groans, and he paused and gave us a long hard stare, a look that insisted upon obedience.

He then restated that the course took five and half years—barring any delays, he was quick to point out. After passing the first Bachelor of Medicine exam it would take another eighteen months to cover the material in Anatomy, Physiology and Pharmacology. These courses would be followed by the second MB exams that would cover all that we had been taught during the previous two and a half years. He stressed that these exams would signal the end of the University of London term and the usual long summer holidays. Following the second MB exams we would become clinical students for three years. This was when we would meet real patients, he added. Once we became clinical students we would have only four weeks of holiday per year and these could not be taken consecutively.

The objective of the Guy's Hospital course was to introduce us to the basic sciences needed to understand medicine. This is what we would get in our first two and a half years. The following three years of clinical medicine were designed to teach us how to communicate with patients, examine them, and organize the appropriate investigations. When necessary we would then treat or refer patients. Dr. Houston stressed that being prepared to ask for help was one of the most important aspects of medicine and this should never be forgotten. He gave us a comprehensive review of the courses we were about to take. His lecture was the first detailed explanation I had been given and I found the prospect stimulating, if not daunting.

Dr. Houston then changed to a lighter topic and encouraged us to participate in the non-academic aspects of university life. He stressed that Guy's had a need for good rugby and cricket players—the inter-hospital rivalry was legendary in London. Then he admitted there were plenty of other activities students could participate in—other sports, art and theatre. Although Guy's Hospital was a self-contained unit, it was part of the University of London. We were expected to become involved in the university as a whole. He told us where the University Administrative Centre was on Gower Street and suggested we have a look to see if there was anything else that was of interest to us.

Dr. Houston concluded his lecture.

"This program is a long haul, ladies and gentlemen, and very stressful at times, but worth the effort. If you look at the people sitting to your left and right only one of you will complete the whole course without failing something. Many of you may require repeating a part of the course with a subsequent lengthening of the total time that you spend with us. A few of you will give up for various reasons, but the majority will complete the course and become doctors. I would like to congratulate you all on getting to Guy's and wish you all the best of luck in the future. Remember that the Medical School Office as well as the academic and clinical staff, no matter how senior, is here to help you. Please don't hesitate to ask us for help when you need it. Most of you will need information at some time or other. Now, if there are any specific questions, I will try to answer them."

A hand was raised by a student who asked, "Sir, what percentage of us will not qualify in medicine?"

"It varies a bit from year to year but you are looking at about ten percent that actually give up for various reasons, not all of which are academic. You are allowed to have two tries to pass the first and second MB exams. Although there are some restrictions on how many times you can take finals, the university is quite lenient about enforcing them and the majority of people who get through the second MB exams finally qualify in medicine. That being said, some graduates never practice medicine."

Another hand went up.

"Yes?"

"With reference to attendance at classes. How does the school know who's in class, and do we have to attend all classes?"

Dr. Houston gave an audible sigh, perhaps of impatience, I wasn't sure.

"Remember, you're now at university and not at school where you had to attend all classes. Here we schedule classes to guide you through the course material. The lectures and practical classes will give you the information that's required to pass the MB exams. Your instructors will also advise you where to find additional information that will complement your class work. You don't have to attend all classes but we expect you to attend the majority. There is a sheet at each class or lecture that attendees have to sign. These sheets are collected and the names recorded for future reference. When we see a student is not doing well we check his attendance record before asking him for an interview to discuss his problems.

"There is a specific curriculum for each subject that you take which is available in the office. And the details of the courses are usually explained at the first lecture. We are aware that you all have different learning techniques and that some of you will find formal lectures tiresome or a waste of time. However, the majority of you will find them of some use. The simple answer to your question is that we expect you to attend, but don't insist, providing you can show that you are progressing successfully. Well, I think that's enough for today. Don't forget to get your schedules from the office. I would like to take this opportunity to wish you all the best during your time at Guy's."

Mike, the student sitting beside me, stood up and gathered his things. "What are we going to do for the rest of the morning? There's nothing else scheduled until this afternoon."

"Have you been to the 'Spit'?" I asked.

"No, I've not really looked around much yet. I came straight from home and just got here in time for the lecture. A cup of coffee would hit the spot."

We joined the stream of students moving towards the exit. The majority of the class seemed to have had the same idea and we wandered across the hospital park to the 'Spit' in small groups. As I talked to the others I discovered that most of the students came from outside of London and, like me, didn't know anyone else in the program. The exception was those who had come from the English public school system. This group represented about a quarter of the class and they rapidly renewed old friendships.

There were only seventeen girls in our class and they soon got together. The remaining students came from diverse backgrounds. There were some from overseas, a few who had already done their National Service, and others who had already completed or tried different university programs. On reflection, I felt I belonged. My fears of being a misfit were groundless.

Right from the start of term, the teachers of the practical classes organized us into small working groups of up to ten. This meant that we often went for coffee and meals together and got to know each other better. During that first term there were four students in my group with whom I began to socialize. Together we settled in to university life. I was interested in playing tennis but discovered I couldn't fit it into my budget, unless I was to give up a meal or two.

I expressed my disappointment to Mike Boundy, whose home was in North London, and Mike Wynne Griffith, who came from Wales and was doing dentistry. They told me they had discovered two squash courts in the hospital that were open to medical students at no cost. Both Mikes had played the game and they decided to teach me. I took to the game with great zeal and it wasn't long before I held my own.

Mike Boundy also tried to interest me in rowing, but I didn't appreciate practicing in shorts in the "tub," a circular pond with a rowing seat set in concrete. The object was to learn how to row by moving the water around the pond. You went nowhere. When I was introduced to this masochistic pastime there was ice floating in the water. The ice and cold made it even more torturous and uncomfortable. Needless to say I never did get as far as rowing on the mighty Thames River.

The three of us also tried out the pool in the nurses' residence. In addition to limited access, it was a small pool and had a low ceiling, like the lid on a coffin, which made it claustrophobic. Later we heard that it was popular with some medical students, but not for the swimming—it provided easy access to the nurses' residence. There were many bawdy rumours about the "goings-on" that occurred there.

Paul and Johnny were the other two students I got to know well in my first year. Paul had ash-blond hair and was part Swiss. He was always immaculately dressed with a rose in his lapel. We both liked chess and spent many hours during our first two years engrossed in the game. He was the better player, forcing me to hone my game.

Johnny was Polish. He and his family had escaped to England during the war via Siberia, India and the Americas. He was an excellent athlete and played soccer for Guy's as well as the university. His other passion was cards and he taught me the finer points of bridge and poker at the "Spit" where we often had our meals, tea and coffee breaks. The "Spit" was so-called because it popped up in the middle of the word "ho**spit**al".

It wasn't long before the two Mikes and Johnny introduced me to the local pub, "The Miller," which was just across the road from the Casualty Entrance. Being lunch it was crowded, but it didn't take us long to push our way to the bar. Since this was a new experience for me, I wasn't sure what I was expected to do.

"Bernard," Mike Wynn asked, with a hint of playfulness in his voice, "what would you like to drink?" He glanced furtively at the other two.

"I'm not sure. Could I have a cider?" This was a drink I had tried before and quite liked.

"What!!" they all exclaimed, laughing.

"What else is there?" I asked, a little taken aback.

"There are three different beers you can order. There's a dark one. There's a light one. And there's a bitter one. All on tap. There are others in bottles, but we can only afford the ones on tap. They're better anyway," Johnny informed me.

"I've never tried beer," I admitted, "what's it like?"

"That's a bit difficult to explain. There are lots of types of beer and they're all different, but most of us drink the bitter one," said Mike Boundy.

"In that case, I'll try it."

We ordered four pints of bitter and took them over to a small table that had just been vacated. "Cheers. May you learn how to drink this stuff," said Mike Wynn, taking a gulp from his glass. I sipped mine and wasn't sure I liked the taste at all. My response must have shown on my face because Mike Boundy laughed and said, "Not too sure about it, eh? It gets better as you drink more. It's a bit of an acquired taste. Where have you been this past twenty years?"

"My father is allergic to alcohol and doesn't go into pubs at all. My mother was brought up a Methodist and only drinks sherry and the odd gin and tonic on social occasions. In fact, this is the first pub I've ever been in!"

Drinking my first beer over lunch with Mike Wynn, Mike B. and Johnny was my introduction to one of the favourite pastimes of medical students. Two pubs were handy to the hospital, The Miller and The George. The George, in an old Elizabethan building just behind the medical school, was considered the more sophisticated of the two. Our pub visits were infrequent. We were all living on limited funds. Mike was right, though, I soon acquired a taste for beer.

Guy's Hospital was situated in a section of London known as the Borough, an older area of South East London, located just south of London Bridge. Parts of the London dock system extended into the Borough. Many warehouses perched on the riverbank and a few snaked into the neighbouring streets. Most of the hospital patients worked on the docks and in the warehouses and most had a broad Cockney accent which was distinctive and hard to understand.

The Borough High Street started at London Bridge and continued on to the famous Elephant and Castle road junction. The narrow high street housed many different kinds of shops including a green grocer, fishmonger, butcher, clothing store, bookstore, small café, a Barclays Bank and even a surgical instrument shop. Several pubs catered to the local population. Many of the terraced, red-brick buildings were two to three storeys and had narrow passageways leading to a rear courtyard or garden. They had been built in the Victorian period or earlier. Snuggled between the Victorian houses stood the occasional white and black Tudor building.

The High Street swarmed with cars, small trucks, double-decker buses, trolley buses, and pedestrians. On most days, wheelbarrows were placed strategically on the pavement and filled with various wares for sale. Some students found accommodation in the vicinity but most, like me, travelled in from other parts of London using the trains, tube, buses or bicycles. But no matter where we lodged, we were accepted and respected by the local community.

Settling into academic work at Guy's was much easier than it had been for me at Nottingham High School. The lectures, most of which I had covered at Nottingham, were well run and there was no pressure, except in Biology. There wasn't much to do in my small room at the digs or at Blackheath, which was a large common with some football pitches and other sports facilities that were used by the local schools. As we were expected to attend classes at Guy's I got into the routine of going into the university daily. Often I would catch the train into London with Elaine whose schedule was much the same as mine. Morton preferred to leave Mrs. Perry's a little later and after the first week we rarely travelled in together.

I continued to wander the tease and maze that was London. During the first few months I stumbled on Senate House, a large concrete structure on Gower Street containing the administrative offices for the whole of the University of London. There I found additional student facilities, notably a cafeteria, reading rooms, a bookshop, some badminton courts and two table tennis tables, but squash remained my favourite sport. Besides, Senate House was a long, inconvenient trip into the West End.

Infatuated. Besotted. Smitten.

Increasingly, Elaine and I spent more and more time together. From Cheshire, Elaine had been in London for over a year and had acclimated to the social life of a medical student. She quickly taught me where the best and cheapest places to eat were, how to navigate the parks, how to get around on the transit system, and where to go to see the latest in theatre and artwork in galleries. One of her favourite diversions was "hospital hops," dances put on by the various Student

Unions. She moved with grace and sensuality and wanted me to partner her steps, her laughter, her abandon. How to dance was only one of many social graces of which I had no understanding. I couldn't feel the music. The beat or the story. In spite of my growing desire for Elaine, I was awkwardly shy around girls and my inability to dance embarrassed me.

We joined the rounds of student bottle parties where I soon learned that too much alcohol gave me gastritis and headaches. Consequently I deliberately stayed within my limits and rarely got drunk during those years. Totally by accident, I was spared the indignity of making a spectacle of myself.

We also went to many London shows on complimentary tickets, available through the Medical School Offices. These tickets were for shows that were just starting up or struggling. This arrangement allowed us to enjoy theatre, ballet and orchestral concerts for free or at a cut rate. Usually the tickets were good ones, for seats in the "stalls." While the bulk of the audience would be in formal evening dress, we dressed casually. And because of our age and dress we were recognized as students and often became engaged in long discussions with other members of the audience about what we were doing or studying. We managed to go to several Henry Wood Promenade Concerts, in the "gods" of course, where tickets were just a few shillings. Only years later did I realize how lucky we were to be treated to some of the world's finest artistic performances.

To my delight, Elaine enjoyed sports. At school, she had played tennis, hockey and lacrosse. She played on the lacrosse team at the Royal Free and the University of London. Lacrosse was a game I had never seen before and I was surprised by how aggressive the games were. It was a rugged sport which perhaps explained why it had such a wide appeal to students.

As former hostellers we both loved walking in the countryside. Before coming to London Elaine had trekked in the Lake District, the Pennines, Scotland and Wales, treks that gave us ample opportunity to compare past hikes and plan future ones.

As our relationship became more intimate we spent more time

together in my room at the digs. Mrs. Perry, who feared we might be ignoring our studies, forbid us from visiting in each other's room. Elaine objected to Mrs. Perry's restrictions. She moved out and into a flat in Hampstead, which she shared with a couple of other students from the Royal Free.

Hampstead was closer to her hospital and more convenient. For her it was a blessing. She required less travelling time. However, the cost and travelling time for me to visit her in Hampstead was considerably more. At the time she was getting ready for the Second MB exams, the most important examinations in the medical course. She told me that stability, peace and quiet were what she needed. In spite of this, we continued to see each other on a regular basis.

The inconvenience of travelling all the way back to Westcombe Park late in the evenings got me thinking that a move to North London, specifically Hampstead, would be a good idea. Over the Christmas holidays I decided to make the change, and luckily located affordable digs in Belsize Park, a fifteen-minute walk from Elaine's flat—its main attraction. The major disadvantages, which I was only too happy to overlook, were that it was on the wrong tube line for London Bridge, required a change in central London, was slightly more expensive and didn't include meals at weekends. It was also smaller, and located in the attic of a four-storey Victorian house. The bathroom was on the second storey. On the positive side, the other boarders were mostly non-medical students enrolled in architecture, law, languages, and the arts who went to different colleges. A refreshing change.

There was one medical student, senior to me, who was studying at St. Mary's. He had a beard and smoked a Sherlock Holmes type of pipe. He used to read the *Times* at breakfast and engage people in philosophical debates whenever he could. He said he was planning on becoming a pathologist, because then the patients wouldn't annoy him with their problems. I found his attitude both amusing and disturbing. I wasn't sure I believed him. Perhaps I didn't want to.

Even with a heavier study load, especially with Elaine facing major exams, my visits to her flat became more frequent. We were often on our own. Her two room-mates were either away at weekends or on call at the hospital. With the freedom to see each other more often, our desire to be together grew, and we became lovers.

One Monday morning after a Biology practical class, Mike Boundy, Mike Wynn and I were having coffee in the Spit when Mike B asked, "How are the studies going?"

"OK, I suppose. I haven't done a lot of review of the books recently," I replied, "but I think I have a reasonable handle on the subject. Why do you ask?"

"Well, we only have eight weeks to go before the first MB exam. I certainly haven't been taking the work too seriously but I thought it might be time to think about it. However, it would be a shame to come unstuck just because we're getting too blasé, and it would certainly spoil the summer if we had to take the exams again in the autumn."

"Good point. Perhaps we should get together and do some form of revision," suggested Mike Wynn.

In the end, five of us met once a week to discuss and question each other about the coming exams. We covered the subject matter and also exam techniques, which was something I hadn't considered. When the exams arrived I felt more confident about them because of this preparation. Our group of five all passed this first hurdle and had the satisfaction of knowing that we'd have no more exams for another eighteen months. At the completion of my first year of medical school, I left on my last trip to see my parents in Nigeria.

I spent a lazy, hot, mosquito-filled summer in both Joss and Kaduna with my parents and Marjory; it was the first time the entire family had spent time together for several years. In late August just before I left Nigeria, Father took me aside and warned me that I was about to start the most difficult part of the medical course and that I would have to hit the books. This extra effort, he explained, was needed as the subjects would be new, frustrating and tedious at times. His most important advice was that I should work steadily, revising throughout each term, and not get into the habit of "cramming" for tests. Especially not for the final exam, he said emphatically.

I was happy to see Elaine and return to Guy's and my medical school friends. At this point in my life I considered my small room in London my home.

Our first scheduled lecture was an introduction to the second MB course and was again given by the Assistant Dean. When I arrived at the lecture theatre I quickly picked out the two Mikes, Johnny Jawarski and Jim, but there were several new faces. To my surprise a few old faces were missing. Dr. Houston arrived promptly at ten o'clock. After looking around briefly he started his speech.

"Good morning, ladies and gentlemen. I would like to congratulate those of you who passed the first MB exam and to congratulate those who have joined us this year as second-year students. Some of the things that I have to say today are known to those of you who were here last year but there is a lot of new information as well, so don't go to sleep."

The new information concerned what we would be doing in the next eighteen months. For the second MB exams we would be covering Human Anatomy, Physiology and Pharmacology. Dr. Houston explained that in order to understand human illness a detailed understanding of the structure and function of the healthy human was vital. In Pharmacology we would study the effects drugs had on healthy people, in order to understand how these same drugs could be used to treat disease.

He talked to us about the ethics involved when working with dead bodies in the anatomy laboratory and stressed that we would be dissecting humans who had, for various reasons, donated their bodies to medical science. He warned us that the anatomy department expected us to be respectful. Any inappropriate behaviour would result in disciplinary action.

He also mentioned that from time to time we would be coming into contact and experimenting with dangerous chemical agents. We were to observe all the warnings and details about how to handle these agents in the laboratories. He stressed that there had been serious accidents in the past and that most of them were because of care-lessness.

"The course is presented to you in formal lectures, practical sessions in the laboratories, and small group projects. In Anatomy you will study the structure and function of the human body. This means learning the names of all the bones, muscles and nerves, how they are attached to each other, and what they do. Then there is the brain, gastrointestinal tract, skin and other soft tissue structures to learn about. You will study the normal histology or the microscopic structure of the body. In Physiology you will study how the parts ac-tually work, which requires an understanding of biochemical reac-tions—the physics of light, electricity, gases and sound. You will also be introduced to microbiology."

He paused for a few moments and glanced around the room be-fore continuing.

There was stillness amongst us I hadn't heard before.

"You will gather from my introduction that there is a lot to learn in the next eighteen months. Are there any questions?"

A hand went up. "Sir, are there any examinations to be taken be-fore the second MB in eighteen months?"

"Yes, some voluntary prize competitions which we hope you'll take. They are good practice and have an honorary and monetary value if you win."

"Then how do you or we know how we're progressing?"

"In the dissecting room you will work in small groups of five to seven and deal with one section of the body at a time. This makes it possible for the demonstrators to identify anyone who is having a problem. As well, the groups as a whole have to attain a good know-ledge of the area being covered and if they don't, the whole group may have to repeat a section. Occasionally we run into students who just can't cope with the course and, after discussion, they usually leave voluntarily. In Biochemistry there is a short exam at the end of the course which lets you know how you are doing and if you need to spend more time in the area. In Physiology the demonstrators are likewise responsible for seeing that you are progressing adequately.

We hope that if you have concerns about your own progress you will come and talk to us. It is only in extreme cases that a student who has attended the course will not be allowed to sit the exams.

Before he left his eyes made another sweep of the room. "If there are no more questions, I would like to wish you all the best of luck. And, above all else, enjoy the course."

It turned out that our second MB class was composed of eighty medical students and thirty dental students. The dental students had to do the same Physiology course as the medical students, but in Anatomy they were only responsible for learning the head and neck, although subsequently they had to do a more detailed study of the mouth, teeth, and related structures. The two courses ran together and were the same length. Mike Wynn was the only one of our small group doing dentistry.

The Medical School Office gave us a list of things that we needed to buy for the second MB courses. These included a supply of white lab coats, required textbooks, and a set of dissecting instruments which consisted of two solid scalpels, dissecting scissors, forceps, as well as blunt and sharp probes. The class was split into two for the laboratory sessions.

On the first day, clutching our new instruments in their clean, green canvas rolls, and wearing our new, well-starched white lab coats, we climbed up the well-worn grey, concrete stairs to the Anatomy laboratory. Although I had spotted signage to the Anatomy and Physiology labs on the upper floors the previous year, I had never visited them.

When we got to the second floor of the four-storey building and passed the doors into the Physiology Laboratory, I smelled a pungent, unfamiliar odour. As we continued to climb, the smell got stronger. At the top of the stairs we faced two solid wooden doors, with frosted glass panels in the top half that were labelled "Anatomy Laboratory, Authorized Personnel Only. Keep Closed." A sickening stench wafted into the corridor.

We entered a long, wide room with a high ceiling. Daylight came in through the skylights, which could be opened by a complex system of rods attached to the walls. There were five waist-high dissecting tables and several bar-type metal stools on each side of the room. Each table had a body on it covered by a white sheet, although on a few tables uncovered feet and hands grabbed the air. The entire scene felt surreal.

Suspended from the ceiling, four or five feet above each table, were two bright electric lights. At the far end of the room there were some shelves with large bottles containing preserved body parts. Once captive in the room we huddled near the door wondering what to do next. At the far end of the room, a door opened and a portly man with a good head of grey hair and piercing grey eyes stepped forward to greet us. Even in his wrinkled white lab coat he looked imposing.

"Good morning ladies and gentlemen. I'm Professor Warwick. Welcome to the Anatomy course you will be taking for the next eighteen months. I realize this is the first contact most of you will have had with dead bodies and that some of you will be concerned about the moral and ethical issues raised by this part of the medical course. We take great care of the bodies and ensure that they are treated according to the wishes of the donors. Preparing bodies for burial has been done for eons. The civilization most recognized for embalming their dead were the Egyptians. Today, many people still have their bodies embalmed, particularly in the United States. If any of you have any serious moral concerns about your willingness to dissect cadavers, please come and see me when I've finished explaining what we're going to do today.

"The Anatomy course consists of a series of lectures that cover the general principles of anatomy and some special areas, particularly histology, the brain, and embryology. You will learn most of the anatomy here in the laboratory and from directed reading. You will have to divide yourselves into groups of not more than seven and be allocated a body. More than one group will work on each body. During the next few months, you will work on several corpses. The dissection is done under the supervision of a demonstrator who will guide you in the process. Each demonstrator will be responsible for several groups, so you will often be working on your own. Be warned that there is a time period set for completing each dissection. Your demonstrator will give you an oral test towards the end of this time to make sure that you are ready to move onto the next area of study. We expect you to work as groups helping each other out as much as possible. Are there any questions?"

"How do we learn the differences between the sexes?" someone asked, trying to be funny.

"When you are dissecting the pelvis we make sure that you get the opportunity to see the differences," Professor Warwick replied, reminding me of a gargoyle watching over the entrance to a new world.

"What's the smell, sir?"

"It's a combination of formaldehyde and phenol. They are the chemicals used to preserve the bodies. You will get used to the smell quite quickly and when it gets very strong we open the windows in the ceiling. Make sure you always have your white coats on when you're working here or you will carry the odour with you when you leave the hospital. It's strongly recommended that you wear rubber gloves while you're dissecting. The chemicals will harden your skin and the smell is difficult to get rid of. —If there are no more questions at the moment, let's start by forming the groups. The dental students should be together since they will only be doing the head and neck dissections."

I was surprised how easily and quickly we managed to divide ourselves up, ready for the allocation of bodies. My group consisted of Mike B., Bill, Jim, Paul, Johnny and me. There were four demonstrators with the professor that day. It didn't take them long to direct the groups to tables and dissection areas. Our group was allocated table four and we were to start on the right leg. When we got to our table we stood for a few minutes staring at the covered body. No one knew what to do. I'm not sure what went through the minds of the others but I felt quite apprehensive. What lay under the sheet was like me and yet not so.

"I suppose we're supposed to take the sheet off first," said Mike.

"Does it say anything in the manual about how to start?"

"Not really. But it does say that we have to look and take notes before starting to dissect," Bill said.

"Well, let's uncover the right leg for a start," said Jim.

Paul carefully folded the sheet up and over to the left revealing the lower part of the right leg. Unsure what to do next, we all stared down at the shrunken, rather shiny, brown-stained leg.

"I wonder what sex it is?" asked Johnny.

"We could have a look," I suggested.

"But that's out of our area," said Jim worried about protocol and rules.

"Oh, let's have a look. We can't dissect a body without knowing if it's a man or a woman and we'll have to give it a name," said Paul. He lifted the sheet up, exposing some very shrivelled up male genitalia nestled in spare pubic hair. "Good grief, he's one of us. Let's call him Fred."

This broke the ice. At that moment, the demonstrator arrived. "How are you getting on?" he asked, nudging between us. "Not very far from the look of things."

"The manual says we have to look, observe and feel before cutting anything and that's as far as we've got. We have a male with a very brown, hairless leg that appears shrunken. The toenails are bleached and broken. The foot is arched and twisted out of shape. We haven't touched anything yet," said Bill.

"Good. My name is Mr. Williams. What are yours?"

After introductions Mr. Williams proceeded to instruct us in how to start the dissection of the leg, which turned out to be a lot more complex than any of us had anticipated. He showed us how to make the first incision in the front of the upper leg to expose the fascia sheaths and how to do blunt and sharp dissections to expose the veins, arteries and nerves without damaging them. Using our books and manuals, he then showed us how to identify the structures he had exposed. We quickly discovered that the foot had twenty-six bones, which were held together by numerous muscles and ligaments. Winding their way through these were the veins, arteries, lymphatics and nerves. All the different parts had specific names and we had to learn the relationships of these parts to each other. Added to this, the bones themselves had many protrusions, hollows, grooves, rough areas and holes, all of which had names that had to be remembered. Luckily, Mr. Williams or one of the other demonstrators was always around to assist us when we were having problems finding the structures we were supposed to identify.

I found Anatomy a particularly difficult subject because of the amount of new vocabulary that had to be memorized. We also had to be prepared to answer questions that described what happened when the biceps muscle contracted, or how a pinprick on the finger got registered in the brain. We were expected to learn what the relationships between various organs were and would be asked questions such as, "What are the relations of the spleen?" A complete answer required knowing all the other structures (bones, muscles. nerves, vessels, etc.) that came into contact with the spleen and the layers of others as one moved away from the spleen towards the head and feet, as well as further in, towards the spine or outwards to the skin.

I found it difficult to grasp this material from reading the written descriptions in *Grey's Anatomy*, the student's anatomy bible, in spite of its diagrams. I learned most of my anatomy in the laboratory actually dissecting out the structures and seeing them in three dimensions. My visual memory and logical thought processes saved me.

The second subject, Histology, the study of the types of cells, was easier to understand. I soon realized that the body was like a building, made up of several different building blocks or cells supported by non-cellular elements such as glues, fluids and gels. The next topic, Embryology, or how the body develops into a human being from a single cell, required one to visualize structures growing and folding in upon themselves progressively. As students, we had to be able to describe what structures had developed at each week of gestation and how this complex process had occurred.

Physiology explained how the body works. In this course we worked on live but anaesthetized frogs, rabbits, mice and one cat. By the time our experiments were completed the animals had to be put down, a practice I found disturbing at first, but gradually managed to accept even though it did sadden me.

We also had to do experiments on each other. My group learned how to take and test blood, how to measure our body's response to mild trauma, as well as test our ability to taste, hear, smell and see. One of our demonstrators was doing research on gastric juices and asked for volunteers. He offered to pay half a crown a session. This was a lot of money, so I offered my services. I quickly learned how to swallow a stomach tube and did so twice a week for several weeks, often leaving the lab nauseated.

Once I had learned the basics of digestion, cellular physiology, nerve impulse transmission, hearing and sight, I found Physiology predictable, understandable and, thus easy to remember. Likewise biochemistry and pharmacology. I soon became a master of arcane information.

The lectures were a different story. Some were phenomenally good. For example, Mr. Williams, the anatomy demonstrator, gave a series on embryology. He had an artistic flair and drew superb pictures on the blackboard to illustrate his topic. He would add colour to get us to remember the content. This technique intrigued me because it revealed something about memory retention and the brain.

Another lecturer, Dr. J.N. Hunt, had the difficult task of covering the physiology of the nervous system. This was an extremely complex subject requiring an in-depth knowledge of the anatomy and electrical transmission of nerve impulses in the central nervous system and brain. At his initial lecture, he came into the theatre, paused dramatically, looked around, and said: "Good morning, ladies and gentlemen. I would like you to consider the following. This morning most of you probably came to the hospital on foot, having used some form of London transport. You walked to the right station, put your hand into your pocket where you had several coins of different sizes and denominations. Without looking, you were able to select the correct coins and put them into the vending machine for the correct ticket. Your walking was done completely unconsciously, but you had to think about the coins in your pocket. Have any of you asked yourselves how you managed this very complex series of actions? In the next ten lectures I will try to give you some idea how you accomplished these feats. But I warn you now, the subject is very complicated."

Unfortunately, other lectures were very poor and boring. Students often slept through them or would skip class and get their friends to sign them in. The Medical School office was most likely aware of this practice, but as long as they were progressing, students were not disciplined.

During the first term back my group spent a lot of time at the books because of the volume of new material to learn. Consequently our social life suffered. At the Royal Free, Elaine was approaching a critical stage of her course work and would soon be writing her second MB exams. Inevitably we saw less of each other.

To balance the intense studying routine of medical school I decided to become more involved in the Guy's squash scene. One of my friends suggested I try out for the hospital team. I went to the trials without a serious expectation of success. I soon found that there was a big difference in the standard of players and that I ranked in the middle. The three top players at Guy's competed at the international level. Two played for India and one for Wales. I enjoyed the trials and felt I could improve.

A couple of days after the trials the captain came up to me in the "Spit" and told me that I had been selected to play on the Guy's second-tier team. He also mentioned that there was a squash professional who came twice a month on Thursday afternoons who would, if I were interested, give lessons for half a crown a session. Although it was a lot of money, I went for several lessons over the next year. Practice paid off. Eventually I was selected to play on the first team.

Selection to the first team meant that I got to play in interclub tournaments four or five times a month for the next five years. It was an excellent way to get a lot of exercise in a short space of time. At Guy's it provided me with the opportunity to meet students in other years, medical schools and many other London clubs.

During those five years I played at Hampstead, Wimbledon, Wanstead, the Jesters, and the Old Merchant Taylor's, as well as at Oxford, Cambridge and Birmingham Universities. During these events I played, watched, or refereed many of the top squash players of the time, amongst them M. Hawkey, R. Wilson, S. Lam, J. Lyon, M. Lyon, M. Oddy, and former world champion, Hashim Kahn.

At different times I was the secretary, vice-captain and captain of the Guy's squash club, positions which came with a few advantages and many frustrations. Ultimately, though, they were jobs I enjoyed doing. My interest in the game continued throughout my life although I had to give up playing competitively in my sixties.

In the latter part of 1954 Elaine was forced to move out of her flat in Hampstead. Her roommates had qualified and were leaving London. She hoped to find new roommates but was unsuccessful. She ended up taking a one-room flat up the hill in Gayton Road. A five minute walk away. Naturally I wanted to be closer to her. Knowing that her old flat was coming available I discussed the opportunity with Mike Wynn who thought we could afford to rent the place if we had another person. Mike found Mick, another dental student, to share the flat and we all moved in as Elaine moved out. The house, a red brick Victorian structure at 7 Willow Road, was built on a hillside and looked out over Hampstead Heath. We entered the basement flat by going down two steps into a closet-sized kitchen. The lounge had a single divan couch, a round table with four chairs, a side board, two easy chairs, and a bay window which looked out at ground level on an unkempt front garden. At night, this space became my room.

The radiators in the flat rarely worked and the gas fire had a voracious appetite for pennies or shillings. We also had the decorative luxury of a few pipes running down from the top floors along our ceiling. The concrete floor was covered with tatty reddish brown carpets. Down the corridor was the bathroom and a separate toilet. Another penny-consuming, gas-operated water heater serviced the tub. We shared these facilities with another flat in the house whose occupant was responsible for keeping the furnace going in order to supply hot water and heating to the whole house. Immediately above us was an "artist's studio." The rest of the three-storey house was divided into small flats, two or three on each floor with shared bathrooms.

Batching was new to all of us. Suddenly we found ourselves cooking, washing dishes, cleaning, doing laundry, dusting, changing beds—doing all the household chores our mothers or landladies had previously done for us. More importantly, we had to learn to live with each other, civilly, in a fairly confined space. Fortunately the three of us soon learned to tolerate each other's idiosyncrasies.

None of us were well off but Elaine's financial circumstances were dire. Her monthly allowance often failed to arrive on time. When she saw us struggling with meals she offered to cook for us, if we provided the food. Without causing any of us embarrassment this arrangement helped ease her financial quandary and we got to eat well. Her presence also benefited us in another way. By this time Elaine had successfully completed her Second MB exams and was an esteemed clinical student who didn't have to worry about exams for a year or so. It meant that she was in the flat most evenings—which pleased me—and started to help us prepare for the serious Second MB exams, which were approaching alarmingly fast.

With the Heath just across the road, Elaine and I often went for walks on the wide-open parkland. It was a splendid place to relax, chat and plan. On a fine day the view of London was magnificent. We could spot St. Paul's Cathedral, Tower Bridge, the Houses of Parliament and even the Monument from the top of the hill. In the opposite direction, Hampstead Village was just a few hundred yards down the road which was where we did most of our shopping at the weekends. Once a month there was an open market packed with fresh goods at bargain prices. Hampstead was a great place to "people watch."

On the next street down the hill was Keats's old house.

One evening, when there was more noise than usual coming from upstairs, there was a knock on our door. At the door stood a solidly built man with thick, curly hair and a roundish, lined face. He wore a greenish brown jacket with a dark velvet collar over an open-necked shirt and multicoloured cravat. Most striking were his thick, horn-rimmed glasses. "Hello, I'm Donald," he said jabbing his finger into the air. "From upstairs. We were wondering if you'd like to join us. We're planning to have a rather noisy party right over you. We don't imagine the floor is sound-proof," he added.

Donald and Lillian's studio was a single room the size of our whole flat. It had windows on both sides which flooded the room with natural light. One corner had been curtained off as a bedroom and there was a stove and sink on the right as one entered the room. The furniture was minimal, consisting of a few battered easy chairs and one settee with colourful throws covering it. Pushed to the side I saw two easels with paintings in progress on them. The walls were covered by oil paintings of different subjects and sizes. The floors were bare wood.

Lillian was short and plump. Long, black hair with a fashionable fringe fell around her oval face. Her dark brown eyes twinkled with an uncompromising surety. She spoke with a French accent, but had been born of Russian parents who had had to leave Russia just before the revolution. Donald had met Lillian when she was in London working as an artist's model. He told us, "Don't mess around with Lillian. She carries a vicious knife in her purse," he said solemnly, followed by a sheepish smile.

The fifty to sixty guests consisted of a few students from the arts, music and language faculties, but most of the people were working, either in the arts field or for the City of London. Their attire was noticeably bohemian. Lillian had invited several friends from Paris, along with her Uncle Boris, who worked as a reporter and chess correspondent for *La Figaro*.

Following the party we got to know Donald and Lillian well. Two or three times a month, a group of us would get together at their place to play chess and other board games. These evenings often ended in lively philosophical discussions on topics from religion to politics and were rarely about medicine and what we were doing at school.

Life in Hampstead was comfortable. The independence Elaine and I had and the time we were able to spend together became increasingly a feast of pleasures and happiness. However, this idyll did not last long. The second MB exams were creeping up on the occupants of 7 Willow Road. After my experience with the G.C.E. and the first MB exams, I thought I would breeze through the second MB. Three months before the exams were to start, their complexity was brought home to each of us during the revision classes we had been advised to attend. I needed to do a lot of serious bookwork. Fortunately I had Elaine and my two flat mates to help. Anatomy worried me the most. I had little trouble visualizing the organs and their relations, but I had a lot of difficulty expressing this knowledge on paper. We had access to old exam questions and I soon realized I had a big problem when I compared my answers to the ones expected. My handwriting was still a problem. For me handwriting was arduous and I actually spent hours practicing this skill. All of us became recluses and did little but revise what we had been taught over the past fifteen months.

Inevitably the exams arrived. The content was divided into three major sections: Anatomy, Physiology and Pharmacology. To become a clinical student we had to pass both the Anatomy and Physiology exams. The Pharmacology was not a requirement but the subject would have to be taken again as a clinical student if you did not pass it the first time. Each subject had two three-hour papers, as well as a practical of three hours. Added to this there was a paper in Biochemistry and a Histology exam where we were presented with slides we had to identify. There were two *viva voce* (oral explanations of a question) to be taken, one in Physiology and one in Anatomy. The papers were taken in the first two weeks of the exam schedule and the rest in the second two weeks. We were all aware that we had to pass the papers. They represented sixty percent of our marks.

On the second Anatomy paper I came to grief. I did not allocate the appropriate time for each question. I remember one of the questions well because I spent over an hour trying to describe the relations of the stomach when it was full and empty, and I couldn't finish the remaining questions. When I walked out I knew for certain I had failed this paper. There was no chance I could make up the loss in the other Anatomy paper.

This predicament made the next week rather depressing and when it came to the final Anatomy *viva* I was not a very happy student. Each *viva* was scheduled for ten minutes and gave the examiners the opportunity to meet the candidates individually. I was the first student in after the luncheon break. A table had been set up in the anatomy lab with three chairs, two for the examiners and one for the candidate. On the table over which a white cloth had been spread lay several anatomical specimens, including bones, some x-rays and jars of dissected body parts. When I went in, Professor Warwick and another examiner, who I did not recognize, were sitting there.

"Sit down, please. Don't be nervous. You are candidate 178?" asked Professor Warwick.

"Yes sir," I replied.

"Well let's see now. Ah, here is something you should recognize," he said as he handed me a skull that had had the vault removed. "Can you tell if it's a male or female skull?' he asked.

"Not for certain, but the general size and the markings where the muscles were attached, which are quite prominent, would suggest a male to me, sir," I replied.

"Hmm, good. Tell me, what goes through this hole?" He pointed to a hole.

"The vagus nerve," I replied.

"What is the vagus nerve?"

"It's one of the twelve cranial nerves and it goes to the stomach carrying both sympathetic and para-sympathetic fibres."

Professor Warwick then proceeded to ask me what went through several other holes in the skull and about the ridges where muscles were attached.

"Very good," said the other examiner. "Come over here a moment." They both got up and took me over to one of the dissected bodies.

"Now, can you show me the recurrent laryngeal nerve?" he asked and handed me a pair of long-handled dissecting forceps.

Fortunately I knew where to find this famous nerve. He then proceeded to quiz me on the rest of the main structures in the neck. This question and answer session continued down the body including the contents of the thorax, abdomen and pelvis. Most of the structures that I was asked to identify I knew. The final batch of questions on the body focussed on the leg and foot.

"Let's go back to the samples," said Professor Warwick. As we walked back to the table I glanced at my watch and was surprised to see that I had been there for over fifteen minutes. The *viva* was only supposed to last ten minutes.

When we got to the table he picked up an X-ray and handed it to me. "Do you know what that is?"

"It's an X-ray of the chest I think." I held it up to the light so that I could see through it. It was obviously unusual because there were some opaque areas in one of the lungs.

"Yes. Let's have a proper look at it," Professor Warwick said as he took it back and put it into a viewing machine standing on the desk. When he turned the light on I was presented with something I had never seen before. It was an X-ray of the chest, but it had some opaque white areas in the right lung, which looked very artificial.

"Well, what do you think this is?" he asked.

"To be quite honest I have never seen an X-ray of the chest like this before. In fact, I have only ever seen a couple of chest X-rays and they didn't have those sorts of white areas on them."

"Any ideas?" asked the other examiner.

"Could the patient have inhaled some radio-opaque material by accident?" I asked.

"Very good. Actually the material was injected to show up the lung structure. This X-ray is called a bronchogram."

They paused and glanced at each other.

"Well, I think that's enough," said Professor Warwick. "You may go now. We seem to have gone a bit over the allotted time. Good luck with the rest of the examinations."

I got up and left the room. When I got out I realized I had been in there for a good twenty minutes. The next two students were sitting on chairs just outside the door and one of them asked, "What the hell were they doing to you in there?

"I'm not sure. They asked me about everything, starting with a skull. Then I was asked to identify all manner of structures in the neck, thorax, abdomen, and limbs. The last question was about an X-ray of the chest called a bronchogram," I replied.

"That's a bit unfair showing you something that we haven't seen before."

"That's what I thought. I suspect I may have failed the papers anyway," I said.

Just then the door opened and one of the demonstrators said, "Next."

So I left wondering how I had done and if there were any chance that I might have recovered enough ground to pass the course. During the next week I had a Physiology *viva* and a Pharmacology practical, both of which went reasonably well. I was still very depressed and worried about the first Anatomy paper. The thought of telling my parents that I had failed and that I would have to wait until September to take the exams again was frustrating and dispiriting.

Results were posted at the entrance to the Senate on Gower Street at noon on the Friday, ten days after the last exam. I went to the Senate building at midday and joined the hundred or so students waiting for the secretary to arrive. Many were obviously quite relaxed and others, like me, were nervous Nellies. Few talked and none of my friends were there so I paced around the periphery of the crowd. No matter how much anatomy I now understood I couldn't stop my knees from shaking and my stomach from feeling it might heave.

Promptly at noon a short man appeared carrying a handful of sheets and a box of drawing pins. "Yes," he shouted to the crowd, "I have the results, but you will have to let me through to the posting boxes if you want to see them." Everyone quickly parted to let him through. He opened the display boxes with a key and started to pin the lists to the cork board. They contained the results for all the medical schools attached to London University, which meant several hundred students' results were listed.

When I eventually made my way to the front I found that our names were listed alphabetically and only showed those students who had passed. The first list was of those who had passed the whole second MB exam. I couldn't find my name on this list. This discovery was a blow but not a surprise. The next box contained Pharmacology results and I couldn't find my name. This was a shock. I thought I had done reasonably well in this subject. The next box contained the Physiology results and to my great relief I was on the list. Finally I pushed on to the Anatomy results, where, to my surprise, I discovered my name—I'd passed!

Sitting in the tube on the way back to Hampstead I had time to think about the implications of these results. The first was that I would be starting on the wards, as a clinical student, in four weeks, and that would be the end of any long holidays for the next three years. It meant that I would be seeing patients, a prospect I embraced—after all, this was what doctors did and what all the hard work had been about. Secondly, I still had to tell my parents about my results. Lastly I would have to repeat the pharmacology exam in October, when I would be on my first firm (ward) as a clinical student. While challenging, this was not the first time I had been faced with retaking an exam. Apart from pharmacology, I would have no more exams to sit for the next two and a half years.

I was at the midway point of my medical schooling. My first two and a half years had been hard work academically and I was glad that I was going to be able to continue the program as planned. I was now twenty-two years old and had been living on my own for two years. I had made some lifelong friends and fallen in love. I had passed two of the major academic hurdles in Medical School and clinical practice was next.

It was not until some years later that I realized how lucky I was to be examined by Professor Warwick, who had taken it upon himself to really try to find out what I did know about Anatomy during my *viva* and used my answers to redress the omissions I had made in the written exam. When later I became a teacher I understood this generous gift he had given me of time, trust and promise, all virtues so much a part of the oath to which I, as a physician and educator, would eventually swear.

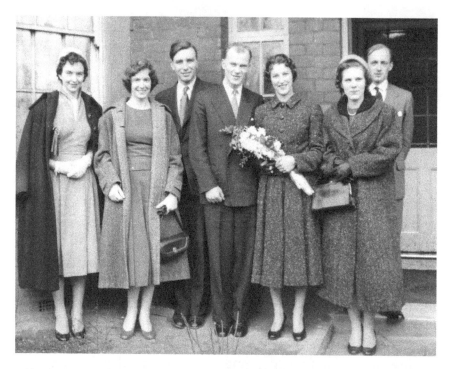

Above: Bernard and Elaine's wedding. Below: Bernard and Elaine, 2018.

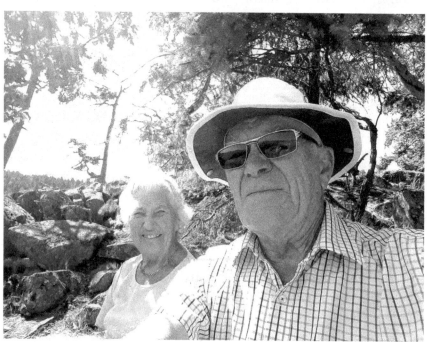

Chapter 7
First Patients: Learning to be a Doctor

After spending the summer holidays in Worksop, I returned to London. I needed to purchase supplies for my clinical courses—a stethoscope, a patella hammer, and two large books: *Hamilton Bailey's Demonstration of Physical Signs in Clinical Surgery* and *Clinical Medicine* by W. Mann. My classes started with a three-month pre-clinical course. The classroom was on the top floor of Hunt's House, which was the medical block at Guy's Hospital. The dental students, including Mike Wynn, had moved to clinical dentistry in the Dental School. There were several new faces in our class of approximately sixty students.

The new faces in our group were students who had completed pre-clinical content as part of a three-year bachelor degree program offered by Oxford or Cambridge. In 1955 Cambridge did not have a teaching hospital to provide clinical teaching experience and the school in Oxford was in its infancy and not large enough to cope with the number of students enrolled in their program.

Our classroom had a desk and blackboard at one end with fifty chairs and fifteen examining couches scattered about. Some small tables had been shoved against one wall and on the other side of the room were several folding, curtained screens on wheels, soon to become familiar pieces of hospital equipment. Our pre-class babble about who had not made it and what we had been doing for the past three weeks was interrupted by the opening of a door at the other end of the room. An athletic-looking, dark-haired man entered the room. An immediate hush followed.

"Good morning, ladies and gentlemen, I'm Dr. Finnegan. Please find somewhere to sit. I will be introducing you to the clinical skills that you'll need when you start your first clerkships in three months' time. First, congratulations on passing the second MB. I hope you'll enjoy the rest of the course. Perhaps the biggest blessing is that you will not have to worry about any major exams for a while. You are now embarking on an intensive course on how to talk to, examine, and assess *people*. You are, of course, excited about seeing your first patients, but you may also be apprehensive about how you are going to approach them. During the next few weeks my two assistants and I will show you how to do this.

"Clinical medicine is a combination of art, science and deduction. Patients are human beings who come to you with a health problem. It is your responsibility to collect their information, interpret it and take the appropriate action. Sometimes this is simple. Responding to a cut finger, for example. Other situations can be extremely difficult, such as when someone presents with hallucinations. To be an efficient clinician you have to have a plan to collect all the necessary information in order to make a diagnosis. Learning how to do this and take action on the information that you collect is what this course is all about. Please organize yourselves into pairs; you will be practicing on each other. I would suggest that the ladies stay together. You will all be doing physical examinations on each other. The class list shows an even number of you, so this should not be a problem."

Since Jim Secubunga and I were standing side by side and had worked together successfully in Organic Chemistry and Physiology, it made sense for us to team up again. Once we had chosen our partners Dr. Finnegan continued: "The outline for the next few weeks is as follows. The first thing we will learn is how to take a clinical history. Once you are comfortable doing this we will show you how to do a detailed physical examination. Once we feel confident that you can do clinical histories and physical examinations safely, and before we go to the wards, we will bring in some volunteer patients on whom you can practice these skills.

"You will also learn how to write down your findings in an organized way on a medical chart. The method of recording information is important because when you arrive on the wards you will be presenting your findings to the firms [as clinical groups were called] and consultants. Don't worry. We'll give you some ideas on how to remember details and present things in a concise, logical manner. Relaying information may seem simple to you now, but under the stress of presenting a patient's history to a group of senior clerks, housemen, registrars and consultants, most of you will feel intimidated. Your seniors will not be trying to trip you up, ridicule or embarrass you, even if you feel this is the case. Their major concern is to clarify what you are presenting so that logical conclusions can be arrived at and further decisions made on the management of the various patients. Your notes in the charts become part of the permanent hospital records and will be there for a very long time, so you want them to be accurate. You will find history records going back twenty to thirty years. Some are extremely interesting since they were written by our senior consultants.

"Here are a few salient points on the taking and documenting of histories. As I've said, you have to be organized in the way you take the history and in what you put to paper. You'll all develop your own way of doing this, which is permissible, providing the end result is complete and clear. Handwriting is important. Please remember, a history which can only be read by the author is useless to other caregivers; others will be looking at your notes years from now.

"The rest of this week will be spent with history taking. Then we'll move on to the physical examination, how to do some basic tests on blood, urine, faeces and how to prepare basic bacteriological cultures. Then we will bring in the volunteer patients to help you hone your skills. Are there any questions?"

A hand went up.

"Yes?"

"Why do we have to learn how to test blood, urine and faeces, particularly the latter? I would have thought the laboratories were responsible for these."

"Collecting specimens is part of your general training. Labs are not always open twenty-four hours a day. Housemen and students are responsible for simpler tests in the case of an emergency or out-of-hours' admissions. If necessary, laboratory staff can be called in to the hospital for more complex testing, but the basics are your responsibility. One reason why this is expected of you is that in the future you may find yourselves working in environments where access to rapid laboratory testing is not available. Being confident and able to do simple tests will be a great help to you and your patients. During the next three years, there are other aspects of laboratory and pathological medicine which you will learn about. This is just a start.

"That's enough talking on my part. Now I would like one in each pair to pretend to be the patient who thinks he is coming down with the flu, and the other to take his history. You have fifteen minutes to do this. Then we will look at some of your efforts."

"Who's going to be the patient, you or me?" I asked Jim.

"Let's toss for it," replied Jim, pulling a coin from his pocket. The toss was 'tails' which meant I became the patient.

"Hmmm, what do I do now? Where do I start?" asked Jim.

"I'm not sure," I said cheerfully. "I'm the patient, remember."

"What's brought you in to see me today?" Jim began, which seemed a reasonable starting place to me.

"I think I might be getting the flu," I replied.

"Oh, and why is that?"

"I was feeling a bit off colour yesterday, played very bad squash, and woke up this morning with a splitting headache."

"Have you noticed anything else, such as a fever or sweating?"

"Not really," I answered, playing the role of a completely uncooperative patient.

"I've written that down," Jim said, a bit flustered. "Now where do we go?"

"I'm not sure, but I think you should ask me about my age and background. I've not been to see you before."

"Good thought," Jim said, and he rattled off a series of questions more like a tax man than a personal physician. "Who are you, how old are you, where were you born and where are you living?"

We continued in this vein for a few more minutes until Dr. Finnegan called us to attention and said, "You've had fifteen minutes, let's see how you got on."

He asked several pairs to read out what they had put on paper. Some had got the patient's details down and a brief account of their complaint. Others had not gathered anything about who the 'patient' was but had details of their previous illnesses and what was bothering them. Some had even suggested taking some aspirin and getting some rest. We soon realized that most of us were at a total loss on how to start taking a proper chronological history.

"I think that's enough for this morning. We're not expecting you this afternoon. Tomorrow we'll get down to some details. Here are some questions for you to think about." Then Dr. Finnegan wrote the following on the board:

1. What is a patient?
2. Why is he or she here?
3. How can I find out what is wrong?
4. After taking a history and doing a physical what should I do next?

"We hope to answer these questions in the next few weeks. See you all tomorrow."

When we arrived the next day we found the following scheme written on the blackboard:

Patient Information (P.I.)
- Name, address, age, phone number, significant numbers, other useful information

Complaint (C.O.)
- The reason why the patient is visiting you
- Should be documented in his/her words

Previous Illnesses (P.I.)
- Details of all his/her previous illnesses including all hospitalizations put down chronologically
- Any medications that he/she is on or has taken recently
- History of allergies

Family History (F.H.)

- Details of his/her marital status, family illnesses (parents, uncles, aunts, siblings, children). Are his/her parents and siblings alive. If not what did they die from

Personal History (P.H.)

- Details of his/her occupation(s), marital status, family, education, drinking habits, drugs, smoking, travel (particularly to the tropics)

History of Present Complaint (H.P.C.)

- Details of what his/her present problem is. How it started, when, how it affects him/her

Social History (S.H.)

- Details of his/her recent social activities
- Specific areas that have to be asked about depending on the type of complaint, e.g. sexual history, obstetric history, psychiatric history

On examination (O.E.)

- General appearance: e.g. nervous, haggard, in pain, shy, old, young, male, female, etc.
- Measurements of vital signs and observations of:
- Cardiovascular System (CVS)
- Respiratory System (R.S.)
- Alimentary System (Al.S.)
- Nervous System (NS)
- Genito-urinary system (G.U.)

Diagnosis and Recommendations

What is your diagnosis based on the above and what do you order for further investigation and/or treatment?

Many classmates started to scribble down the scheme before Dr. Finnegan arrived; others just read it and discussed it with their partners.

"It looks as though there is more to this taking a history than I first thought," Jim said, stroking his chin between his thumb and two fingers.

"I was just thinking that to put all my details down on a sheet of paper would take quite a long time and would cover two to three sheets," I said. "If we have to do it on all the patients we see we'll be spending a lot of time writing."

"I wonder when we'll have time to write all that information down, and where does one do it?"

"I think we'll be doing it on the wards as we take the histories from the patients."

Dr. Finnegan arrived. "Good morning. I see you've seen the scheme on the board. It's just an outline of what we expect you to gather from patients when you first meet them. As you have probably noted, it's fairly comprehensive. We expect all of you to think through these questions when you see a patient for the first time. It will seem tedious and at times irrelevant, but you'll be surprised by how important attention to details can be. Sometimes they might be life-saving. That's why we allow three months to teach you how to take histories and do physical examinations properly."

I think most of us thought three months were a long time to spend learning how to do this seemingly simple task, but the time went by fast and there was a lot to know. We spent the first two weeks learning about and examining each other, which in itself was quite illuminating. Next we learned how to take down the details of what patients could present with and how to use this information as a guide to what might be wrong with them. The significance of the initial information presented to us became apparent and certainly remained engraved on my brain throughout my medical career. Dr. Finnegan stressed that the format could be altered to suit an individual physician's requirements depending on the speciality they chose to follow or the patient they were examining. The taking of surgical histories might appear to be different from medical histories but the fact remained that a good physician always thought about the whole patient. Each individual point in the history needed to be considered and noted. For example, if a patient with a broken leg also had a heart condition such detailed information could be vital. If a general anaesthetic were given to such a patient the outcome could be fatal.

As a class we started to learn how to observe people by looking at our partner's posture, general looks, build, deformities and mental attitudes. We examined each other starting at the head and ending with the feet. We opened our mouths and looked at each other's tongues, teeth, and tonsils. We listened to our lungs and hearts, and palpated our abdomens. Using our new equipment and knowledge we tested our nerve reflexes. Jim and I watched our eyes move and assessed how well we heard sounds. After using a test for colour blindness, we decided that we were both normal, which was a bit of a relief. Interestingly, we recorded the general health of hands, fingers and nails. Hands can be pleasantly cool, hot and sticky, or freezing. Each state could indicate an underlying illness or condition.

The basic medical tests we learned and practiced on each other ranged from how to take blood pressure without hurting your partner's arm to finding pulses in various parts of the body. Once we found these pulses we had to learn how to count and record them. We used an otoscope to look into our ears and discovered that looking into eyes with an ophthalmoscope was not easy. Lastly, we had to learn how to take blood from each other. This was a daunting task for many of my classmates. It's hard to find a vein when your hands are shaking, let alone puncture the vein and withdraw enough blood for a complete blood count.

Attached to the classroom was a small laboratory with four workbenches, sinks and microscopes. When we were all present, the space was a bit crowded. It had the characteristic smell of a medical laboratory—the odour of chemicals mixed with boiled urine and faeces. Once we had mastered venipuncture we took the samples of our blood and learned how to prepare slides using different stains in order to see different things. We centrifuged the blood to separate the layers of red blood cells and plasma. We looked for normal and abnormal white cells in the plasma and learned how to do red and white cell counts. We tested our urine for proteins by heating it to its boiling point and adding Biuret reagent. We added Benedict's solution to test for the presence of sugar and mixed a sample with a strong acid to test for the presence of ketones. We plated out microbiological specimens and studied them under the microscope. The most offensive task was looking for ova and parasites in samples of fresh faeces. Few of us had ever been faced with these embarrassing or unpleasant tasks. We had many laughs and the occasional scare, especially when one of us splashed concentrated acid about. The instructors were very conscious of the risks we took with toxic materials used near our eyes; they repeatedly stressed the safety rules.

Two little books reviewing how to take a history were given to us by our instructors midway through this initial phase. The red book was for surgical cases and the black one for medical patients. They were small enough to fit into a lab coat pocket easily. Many of us found them invaluable during our first few months on the wards.

The first volunteer patients arrived when our instructors thought we were proficient enough not to harm them. The volunteers were people who had been seen in the hospital for some medical or surgical condition and who had clinical signs and symptoms. They had been asked by representatives of the Medical School if they would be willing to come to our classes to have their histories taken and to be examined. Most of the volunteers were locals who had a variety of chronic illnesses. Many were loyal supporters of the hospital who wanted to do something to help educate young doctors. Some had been coming for years and enjoyed their visits, while others were new with acute conditions that would soon be treated. Some were inpatients who had been brought over in order for us to see a specific symptom. An example of this was a patient with petechia, which looked like a rash but was the result of small blood vessels bleeding under the skin.

The volunteers were prepared for our questions and examinations. We were broken up into groups of two or four depending on how many patients were available and the patients' conditions. We were suervised very closely and occasionally warned not to ask certain questions or do certain tasks. The volunteers received little remuneration for their time and it was only years later, when I became involved in medical education, that I fully appreciated the immeasurable value that these patients had contributed to my education.

During the last few weeks, before we were divided into our various firms (clinical groups), we saw patients with abnormal blood pressures, irregular heart rates, abnormal heart sounds, strokes, amputations, enlarged livers, enlarged spleens, glass eyes, deafness, partial blindness, respiratory failure, and jaundice, to mention a few. The experience was invaluable and allowed us to become comfortable talking to and examining strangers suffering from extreme medical problems.

Throughout our pre-clinical time we learned how to look up medical problems in the library and in the textbooks we had purchased. These tomes were detailed and covered large sections of medicine and surgery. However, finding details of specific illnesses required a bit more direction. In certain cases we were sent to the library to find up-to-date information in the many different medical journals. The danger here was that while flipping through pages in these publications it was easy to become distracted by more interesting topics.

We were strongly advised to visit the Gordon Museum, which had opened in 1905. This macabre museum of some 5,000 preserved medical specimens, stored in glass jars with brief details of patients' histories and a description of their pathologies, was situated in the Medical School. Architecturally the museum was Victorian. It had four floors in four sections. On the ground floor there were displays of wax models showing various anatomical dissections in lurid detail and colours, all illustrating different regions of the body. These superb models were similar to the wax models on display at Madame Tussaud's. On the walls of these rooms, paintings of famous Guy's surgeons and physicians hung beside pictures of some very bizarre medical and surgical conditions. One room was set aside for research and another for special exhibitions.

On the second, third and fourth floors, accessible by a central spiral staircase, there were four galleries constructed from wrought iron and glass. Each gallery was lined with shelves which housed labelled medical specimens in jars of preservatives. In front of each group of specimens there was a box attached to the wrought iron railings. This contained a loose-leaf folder with details on each specimen.

The galleries were just wide enough for two people to pass each other.

The specimens were grouped into different categories to illustrate regional diseases or conditions. The popular medico-legal section, which was on the top floor, had some very graphic specimens of murders, gunshot wounds, burns, rapes and assaults. I found I could learn and assimilate information from these specimens easily and I spent quite a lot of time in the Gordon Museum over the next three years.

During the last week of our pre-clinical class we were assigned a ward and given instructions. We were all very nervous but excited to start this new phase of our training. I was assigned to the Sam ward, which was a surgical floor where I was told to report to the Sister in charge on the first day. When I got to her office the door was open. I could see a fairly tall, middle-aged lady in a dark blue uniform standing behind a desk looking at a patient's chart. I knocked timidly on the door and she looked up at me over the top of her reading glasses.

"You must be one of the new students. I'm a bit busy at the moment, but Staff Nurse Brooks will explain what you have to do and which patients you have been allocated. You'll find her down the male ward on your right. She's the nurse with the pale blue uniform and the dark belt. Don't be nervous; we'll help you as much as we can."

The ward was long and open with sixteen metal-framed black beds on wheels down each wall. The floor was a grey mottled stone and highly polished. Several large windows lined either side of the ward and its end. Each bed had a high curtain rail around it so that the patients could be screened off when necessary. There was plenty of room down the centre to move beds when necessary. Most of the beds were occupied and several had their curtain screens drawn.

I was pleased to see that most of the patients looked reasonably cheerful. A few were asleep and others were reading. Next to each bed there was a fairly comfortable looking chair and a small bedside table. At the end of the beds there were tables on wheels for eating meals and storing personal items. Over the head of each bed was a light attached to the wall and some of the beds had hand grips suspended on a light chain which patients could use to help pull themselves up. Hanging on the end of each bed was a clipboard with a record of the patient's temperature, blood pressure and pulse. Glancing at the clipboard gave one a quick assessment of how the patient was doing before speaking to them. The nursing sisters, nurses, physicians and consultants would keep an eye on these charts as they walked down the wards. The clipboards were kept up to date by the nurses.

I spotted a nurse at the end of the ward and walked toward her, feeling self-conscious, as if I were an imposter. On the way I recognized several different smells—the disinfectant Dettoll, which gave off a powerful whiff as I passed one of the curtained-off beds, and the smell of sepsis, an infection, which I had first smelled during my time on the wards in Nigeria. "Staff Nurse Brooks?" I asked.

"Yes, can I help you?"

"Sister sent me to find you. I gather you have a list of the patients for the new students."

"Yes, I have the list here," she said, consulting her clipboard. "What's your name?"

"Binns."

"Let me see, Mr. Binns. You have been allocated Mr. Cochran, in bed 30, and Mr. Welsh, in bed 17. They are both post-ops so you won't have much to do today. You should go and see Mr. Bright in bed 6. He needs some blood collected for the lab. I'll show you where to find everything if you come along with me." She started off down the ward towards the exit with me tagging along behind.

Just outside the ward she entered a small room on her right, containing many shelves and a small table. Some of the shelves were filled with items of linen. I quickly located the shelf that held rows of sterile specimen bottles and jars designed specifically for collecting urine, sputum and faeces. On the next shelf up, there were syringes of different sizes, a few rubber tourniquets, bottles of alcohol, and cotton wool swabs.

"You'll need two of the test tubes from over there, one with a red and the other with a blue top, some alcohol, swabs, and a tourniquet. The sterile kidney dishes with Wasserman needles are over here. They are wrapped in a clean cloth. We would appreciate it if you could keep blood off the cloth. We have to clean it after you finish. Is this the first time you've taken blood on the wards?" she asked.

"Yes."

"Then I'll come along with you. Mr. Bright is a nice older man of seventy who is here for some investigations for the stomach pain he has been suffering for the past few months. The doctors are not sure if he has an ulcer or cancer and they have requested several blood tests to monitor his haemoglobin. Mr. Bright is almost totally blind so you'll have to tell him exactly what you are going to do and how he can help you. The houseman has filled out the forms for you. You'll be pleased to know that Mr. Bright has good veins," Nurse Brooks said, her voice soft and reassuring.

We arrived at Bed 6.

"Good morning, Mr. Bright. I've brought Mr. Binns along to take some blood from you. He's the student who will be looking after you while you are on the ward."

"Nice to meet you, Binns. I hope you know what you're doing," he said looking vacantly between us. "You know I can't see, don't you?"

"Yes, Nurse Brooks told me about that. I'll explain what I'm doing as we go along."

While I explained that I needed an arm exposed, that I would use a tourniquet and that I would then put the needle into a vein to get blood, Nurse Brooks drew the curtains round the bed. The procedure was not new to me. I had drawn blood from Jim several times. It involved putting a Wasserman needle, which has a large gauge, into the vein and letting the blood drip into the test tube. A kidney dish was used to catch any blood spilled when starting the collection or when changing tubes. While I had performed the procedure before, this was the first time I had done it on someone I didn't know and who wouldn't appreciate my failing to get blood the first time. Thankfully, Mr. Bright could not see how shaky my hands were, nor how profusely I was sweating. As it happened things went well.

Nurse Brooks took the blood samples from me. "Thank you, I'll send these samples to the lab. Mr. Bright's chart is in the trolley over there by the wall. He needs to have a history taken. If there's anything else you need, let me know."

With that she walked away down the ward before I could thank her. I then turned to Mr. Bright. "If you don't mind, I'm going to get your chart and ask you a few questions. I've been asked to write out your full history."

"One of the doctors has already done that. Do you have to do it again?"

"Yes, that would have been the houseman. He would have written a brief history, which is at the head of your bed with the orders for the day. I have to take a more detailed one and write it up in the chart. It shouldn't take too long," I explained

"Well, I won't be going anywhere, will I?" he said, crossing his arms over his chest.

I got his chart and then went through the list of questions we had been taught to ask. I made some notes on a blank sheet of paper so that I could remember the details of his history and only had to consult the little red book a couple of times. I continued to be relieved that he couldn't see me.

Mr. Bright is seventy-two years old and has been having abdominal pains for the past three months. These are new. He hasn't had anything like it in the past. Apart from his eyesight, which had started to deteriorate three years ago, and an appendectomy when he was a child, he has always been well. He has been feeling tired and weaker during the past month. He has had some nausea but no vomiting. His appetite is not good and he feels he has lost some weight. The pains are in the pit of his stomach and come and go. He describes them as spasmodic. The pains wake him up at night but he has found that a glass of milk helps.

He is not on any medications from his doctor for the pains or anything else. He is married, lives with his wife and they have three children who are all well and have left home. Mr. Bright regards himself as an active person who goes for long walks with his wife three or four times a week. He goes to the pub once a week on Saturday evenings and has a couple of beers. He is a non-smoker. Losing his sight was very distressing but with the help of his wife and the Blind Society he is coping quite well.

Having got this oral history I proceeded to examine him. Apart from his raised blood pressure, his appendix scar, his blindness and the fact that he was thin, I couldn't find anything wrong with him. When I'd finished he asked the inevitable.

"Well, Doc, what do you think's the matter with me?"

I answered honestly: "I'm new to this as you know and I really haven't a clue. There are several possibilities. We hope that the tests we'll be doing in the next few days will help us come up with an answer."

"That's what you all say," he said, shaking his head. "I guess I'll have to wait, then, won't I?"

"I have to be off now," I said, unsure about how to answer him, "but I'll be back tomorrow. I'll probably have some more questions for you then. Mr. Grant-Massey will be doing rounds on Wednesday by which time I should know more about the tests that have been done."

Then I sat down at a desk near the entrance to the ward and wrote out all I had gathered from our talk, and added a few of my own thoughts on what might be wrong with Mr. Bright. All I could think of simply confirmed what the doctors had already diagnosed—that he might have a stomach ulcer or some sort of abdominal cancer.

I had time to introduce myself to the other two post-operative patients assigned to me before going to the female ward. One was a young man who had had an inguinal hernia repaired two days ago and was still experiencing quite a lot of pain. The other was a six days' post-op partial gastrectomy, who was doing well. In the ladies ward I had been allocated a patient with gallstones. She was to be operated on the following day and still needed a lot of things done. I discovered that I was expected to help move her to the theatre and to stay in the operating room during the surgery. As a junior clerk I was not expected to scrub up. Even so I was going to be busy.

My first official "ward round" with Mr. Grant-Massey was not for two days but I knew that I would be expected to present a complete history for Mr. Bright. This meant memorizing everything I had gathered including the results of all the tests. I had to be prepared to offer the most likely diagnosis as well as an alternative possibility. Some homework would be required if I wanted my secondary suggestion to be plausible.

Each firm was led by a consultant or surgeon. Firms were usually large, consisting of four junior dressers (a term used for surgical students), four senior dressers, two houseman (newly qualified doctors), two registrars (doctors in specialized training) and a senior nurse. Any student with free time was expected to attend other consultants' rounds. The "grapevine" was good at letting students know when interesting cases were to be presented.

On the appointed day, my firm met at ten minutes before ten outside the ward. "Binns, we will be presenting Mr. Bright today. I hope you have the history and results ready," the houseman said to me.

"I think I'm ready. I have the blood work, urine results, and some X-ray reports," I replied.

"Good," he said before I could raise questions about anything else I might need. "Don't be nervous, Mr. Grant-Massey is a gentleman."

Just then the door to Sister's office opened. Out stepped Sister, followed by a portly man, with thinning hair and wearing glasses.

"Good morning, gentlemen," he said as he reached the group. "What have you got for us today, Sister?"

"There are two post-ops to see. Mr. Bright, who is new, needs to be assessed. Who would you like to see first?"

"Let's see the post-ops first, Sister," instructed Mr. Grant-Massey.

We all followed her into the ward, which was immaculate with all the patients in neat and tidy beds. They looked as if they were about to be inspected by a commanding officer at a parade. The patients' eyes followed us with interest as we walked down to the first post-op.

"This is Mr. Green who had a hernia operated on five days ago and who is doing very well," said Sister.

"Which junior dresser has been looking after Mr. Green?" asked Mr. Grant-Massey.

"I have, sir," said George Williams, a fellow classmate who not unexpectedly was clearly uneasy about being selected first. Any one of us would have felt the same way.

"Well then, tell us about Mr. Green."

George took a deep breath and started his description: "Mr. Green is a twenty-six-year-old dockworker who noticed a painful swelling in his right groin a few months ago. It used to come and go, but gradually got worse and became a constant annoyance which started to interfere with his work. He went to see his doctor who sent him to us for assessment and treatment. We discovered he had a right inguinal hernia which was operated on five days ago. His post-operative recovery has been uneventful and he is just about ready to go home, sir."

"What sort of hernias do you know?" asked Mr. Grant-Massey.

"There are two types of inguinal hernias. Direct and indirect. Then there are femoral hernias and umbilical hernias," said George expanding on his explanation.

"Are there any other abdominal hernias that you have read about?"

"No, sir," replied George.

Mr. Grant-Massey looked at the next student in line and asked him the same question.

"There are some called internal hernias," suggested Brian rather timidly.

"Yes, do you know anything more than the name?"

"Not really," said Brian.

"Can you expand on internal hernias?" asked Mr. Grant-Massey of another student.

This method of questions and answers continued until everyone present, including the guests and registrars, had added to the body of knowledge about the patient and about all kinds of hernias. Specific nursing questions were directed at Sister, but her answers were never questioned. From this first session I learned that there were inguinal, femoral, umbilical, obturator, internal, incisional, hiatus and lumbar hernias. The anatomy and presentations of these hernias were discussed. The rarity of some was stressed. At the end of the session, Mr. Grant-Massey gave a brief summary and made some general comments on the subject. With a relatively simple topic, like hernias, the lecture and discussion could be as brief as twenty minutes or so. If the patient had been seen in the last few days and the surgery reviewed, then complications and future management would be questioned and discussed. Sometimes two hours or more could be taken up with one topic.

When he had exhausted the topic of hernias, Mr. Grant-Massey turned to Mr. Green: "I think you will be ready to go home tomorrow and we hope that the repair is a success. We would like to see you in six to eight weeks to make sure that all is well. Sister, or one of her staff, will give you instructions about what you can and can't do when you get home. You will have gathered that there are a lot of different kinds of hernias. Yours was a straightforward one and you should not have any further problems. Thank you for coming to Guy's and letting us teach our students about your hernia. Have you any questions?"

"Yes," he said, and paused to clear his throat, "what's the chance of my having another one of these?"

Mr. Grant-Massey turned to the registrar and said, "How would you answer that question, Mr. North?"

Mr. North, who had done the surgery, said: "We looked for evidence of a hernia on the other side and couldn't find any. However, there is a five to ten percent chance that you might get another one on the other side and a small chance that you might have a recurrence on this side. You can reduce the chances of this happening again by keeping yourself physically fit in the years to come."

"That sums it up, I think," said Mr. Grant-Massey. "If there are no more questions let's see the next patient. Lead the way, Sister."

"Mr. Bright is in Bed 6, sir, and is a new patient who came in two days ago."

On our way to Mr. Bright's bed I saw Mr. Grant-Massey stop and wait for the nurse who was pushing the trolley with the charts. He picked out Mr. Bright's chart, opened it, and started to look at the history I had written.

"Who's looking after Mr. Bright?" he asked.

"I am," I said.

"And what's your name."

"Binns, sir."

"Did your father train at Guy's? I seem to remember the name," he said, after a brief pause.

"Yes, sir."

"What did he end up doing?"

"He joined the Colonial Service and went to the Falkland Islands for two years; then he was in the Indian Medical Service and Chinese Turkestan during the war. He's now in Nigeria, sir," I replied.

"Yes, I remember him now. He was a clerk when I was a senior dresser here many years ago. We were in the Middle East together but never actually met. He was I.M.S. and I was Royal Army Medical Corps. Remember me to him when you see him next. Now, tell us about Mr. Bright."

I presented Mr. Bright's history as well as I could from memory being careful not to digress from the scheme that we had been taught.

"So, in summary we have a seventy-two-year-old man who has recently developed periodic central abdominal pains, lost some weight, and is generally feeling under the weather."

"Yes, sir."

"That doesn't really give us much to go on does it? Has he been jaundiced?" Mr. Grant-Massey asked.

"No, sir."

"Why would I want to know about that?"

"Jaundice would suggest gall bladder disease, sir," I replied.

"What's his appetite been like?"

"I'm not sure, sir."

"Well, let's find out." He turned to the patient. "Mr. Bright, have you noticed any change in your appetite lately?"

"It's not been good, especially for fatty foods. They seem to make the nausea worse."

"Have you had any diarrhea or constipation recently?"

"Now you ask, sir, I've had some diarrhea recently, but it was not that bad. Just a bit loose. I thought it might have been something I'd eaten."

"Have you felt bloated or noticed any abdominal swelling associated with the nausea?"

"No, sir."

"Binns, why would I ask about that?"

"I'm not sure," I replied.

He then turned to the student on my right.

"Have you any ideas?"

"He would be distended if he had an obstruction, sir."

This question and answer discussion continued round the group until all causes of abdominal pain had been exhausted. Mr. Bright did add several facts I had missed, but since it was my first day doing rounds I was spared any ridicule.

"Good, Mr. Binns, I think we've exhausted the history. What should we do next?

"I did an abdominal examination, which was not very helpful, sir. I was unable to find any masses or localizing signs."

"Let's see if I can find anything," Mr. Grant-Massey said and Sister prepared Mr. Bright for an abdominal examination by making him lie flat and exposing his abdomen.

"Mr. Binns, what is the first thing you do when you examine an abdomen?"

"Feel if it is soft or hard, sir."

"No. You look at it. The last thing you do is touch it. What are you looking for?"

"Scars, sir," I said hesitantly, trying unsuccessfully to look Mr. Grant-Massey in the eye.

"Yes, he has an old appendix scar, but we knew about that from the history. What else?"

"Colour of the skin, sir."

"Anything else you can think of?"

I was all out of ideas, but Mr. Grant-Massey let me off the hook. He turned to the next student on my right, "Any ideas?"

"Is there any peristaltic movement visible, sir."

"Yes, anything else?"

"Any bruising or staining, sir."

"What do you mean by staining? Has he been painting himself?" asked Mr. Grant-Massey.

"Well, sir, sometimes people put hot water bottles over a sore area and this can cause brownish staining of the skin. It takes a while and indicates that the patient has been having chronic pain in that area."

"Very good. Where do you usually see this staining?"

"Over the left lower quadrant or the hips," replied the student, whom I didn't recognize.

"And what causes the pain in the areas you have mentioned?"

"Diverticulitis and chronic hip disease, sir."

"Yes, but I don't think that's relevant to Mr. Bright, do you?"

"No, sir, I don't think so."

He turned to the next student. "Mr. Jones, have you any other ideas about what we might observe in an abdomen in a patient who is complaining of abdominal pains?"

"Distension, sir?" he said rather quietly.

"Yes. Is there any here?"

"Not that I can see, sir."

"Mr. Jamison, you will be taking the finals soon. If there was distension here what else might you observe?"

"Peristaltic movement can be seen in obstruction sometimes and if there is a lot of gut activity you can sometimes hear gurgling noises, sir."

"Yes, yes, good. Now, Mr. Binns, you have learned that looking and listening before you touch is a very important part of the examination of the abdomen. If you don't observe and listen you may miss some vital bits of information. In Mr. Bright's case, there are none of these signs so we can proceed to the examination. There are several things that you have to do while palpating an abdomen. The first is to run your hand very gently over the whole abdomen, thus." And he showed what to do. "From this you can get an idea of the softness or hardness of the abdomen. If you are watching the patient's face and you touch a sensitive area, you will see a reaction, so be warned to be careful while palpating that area. Once you hurt a patient, examination is much less productive because they tighten up their muscles reflexively. Once you have done the gentle palpation you can go to the more detailed palpation for specific abdominal organs, such as the liver, gallbladder, kidneys, spleen and masses that should not be there. Finally, you palpate more firmly to see if there are any areas of tenderness or rebound tenderness." All of the above examinations he demonstrated while he was talking.

"Thank you, Sister. You can cover Mr. Bright up now. I presume the registrar has done a rectal?"

"Yes, Mr. Grant-Massey," interjected Mr. Bright to make sure there was no doubt.

"There was nothing to feel in the abdomen today. Now, Mr. Binns, what are we going to talk about next?"

"The usual screening tests of his blood, urine and a chest X-ray have been done, but all the results are not back yet," I answered. "The blood test shows that he is anaemic, his urinalysis was normal and the chest X-ray was negative. A cholecystogram and barium meal and follow-through have been ordered but not been done yet. The occult blood test results have not come back."

"What do you think the tests ordered will help us find?"

"The barium meal and follow-through X-ray should help with the diagnosis of stomach ulcers or problems with his duodenum. The occult bloods will show if he is bleeding from his gastro-intestinal tract, and the cholecystogram should exclude any major gallbladder problems."

"What do you think is the most likely diagnosis, Mr. Binns?"

"A gastric ulcer," I replied tentatively. It was my best guess, although to be truthful, I really had no idea.

His questioning moved away from me and with the rest of the firm he explored other possibilities. These included neoplasm of the gastrointestinal tract and other abdominal organs. Even possible non-physical causes of Mr. Bright's symptoms were discussed. At the end of an hour many aspects of abdominal pain had been touched on. A few days later, once all his tests came back, it turned out that Mr. Bright had a duodenal ulcer, which responded quickly to medical treatment.

As surgical clerks we had to attend one consultant and one registrar ward round a week. The registrars' rounds usually concentrated on basic medical topics and focussed on how to think about and analyse patient data. They were good because they usually covered one subject in depth. There were also two outpatient clinics a week. These were held in the Outpatients Department which was above the Casualty (ER) Department on the other side of the Hospital, immediately opposite the Pub. The building was old and a bit of a rabbit warren. It consisted of several examination rooms and a larger consulting room where Mr. Grant-Massey would see new patients or patients with problems with which the registrars wanted his help. As clerks we spent a lot of time with Mr. Grant-Massey. The sessions in the Outpatients Department tended to be practical. Because there would be only three or four clerks, the houseman, registrar and consultant, we were asked to participate. The houseman would do the presenting and we got hands-on experience examining patients with clinical signs and symptoms.

On the surgical firm there were two operating sessions a week. We were expected to attend all operations on the patients we had been assigned. As junior dressers we had to help with the transport of patients on stretchers either to the theatres or other parts of the hospital, such as the X-ray, physiotherapy, and radiotherapy departments. If one of our patients died and needed an autopsy, clinical students were expected to present the case histories to the pathologist. When a patient with an unusual illness or disorder died the required autopsy was attended by the whole firm.

Clinical talks were given in the main lecture theatre once or twice a week by various clinicians from different departments. Each speaker presented a specific specialty topic. About once a month famous visitors from other medical schools or from overseas would present topics. These guest lecturers usually explored cutting-edge research or suggested new approaches to old problems. We were required to sign in for at least one hundred of these lunchtime lectures during the three years of the program, although I don't think anyone ever feared that our attendance was actually being tracked.

One morning several weeks into my clinical clerkship I heard that the famous Guy's Hospital pathologist, Dr. Keith Simpson (1907–1985), was going to perform an autopsy at one of the lunch-time lectures. He was renowned for his post-mortems on high-profile murder cases. These included the 1949 Acid Bath Murders committed by John George Haigh on which Dr. Simpson pioneered the use of forensic dentistry to identify the victims. Dr. Simpson's pathology research also increased the awareness of battered baby syndrome. He was the first forensic pathologist to be recognized by the Home Office when he was awarded the Commander of the Most Excellent Order of the British Empire (CBE) in 1975.

Since I had not seen an autopsy before I thought it was time for me to attend one. The post-mortem room was between the Nurses' Home and the Dental School, near the surgical wards. It was well shielded from the outside world by a short corridor. When I got into the large rectangular room with its tiled floor and high ceiling, I found two autopsies in progress, surrounded by several students and physicians. There was a ceiling skylight and numerous powerful lights suspended over the centrally placed stainless steel autopsy tables. At the far end of the space there was a closed door with two shrouded trolleys against the wall.

The tables were long with a sink at one end and two taps at the other. Attached to one of these was a short red rubber hose. Situated next to each table there was a large wooden chopping board on which were placed the organs of the body when illustrating significant pathology. Alongside the chopping board were several knives, scalpels, dissecting forceps, grasping tools, and saws lined up ready for use. Two large sponges were at hand to mop up blood and other materials. By the time students arrived the bodies had been uncovered and placed on their backs with a wooden block under their necks. A cardboard hospital identification label was attached to one of the great toes.

On the wards I had become accustomed to the smells of sepsis, bad breath, urine, faeces, and other body odours. Even so, there the odours were often masked by the smells of antiseptics and other scents (deodorant sprays did not exist at that time), and I had not experienced the characteristic smell of freshly cut tissue that was beginning to decompose. (On this particular day the bodies being autopsied were fresh, so the smell was not strong, but on other days it was almost intolerable. The worst odour came from autopsies being done on decomposing or badly burnt bodies.)

Dr. Keith Simpson was a slim, bald man who stood very straight and spoke in a quiet, clear voice. He stood at one of the tables with the body of a large white male in front of him. "Good morning gentlemen. Today we have a coroner's case as well as a hospital patient to show you. This is Mr. Sylvester, about whom we know very little. He worked in the City at a sedentary job in one of the big offices. Yesterday he was having lunch with his girlfriend when he suddenly complained of severe pain in his neck, after which he quickly became unconscious and collapsed onto the table. By the time the ambulance arrived there was no pulse and efforts by the ambulance people to resuscitate him failed. On arrival at Guy's it was determined that he was dead. He does not seem to have any relatives in London and the police are trying to contact his mother. We have no medical history available and need to determine the cause of death."

He looked up at the student standing next to me. "What observations would you like to make about this man?"

The student paused for a moment, looking at the body spread out in front of him. Then he said, somewhat cautiously, "We have a large, slightly overweight man who looks to be about fifty years of age. There is a lot of bluish staining on the side of his face and down the back of his thighs, buttocks and back. There is no obvious trauma, or cuts other than the one you have made. I can't see any surgical scars on the abdomen or chest. Apart from being a little overweight he looks quite fit and well-nourished."

I wondered what the next question was going to be as there was a fifty-fifty chance that it would be directed at me and I really had no ideas about what might have happened to the man.

"Yes, that's a good start. The blue staining you see is related to post-mortem changes. Surgical scars can give us clues about what illnesses a person may have had but not in this case." To my relief Dr. Simpson turned to the student standing in the opposite direction to me and asked, "In a case like this, are there any special things that you would look for before starting an autopsy?"

"After looking generally at the body for any evidence of trauma to the head or other wounds, I would look in the mouth and throat to see if there was any airway obstruction. People do occasionally suffocate on food," a senior student offered.

"Good. We looked and found no food in his mouth or throat. What other ideas have you about how or why a relatively young person can just collapse and die like this man did?"

"The common causes are heart attacks and strokes," replied the student.

"Yes. We usually use more formal medical terms here but you're right." He stood back a bit and looked round the assembled audience and asked, "Any other ideas?"

There was a long pause before someone at the back said, "Poison, sir?"

"Yes, but it's unusual to drop dead from a poison like this man did. There are a few poisons that will act that quickly but the patients will usually show other signs of poisoning like having a convulsion or complaining of abdominal pain before collapsing. All this man complained of was a pain in the neck. Poisoning is something that one has to bear in mind, though."

At this point Dr. Simpson smiled. I think he was enjoying this moment because we were having such difficulty solving what for him was the simplest of mysteries. "Anything else you can think of? It's a very silent and fairly common problem?"

"Pulmonary embolus, sir," one of the more senior members of the audience suggested.

"Yes, that covers most of the common things. So now let's have a look and see if we can determine if that event happened here."

The autopsy started with the removal of the heart and lungs, then the liver, spleen, kidneys, and, in this case, the stomach, after carefully tying off both ends so that the contents could be looked at separately and sent for analysis. The rest of the intestines were put down at the bottom of the table to be opened later. Dr. Simpson did not take out the brain but it would be looked at in due course. He picked up the lungs and put them on the chopping board, showed us both sides and then asked, "Who would like to describe these to me?" There was a long pause so he looked up and addressed the gentleman who had suggested the poison idea. "Well, Mr. Johnston, what do you think?"

"May I ask what they weigh, sir?"

"Good question." After weighing them on the scale at the head of the table, he said, "950 grams, which is normal for a man of this build. Why do you ask?"

"If the lungs were heavy, the cause of death could be fluid retention or neoplasm. To me the lungs look very normal for a man who has lived in London. They are grey with a lot of black specks over their surfaces and are uniformly shiny. There are no dark areas suggesting emboli. Do they feel uniformly soft, sir?" he asked.

"Yes, and the cut surfaces are not showing any pathology," Dr. Simpson said as he proceeded to slice the lungs up in layers with a long, sharp knife. "There are no large ante-mortem clots in the pulmonary vessels. Let's have a look at the heart next. It weighs 350 grams, which is a bit heavy but it looks normal on the outside. The pericardium did not contain any blood-stained fluid and was again perfectly normal. There is no bruising of the heart muscles, the coronary arteries show some evidence of atherosclerosis, but the main branches are clear of blood clots or emboli," he said while illustrating these points. "The aorta has quite a lot of atheroma in it as you can see, here," he said, pointing to the raised plaques.

"Is there anything else unusual here, Mr. Johnston?" he asked, again looking up with a slight smile forming at the corners of his mouth.

Mr. Johnston moved forward a bit to get a better view. "There is an unusual amount of blood clotted in the aorta, but it could be post-mortem, sir."

"Yes, but when you look at it carefully it is not a typical post-mortem clot. It is fairly firm to touch. If it is ante-mortem then it could be the cause of death. In a few days, histology will be able to confirm when and where the clot developed. This is quite an unusual case as I'll show you. To see what happened to this man we will have to remove the aorta intact which is done by first cutting through the diaphragm. Then after dissecting out the abdominal aorta, we cut the aorta across at the origins of the femoral arteries. After that we can lift the whole vessel forward and cut the various branches as we go along. While doing this carefully we can see if there are any obvious changes to the aorta." He did this very deftly while explaining what he was doing.

When he got to the renal arteries, he said, "Ahhh! Here we are. You can see where the vessel suddenly gets larger and has a bluish colour to it. This is probably where the trouble started. I will remove the whole aorta so that we can have a good look at it. You can see that the vessel in the upper portion is enlarged. When we cut across it the reason becomes obvious as you can see here. The wall of the artery has split and there is a clot in it which partially blocks off the main vessel. This is a dissecting aortic aneurysm which can occur quite suddenly and rapidly, with early collapse and death because the aorta becomes obstructed and there is no blood returning to the heart. Sometimes it can be quite a slow process with repeated episodes of pain, suggestive of coronary artery or gastro-intestinal disease. I think we can safely say that Mr. Sylvester's pain in the neck, collapse and death were all related. Let's go and look at the other case which is very different."

We all gathered round the other table on which there was a very emaciated, old-looking lady whose body was severally jaundiced.

"This patient is interesting because she illustrates how much pathology can be present without death occurring. She was only fifty years old at the time of death. Two years ago she was diagnosed as having an ovarian cyst, which was removed at the time of a hysterectomy. Unfortunately the pathology came back as an ovarian carcinoma and she then received pelvic irradiation. At the time of death she weighed 45 kilograms and was very jaundiced as you will observe. A few weeks ago she was admitted to hospital for terminal care and she died peacefully yesterday. She was still walking around a month ago which is quite amazing when you see how extensive her disease is. Would any-one like to hazard a guess as to what finally caused her death?" he asked.

"Pneumonia," someone muttered.

"Yes, that's the usual thing," said Dr. Simpson.

He then showed us what pneumonia looked like, but pointed out that this lady's lungs were studded with white abnormal tissue which was quite hard to cut. These malignant deposits varied in size from a pinhead to two or three centimetres in diameter. The malignant de-posits had spread all over both lungs and would have interfered with her breathing, yet she had survived for over a year. He then showed us that the deposits were also on and in the heart, pericardium and pleura.

"Now, when we look at the other organs we see that they are all involved to some extent. The jaundice suggests that there is involve-ment of the liver, so let's have a look." He picked up the liver and put it onto the block.

"It weighs 2,000 grams which is heavy. Mr. Jones, you have not said much today. Would you like to describe what you see here?"

Jones moved closer to the table and looked at the liver. "It's a very unusual shape because of the large white nodules that are present just below the surface of the capsule. The liver tissue is dark brown and stained yellow. There are some nodules around the gall bladder and the cystic duct."

"Yes, her jaundice was probably caused by obstruction of the cyst-ic duct as there seems to be a reasonable quantity of normal-look-ing liver tissue. These white nodules are all malignant deposits." Dr. Simpson then proceeded to slice up the liver to show how extensive the involvement was.

"In fact, every organ, including the skin and muscle, has malig-nant tissue. The origin of the malignancy, an ovarian cyst, was re-moved two years ago and cannot be shown. I think this patient illus-trates how resistant the human body is to disease. However, our other case this morning showed that a small break in a vital organ can cause death very suddenly. One of the smallest pathologies that can cause death is a tiny clot in the coronary arteries or cerebra-vascular vessels. Well, gentlemen, I think that will be enough for today. Thank you for coming. I hope it was a valuable experience."

Dr. Simpson was an excellent lecturer and teacher; his lunch-time lectures were always packed and were often about medical, legal or unusual pathological topics. After the initial desensitisation, which most of us needed to get past—the odours and the sight of seeing a human body gutted and cut into pieces—I found that attending autopsies was a dramatic and stimulating aid to my learning.

As the three months of the surgical firm progressed our involvement in the theatres increased. In the beginning, we just had to stand, watch and listen. This was sometimes awkward. There were a lot of people in the operating theatres. The nurses were often bringing in sterile items and we had to keep out of their way or receive a serious reprimand. It also got boring. With a consultant, two assistants, a nursing sister, her assistant and the anaesthetist and his assistant all working around the patient one could not see much. There were a few footstools on which to stand, but it was still difficult to see over and around the crowd. Mr. Grant-Massey would tell us what he was doing and once in a while stand back so that we could have a look, while being careful not to touch anything. The other alternative was to go up into the gallery above the theatre where the view was much better. Unfortunately the galleries were glassed off and it was not possible to hear what was being said. Also, Mr. Grant-Massey would not know that we were there and might think we were disinterested.

Our firm was on "take" every fourth week. This meant that we were responsible for any emergency admissions during this time. As students, we were "on call" to cover these admissions at least twice during our term on the firm. This meant being in the hospital for the whole week and admitting patients as they came in, either directly to the wards from their family practitioners or through Casualty. In the latter case we often had to go to Casualty to see them. We students usually worked in pairs and had bedrooms on the top floor of Hunt's House. Adjacent to these rooms was a small laboratory where we were expected to do routine lab tests. The housemen and on-call registrars also lived in the hospital. They were housed in Baker's House, which was part of the "Spit."

When we arrived on the ward we would be told about the newly admitted patients. We were expected to see them as soon as possible. Often we were very busy at night and would not get a normal sleep, and yet we were expected to continue with our regular clerkship duties during the day. The on-call experience also introduced us to surgical emergencies. These operating sessions tended to be challenging because students were often asked to assist with the operation. Fortunately, because it was off hours, there were fewer people in the theatre. These encounters were a mixed blessing. While we saw acutely ill patients for the first time, some cases could also be very stressful. However, the nurses were less senior at night which permitted more interaction between the nurses, doctors and students. Consequently students became more familiar with nursing responsibilities on the wards.

During my three months on the surgical ward, under the guidance of Mr. Grant-Massey, I was introduced to the basics of surgical practice and saw patients with many different conditions. Even though patients often came in with a similar diagnosis, for example, "for a gastrectomy," no two patients were identical. The more I got to know the patients the more the differences became apparent. There were several occasions when very sad and tragic situations came to light and I was introduced to the compassionate aspects of medical care. I learned how to interact sympathetically with grieving relatives.

The medical clerkship was run in a similar manner to the surgical one, but generally there were more members on the firm, about fifteen, and a lot more time was spent on the wards taking histories. Consultant medical rounds were notoriously long, often going on for four or more hours. My medical clerkship began in January 1956 on Dr. Boland's and Dr. Baker's firm. The junior clerks were responsible for Dr. Boland's patients and the senior clerks Dr. Baker's. We did, however, have to go to both consultants' rounds and thus got the benefit of both consultants' teaching. Although Dr. Boland's special interest was chests, we received input about other specialties by attending other consultants' rounds, frequently in our spare time.

The entrance to Hunt's House and the medical wards was opposite the Medical School. The front doors opened into a hall where the firms used to gather to wait for the consultants to arrive before rounds started.

Our firm's ward was called Addison and was situated on the first floor. It had a similar layout to the surgical wards, but, with fewer windows, was not as bright and airy. Attached to the ward there was a balcony which had been converted into a tuberculosis unit with eight beds. The area was glassed in but the windows were rarely closed. It was policy to keep these patients in as airy a place as possible. In the winter months they could often be seen wearing overcoats in bed to keep warm.

There were three levels of student seniority in the firms, one for each year of the teaching program. The senior students, who were soon to take finals, were expected to help the other students when necessary. Some actually taught the junior clerks about simple medical problems. Tutoring was an effective form of revision and good preparation for final exams.

Our medical clerkship lasted three months and each of us was assigned four or five patients to look after at any given time. A few patients stayed on the ward for up to two weeks and some came in terminally ill and died. Most of the patients admitted to the ward were seriously ill and came in because they could no longer be looked after at home by their family doctors. Others presented diagnostic problems that necessitated hospital admission. By the end of this three-month period each student was personally responsible for approximately forty patients. We were, however, privileged to actually see, hear and learn about, and examine specific clinical findings on several additional patients.

As medical clerks, talking to, examining and collecting blood from patients soon became routine, but the human interest and personal problems that patients presented with were frequent challenges, some of which left indelible memories. One challenging example for me was a sixteen-year-old school boy who was admitted with tiredness, a little shortness of breath on mild exertion and some episodes of sweating. He was the only son of a middle-class family and the "apple of their eye". He was a very bright student who was preparing for the General Certificate examinations in the hope of going on to university. He wanted to become a doctor. His major concern was that he was having difficulty concentrating on his studies.

Initial examination showed him to be of average build and above-average intelligence. He answered questions well. He had no previous serious medical history. This was the first time he had been in hospital. When he arrived his pulse was marginally raised and he had a slight temperature. He looked pale and a little tired for someone who was sixteen years old. He had been admitted to the medical ward because he was too old to go to the Children's Hospital. The admitting doctor thought he most likely had a viral infection, which is what he was being investigated for.

On a Friday morning during Dr. Hardwick's rounds—he was one of the consultants—there was much discussion about the different diagnoses, which included various types of infections. During his chest examination, Dr. Hardwick mentioned that he thought he could hear a very faint systolic heart murmur but that it was probably not significant in a young boy. And yet a long list of investigations was suggested which included blood, urine and stool cultures, an electrocardiogram, a chest X-ray and a sputum sample for tuberculosis.

Dr. Hardwick concluded the round by saying, "Here we have a young man who has recently noticed a change in his physical fitness and who is becoming tired rather easily. Clinically there is little of note so we have to look into things in more detail. The chances are that he has a viral infection which will get better soon and we'll never know what the problem was. However, as this has been going on for a few weeks and seems to be a serious concern to him, his parents and their family doctor, we admitted him for further investigation. We will talk about him again at Wednesday's rounds. I think that will do for today. Have a good weekend."

On Tuesday the clerk who was looking after the boy told me the young man looked terrible.

"What do you mean?" I asked

"He's pale, lethargic, is breathing fast and his pulse is over 100 while resting in bed."

"Is there anything else? Does he have any pain?" I asked.

"Not really, but he has a few peticheal haemorrhages on his arms. His temperature is a hundred which is a bit high. Sister does not like the look of him, either."

"Are any of the test results back yet?" I asked.

"His haemoglobin is a bit low at eighty percent; his white cells are up a bit with a differential suggesting an infection; his chest X-ray suggests that his heart might be a little enlarged but the electrocardiogram is essentially normal."

"What does his chest sound like?"

"I can hear the murmur that Hardwick heard at rounds on Friday and there are these peticheal haemorrhages that seem to be new. I missed the murmur the first time but it's quite loud now."

"None of that seems to be very conclusive. Have they started him on any treatment yet?" I asked.

"No. They're waiting for the rest of the tests and for Dr. Hardwick to see him."

At rounds on Wednesday we went to see the boy first. The first thing that struck me was that he looked much worse. He just lay there, was extremely pale, was breathing rapidly and his neck veins were engorged. Dr. Hardwick went to the bedside and asked, "How are you feeling today, Brian?"

"Not too well, just very tired and a bit short of breath. I could hardly get out of bed this morning and was very glad to get back."

"Have you noticed any pain?"

"No. Only a little tightness in my chest."

"Let's listen to your chest for a minute. Can you help him, Sister? I want to listen to the front and back," said Dr. Hardwick.

Once Sister had got Brian sitting up in bed with his pyjama top off, Dr. Hardwick picked up Brian's hand, looked at his palm and his forearms, noticed the peticheal haemorrhages, felt his pulse and asked, "Have you had these spots before?"

"Yes, I noticed them about a month ago. They don't last long. What are they?

"They are miniature bruises. Let's listen to your chest again,"

Dr. Hardwick first percussed the front and back of Brian's chest and listened to it closely. Following this he asked Brain to lie back so that he could examine his abdomen. I noticed that he felt the liver carefully. Dr. Hardwick didn't say anything until he had finished. Then slowly, almost deliberately, he turned to thank Sister. Slowly he shuffled around to face us and asked the clerk who was looking after Brian, "Have you noticed any change in Brian's chest findings since Friday?"

"Only that the murmur is easier to hear now."

"Yes. It's become quite noticeable and certainly suggests active pathology. He is a lot sicker than he was on Friday. I think we better start him on treatment with penicillin today. I don't think we should wait for the blood cultures to come back. The penicillin should make you feel a lot better, Brian, but it will mean some injections in your bottom."

"That won't worry me as long as it makes me feel better." He tried to smile.

"We've taken enough of the young man's time. We better go and see another patient, Sister," said Dr. Hardwick, patting Brian on the shoulder. We all moved off down the ward. At the end of the round, when we were all gathered in the corridor, Dr. Hardwick turned to us and said quietly, "Brian is very sick. He has got sub-acute bacterial endocarditis and there has been a sudden change in his aortic valve this week. His liver edge is palpable. He may be in early heart failure. Let's hope the penicillin controls the infection of the valve."

When I went into the ward two days later I noticed that it was very quiet and that Brian's bed was empty. I looked around to see if he had been moved but couldn't locate him anywhere. The clerk who had been in charge of Brian came into the ward. He looked sad and depressed.

"What happened to Brian?" I asked.

"He took a sudden turn for the worse late last night and died about three hours ago. His parents just made it in time. I think Dr. Hardwick wants to talk to us at rounds about what happened."

"Are they going to ask for a post-mortem?"

"I think so, but it won't be until tomorrow if they do one."

When Dr. Hardwick arrived he met us in the corridor outside the ward.

"Gentlemen, we have just witnessed a tragedy. Young Brian died suddenly during the night. He became very short of breath and his heart stopped. We did everything we could to resuscitate him, but he did not come round. The most likely explanation is that one of his valve cusps broke. When a cusp breaks the valve no longer functions properly and the heart overloads and goes into arrest. The reason for the cusp breaking would be the infection weakening and eroding the delicate valve supports. Brian's condition was an acute bacterial endocarditis rather than the more common sub-acute disease. He may have had a mild congenital malformation of his heart valve which predisposed him to the infection. These valve infections occur because we all have periodic transient episodes of bacteraemia. The common bacterium that causes sub-acute endocarditis is *streptococcus viridians* which rarely causes other infections and is a very common resident of the mouth and nasal passages. Acute bacterial endocarditis is more often caused by *staphylococcus aureus*. We have asked for a post-mortem examination and if there is one I think you should all attend.

"The unexpected death of a young healthy man is a tragedy, especially for family and friends. For some of you this will be a first experience, others will already have seen this sort of event in your very short medical careers. There will be one or two of you who have had personal experiences similar to Brian's family. A major part of your medical training is to observe these events, assess the impact on the family and advise them as best you can, sympathetically.

"You will find that people vary a lot in how they are affected and how they respond. It is one of your jobs to be aware of the community services available and to direct patients and families to this help. This includes district health services, financial aids, religious counselling and funeral services. In hospital we have a whole department that deals with most of these problems but in general practice you will be the person responsible for knowing how to get this help. This sad event will be the first of many that you will have to experience in your medical careers, but remember, although you may be experienced, it is often a first for the relatives and thus very stressful. Have any of you got any specific questions that you would like to ask?"

"Sir, how does one approach the relatives of a family in these stressful circumstances and, at the same time, make a request for a post-mortem?" asked one of the junior clerks.

"You will find that talking to relatives about these problems is easier than you imagine. Most want to know exactly what's happened. And when there is any doubt in our minds, being truthful is the only approach. Sometimes there is no choice for the relatives. For example, when an autopsy is required for medical-legal questions or when the cause of death cannot be ascertained. Finally, in a teaching school, it's important to explain to the family the immense value that post-mortem examinations have as a teaching tool. There are some relatives who will refuse examination on personal or religious grounds and these have to be respected." He hesitated and calmly looked from face to face. "I think that's enough on that subject. Let's see what Sister has for us today." After finishing his speech, Dr. Hardwick led us into the ward for another three hour round.

The death of this young man was my first exposure to the tragic side of medicine, the side that faced the daily and unfathomable reality of death; the mystery medicine would never fully understand. Up to this time I had been either fortunate enough to avoid a face-to-face confrontation with death or I had been deliberately sheltered from this kind of emotional experience, except in the case of my pigeons. Optimistically, I had assumed Brian would recover. Now doubt seeped in. As I continued my medical training I constantly came into contact with human stories that were often tragic and over which I—or my colleagues—had little control. These encounters showed us that doctors and technology were not able to fix every medical condition, and we slowly came to accept death as part of life. We also learned that it was not healthy to dwell on these events—one could be consumed by them and unable to focus on the urgent problem of helping the living.

On a Saturday afternoon, a few weeks after Brian's case, a young twenty-six-year-old father of three was admitted to our ward because he had collapsed at a football match, which he was attending with his five-year-old son. He had convulsed and then gradually regained consciousness, but he was still disorientated when he arrived in the Emergency Department. Although there was no previous history, the Emergency staff thought that the most likely cause was epilepsy and that he should be admitted for observation, investigation and treatment. Further examination and routine investigations failed to show any specific diagnostic pointers, but the young father did have a low-grade fever and a slightly raised white cell count. On Sunday morning he was well and was told that he would be going home on Monday after some X-rays, further tests, and a consultation with a neurologist.

That evening he became confused again and the neurologist was called in to assess him. Based on his assessment the neurologist recommended that a neurosurgeon be consulted as soon as possible in the morning. By the morning the patient had lapsed into a semi-conscious state. The neurosurgeon thought that the patient might be suffering from a brain tumour or abscess and that he should be operated on as soon as possible. Surgery confirmed this diagnosis and the neurosurgeon found and drained an abscess. Unfortunately the outcome was again tragic; the patient died on the operating table.

This case was significant. A subsequent investigation raised questions about the quality of medical attention patients received on weekends. The timing of consultations and general medical and nursing coverage over weekends was discussed in detail. Many of the staff were concerned that if the patient had taken ill on a Monday and not on a Saturday he would have survived. The event was a very important learning experience for me. I became aware that people who got sick or injured during the off hours, that is, at night, during holidays or on weekends, might not get the best treatment, in spite of the efforts of the on-call staff.

Another noteworthy case I had to present at rounds was that of

Mr. John Stone. He was fifty-two and had been admitted to the ward because of jaundice and confusion. When I took his history I failed to recognize that many of his answers to my questions were fabricated. In fact, he gave a very plausible story about his life and occupation by piecing together memories that were several years apart. However, the answers that I got to questions about his youth were accurate and consistent. He had spent many years in the British Army and had attained the rank of Sergeant-major. He had been a good boxer, winning an army middle-weight title before the Second World War. He saw active service and then retired at fifty.

When I asked him about his early drinking habits he said that he used to drink several pints of beer most nights and at weekends—the beer often fortified with hard liquor. Apparently his drinking had gone on for several years, but he stressed that he had stopped drinking. According to Mr. Stone, he should not have been admitted to hospital and he kept asking me why he was there. My examination revealed a middle-aged man who was a little overweight with a ruddy complexion and rather coarse skin. On examination the only significant finding was a slight jaundice. The blood tests suggested that his liver functions were abnormal; his bilirubin was high and he was a bit anaemic. My conclusion was that he was probably suffering from hepatitis with an associated confusion.

At rounds, when Dr. Boland came to Mr. Stone's bed, Dr. Boland's face lit up and he chuckled. "Good morning, Mr. Stone, how are you these days?" he asked.

"Not sure why I'm here this time," Mr. Stone replied.

I knew at that point that I was in trouble because I had not gone looking for an old chart and was not aware that Mr. Stone had been admitted under Dr. Boland before.

"Who is Mr. Stone's clerk?" asked Dr. Boland as he looked round the gathered firm with his one eye.

"I am sir," I said.

"Ah, now tell us about Mr. Stone then."

I gave a brief résumé of my findings and what I thought the problem might be.

"Hmm, he is a bit jaundiced but did you notice anything else when you were talking to him?" Dr. Boland asked.

"He seems to have had quite an interesting life in the Army, sir."

"Yes, that's true. But was there anything you thought was unusual about his history?"

"No, sir."

"Mr. Stone, how old are you?"

"Forty-six," Mr. Stone answered convincingly.

"Are you sure?"

"Yes, sir."

"Hmm, what day is it today?"

"Tuesday, sir"

It was, in fact, Friday, but anyone could make that mistake, especially when in hospital, I thought.

"Do you know what month and year it is?" asked Dr. Boland.

"Of course I do. It's 1950 and November, sir." He was a long way off on this little detail. It was actually September, 1956, and I realized I had missed something important. Something critical.

"Where do you live now?" Dr. Boland continued.

"Wanstead, sir."

I knew that was wrong as his admission chart clearly stated that he was living with his wife in the Boroughs and had done so for the past twenty years.

"Perhaps we better have a look at your tummy. Sister, can you help him?" asked Dr. Boland.

"I don't think you will find anything interesting there," said Mr. Stone as he lay back and pushed the bed covers away with Sister's help.

Dr. Boland then looked at the exposed abdomen and after a pause gently palpated it. When he had finished he looked around at me and asked, "Did you find anything unusual when you examined Mr. Stone's abdomen?"

"I thought I could just feel the liver edge, but I wasn't sure, sir."

"Come over and try again. I'm sure Mr. Stone won't mind, will you Mr. Stone?"

"Not in the least," he said.

I moved over to the bedside and put my hand out to feel Mr. Stone's abdomen.

"Stop, not yet. Have a careful look and ask him to take a big breath, before you put your cold hands on him," said Dr. Boland.

So I stood and looked, and then asked Mr. Stone to take a deep breath. I really couldn't see anything unusual and, more frustratingly, was not sure *what* I was supposed to see.

"What do you think? Dr. Boland asked.

"I can't see anything unusual, sir," I replied.

"How about anyone else?" Dr. Boland asked, looking around.

"From this angle and with the light coming across the abdomen I think I can see fullness under the right rib margin which comes down when he takes a deep breath," one of the senior dressers said quietly.

"Yes. It's a little unusual to be able to see it, but you will if you learn to take time to observe carefully before putting your cold hands on a patient's abdomen. There are other things that you will see from time to time. These include peristaltic movements, lumps, scars that surgeons have left, bruising, heat pad stains and, as in this case, jaundice."

He gave me a somewhat quick and unnerving glance.

"Mr. Binns, you can palpate Mr. Stone's abdomen now."

I proceeded with the abdominal examination, being very careful to follow the directions that we had been given. It was possible to feel Mr. Stone's liver edge, which I hadn't really been sure was there previously, but knowing that it was there made it easier.

"So, you felt the liver edge, Mr. Binns?"

"Yes sir, it is clearly palpable now."

"Good. I think that will do for today, Mr. Stone," said Dr. Boland. "Let's go onto the next patient, Sister."

After seeing three other patients we all moved out into the corridor between the wards and were given a bit of a debriefing by Dr. Boland.

"Mr. Stone is a very interesting man. He is still relatively young and is having a major problem remembering recent events. To cover this up he invents things and can get away with quite a lot until he is asked very specific questions. He has jaundice and an enlarged liver which is easy to feel. His history of heavy drinking in the past is very significant and he presents as a patient with early alcoholic liver cirrhosis and alcoholic encephalopathy, sometimes known as Korsakoff's Syndrome. Although he has stopped drinking, the prognosis is not good for either pathology as neither condition will improve and will, in all likelihood, slowly worsen. If he starts drinking again things will progress rapidly. He has been admitted for further investigation and assessment to see if he can still cope at home. His wife is working and he is left on his own a lot of the time. We have asked one of the psychiatrists to see him for advice on his mental state and further management."

Another disease we had to cope with was tuberculosis, where patients were kept in a room more like a greenhouse with windows all round and a glass roof. The idea of treating the disease with a triple-antibiotic management of streptomycin, P.A.S. and Izodiadine was in its infancy. The usual methods of treatment in those days included artificial pneumothoraces, surgically collapsing the lungs, instilling kaolin into the pleural space, and rest in hospital.

These patients were remarkably cheerful and the majority were young adults. Because of the infectious nature of the disease, we were cautioned about going onto the ward and had to use masks and take other precautions. Ninety percent of us had already had a primary infection with TB. Those who hadn't had been vaccinated prior to coming onto the wards.

One patient prided himself on his oratory capabilities and was a regular speaker at Hyde Park Corner during the summer months. When he took a turn for the worse or the weather became inclement, he would be readmitted. As one of our consultants put it, with a hint of annoyance in his voice, the man was highly infectious and spent the summer spraying his audiences with tuberculosis bacteria. The man was a health hazard. Social Services and the Public Health authorities had tried to stop this activity but there were no legal procedures available to forcibly confine him to hospital. At the time this was only true for smallpox or the plague.

By the end of my first year, I had completed four firms. Two medical and two surgical. I had taken approximately 280 histories from patients, and seen many others who were discussed at rounds. The routine was tiring and demanding. We usually went to the hospital every day between 8 a.m. and 9 a.m. and would not leave until about 5 p.m. We were not expected to go in at the weekends unless we were on call, but often did to check up on patients.

During that first year I saw or was taught about most general medical and surgical conditions. Many were very rare. For example, I saw patients with tertiary syphilis, anthrax, elephantiasis and some tropical skin conditions. The in-depth teaching I received was considerable. Common subjects were covered repeatedly to reinforce the conditions and to illustrate the many different facets of presentation, progress, prognosis and management that clinical medicine requires. Some students felt the teaching was a bit too repetitive and that the information could be equally well learned from books. Personally, I did not feel this was the case because of the uniqueness of both the people and the progression of their illnesses and injuries.

One criticism I frequently heard about learning medicine in a hospital setting was that it did not really prepare us for general practice, which was the goal of most of the students. Our instructors were aware of this and attempted to bring this aspect of medicine to our attention. Some of them had been in general practice before becoming consultants and could call on their experiences to help prepare us for that role. Besides, we were assigned a brief spell in general practice in our second year when we had to spend two weeks living in with a General Practitioner. During this time we were expected to go to all the GP's surgeries (office sessions) and attend all house calls, which were a major part of general practice.

While our time as medical students in the clinical practice years consisted of intensive patient schedules at the hospitals, with long and often exhausting hours, we still did not have the commitments of full-time practicing physicians. We had a social life, and mine was typical. I continued to play squash on a regular basis. At the new Student Union facility in the hospital, I played card games, board games, snooker, table tennis and socialized at the bar. I even managed to squeeze the occasional chess match into my hospital activities and once a week played at Donald's in the flat above us at Willow road.

Elaine and I continued to go to complimentary theatre shows and orchestral concerts and several times arranged to attend the Henry Wood Promenade Concerts. Together we took in most, if not all, of the permanent art galleries and spent hours wandering around the famous sites of London. I loved to escape into the British and Science Museums which were filled with objects and exhibitions that held, for both of us, endless promises of adventure and discovery, both familiar and odd.

Arranging holidays together was difficult, but Elaine and I managed to get to France for two weeks of hitchhiking in 1956. The cheapest ferry was from Hastings to Boulogne at a cost of seventy shillings each. We were lucky and got a lift to Paris on the first day. We spent the night in a tent in the Bois de Boulogne, but in the morning discovered that breakfast was going to be expensive—we only had twenty pounds between us—so we headed out and hitchhiked down the Loire Valley. We then circled back to Boulogne along the Brittany coast. On another trip we flew to Switzerland to visit with Edith and Walter, teacher friends of Elaine's. On this occasion we took the cable train to the summit of the Brenner Pass and cycled down the other side, warm summer air brushing against our hands and faces. For a brief time carefree. It was stunningly beautiful and some of the vistas reminded me of my climbs over the Himalayas—the sudden shift, again, from a horizontal to a vertical world.

In 1956 my father came to London for nine months to do the Diploma of Public Health course. He was preparing to return to England after his next tour of duty in Nigeria. My mother came with him. This gave Elaine a chance to get to know my parents. It was also the first time since leaving Nottingham that I had spent time with them as an adult. I was surprised by how well they accepted our new relationship. They bought a car while in London and left it for me to look after when they returned to Nigeria.

When we could spare the time from our studies, Elaine and I visited her parents in Frodsham as well as my extended family in Worksop. Easter, Christmas and Whitsun holidays were split between the two places.

Our second year on the wards was also organized into three-month firms, during which we covered the subspecialties—obstetrics, gynaecology, paediatrics, ear, nose and throat, eyes, psychiatry, dermatology and anaesthesia. For some of these subspecialties we had to go to satellite hospitals, such as the Evelina for paediatrics and St. Olives for anaesthesia and ENT. The time spent in each specialty could vary, but it was always a minimum of four weeks. Some specialties were taught during the same three month block: for example, dermatology, psychiatry, and eyes. Learning to give anaesthetics safely received special emphasis. At the time junior house staff in hospitals around the country were responsible for giving short anaesthetics in casualty departments which could be a frightening and hazardous situation for both patients and staff alike. I only appreciated how good my training was when years later I was faced with giving an anaesthetic in Uganda.

Obstetrics and Gynaecology was a major subject. We spent four weeks at Guy's and four weeks at a peripheral hospital. District midwifery was being phased out and not many students actually delivered babies at home. Some students went as far as the Rotunda Hospital in Dublin for their midwifery experience. They returned with some fanciful tales, seemingly more imaginative than scientific, about district midwifery and how it was practiced there. I wondered if they had been sprinkled with fairy dust or had taken a Guinness tour instead of attending to their duties but all gave a passionate defence of what they'd observed.

We were divided up into groups of two or four for our obstetrical experience. Mike Boundy and I ended up in Farnborough which is just south of London. Farnborough maternity unit was quite large. There were two consultants. It was also a midwifery training school and medical students were part of this program. During our training we had to deliver a minimum of forty babies and, as we were in competition with the midwives to get our quota of deliveries, we got to know the student midwives well. We were expected to participate in all the duties that the midwives performed which included giving enemas, cleaning up after deliveries, making beds, collecting specimens and checking up on the patients and the babies afterwards. We soon learned that getting on with the female students could lighten our duties considerably as they would take pity on us and help with some of these duties.

Students were expected to go to the operating theatres to assist with both elective and emergency gynaecology cases. Here I witnessed surgeries for ectopic pregnancies and twisted ovarian cysts. I also assisted at several abdominal and vaginal hysterectomies, learned how to perform a diagnostic dilatation and curettage, and how to evacuate a uterus after an incomplete miscarriage.

I was lucky to see a set of twins being delivered as well as a breech presentation. A couple of times I was shown how to use obstetric forceps. I witnessed several forceps deliveries and was the second assistant for three caesarean sections. During my time on obstetrics I helped to look after a young woman with pre-eclamptic fits. Sitting watching a semi-conscious person in a dark room waiting for the next fit to start was traumatic and brought home the dangers that can accompany pregnancy. During this time, I watched mothers suffer through the sad and haunting agony of stillbirth and neonatal death. My exposure to these lesser known tragedies was heartbreaking, but important to see as a doctor-in-training. For me, sharing their loss and their grief enlarged my capacity to be human.

Emergencies in obstetrics were very stressful because two lives were at stake, typically during the sudden onset of acute fetal distress. One minute all was well, with the happy expectant mother labouring in moderate comfort, and the next moment everyone was worried whether the baby was going to survive long enough to be delivered. The patient had to be moved to the theatre while the anaesthetist, surgeon, operating staff and paediatrician all had to come in immediately for the delivery. Time and speed became critical factors. Any minor delays might be life-threatening to the baby. It was impossible to keep these concerns from the mother, so understandably she became upset and frightened. The mother's safety was also paramount. Often patients might have been eating and drinking fluids before coming into hospital, which presented the anaesthetist with potential complications. The entire drama became tense, scary and of the greatest urgency for everyone concerned.

For paediatrics we went to the Evelina hospital, a specialist children's hospital close to Guy's. At Evelina I saw both outpatients and inpatients and was expected to clerk the latter. My time there coincided with the winter flu season so I had to work in the steam room. This room had ten beds and cots enclosed by glass. It was kept at a humidity level of one hundred percent and at a temperature distinctly higher than the rest of the ward. The goal in this instance was to relieve the symptoms of children with croup. Admitted with severe respiratory distress, these children were often blue because they could not get enough oxygen into their lungs. They recovered rapidly in the steam room and with the application of oxygen. Some children were sent there to have their asthmatic attacks treated; they also improved in the hot, humid conditions.

A ten-bed children's ward was designated solely for treating the complications of primary tuberculosis. I saw children with collapsed lungs, abscesses, peritonitis and one child who had been diagnosed with TB meningitis. Most of these children were severely ill and if they did not respond to treatment were not expected to live. The ones who did survive were likely to be handicapped for life with brain damage or other long-term medical issues.

Other children's wards treated patients with complications from infectious diseases such as mumps, measles, chickenpox and whooping cough. To prevent the spread of these diseases, we followed stringent isolation protocols.

Acute rheumatic fever was another common reason for admission to the hospital. Rheumatic fever was a complication of a strep throat infection which could damage the valves of the heart and cause heart failure. The severity and implications of this infection were brought to our attention in graphic detail far too often.

We assisted juvenile diabetics (those with type 1 diabetes) who presented with major medical symptoms and needed continual follow-up with blood and electrolyte tests after they were stabilized. Although insulin was available, it was derived from pork and beef pancreases and many patients developed intolerance to it. Monitoring blood sugar levels on a daily basis back then was much more difficult than it is today. It had to be done using urine tests for sugar; blood tests took longer to get back. Long-acting insulins were just becoming available and all treatment methods were individualized.

In the mid-1950s, despite a massive immunization program undertaken as soon as the first polio vaccine was made available early in the decade, polio or infantile paralysis was still prevalent and there was a ward for patients recovering from this viral infection. Those children requiring respirator support were transferred to the polio unit.

The surgical side of paediatrics dealt predominantly with ears, nose and throat problems. I helped remove a lot of tonsils and adenoids.

There was a small neurological-surgical unit which I found especially depressing because the outlook for these children was so grim. Even more depressing was the chronic care hospital for children at Carlshalton, where I spent a week in September when the blue skies were at their clearest and the summer harvest was most abundant.

Carlshalton was an old, dark grey stone building, with a large wooden gate entrance which was usually closed. There was a smaller pedestrian door to one side. Damp concrete corridors led to the wards. The chronic care section housed approximately a hundred patients in four wards. One ward was reserved for girls between ten and sixteen, with incurable rheumatic heart disease. Because of their heart failure, these girls could not get out of bed without becoming short of breath.

When listening to their hearts it was possible to hear all the murmurs that damaged heart valves can produce. None of these girls was expected to live more than a few months and yet they were quite cheerful. The additional wards in this hospital housed mentally challenged and terminally ill children with muscular dystrophies, hydrocephalus, microcephalus, spastic palsy, and other untreatable illnesses.

The week I spent on these wards was my most depressing as a medical student. There was nothing medicine could do to treat damaged heart valves. The simple truth was that the girls were all going to die. A common bacterium (strep) had migrated from their throats into their hearts and damaged them. Each day I realized only a special kind of person could find their calling in this field of medical care.

The arrangement at Willow Road continued with Elaine coming down from her flat up the road to help with cooking and running our place. She also found it more comfortable to study in our sitting room than her own flat, which was small and damp. We always had a lot to talk about; and when we didn't, we welcomed each other's silences and the promise of new discoveries to come. One evening, in January 1957, a few months after my parents had returned to Nigeria, we were alone in the flat and I decided this would be a good time to speak my heart.

I could foresee a time, once Elaine qualified, in about a year, when we would be separated. She would be doing house jobs while I continued my studies—a dismal prospect. I feared that, once apart, we might never get together again. I wanted to get married and live together as a married couple.

That evening I steeled my nerve and popped the question.

"Will you marry me?"

After quite a long pause, which got me wondering if I should have kept quiet, she said softly and coyly, "Yes."

I was taken aback by her hesitation, but relieved. And delighted. I rushed on to my next question, perhaps a little too hurriedly.

"When do you think we should get married?"

"That's more difficult to answer," she said. "When did you have in mind?"

"You have one more year to go, and I have two, before I qualify. Once you qualify you'll be off to do house jobs and I'll be here. Then it'll be my turn to do house jobs. I was thinking it could be a stressful time for us and that any long-term wedding plans could run into scheduling problems. Perhaps we should get married sooner rather than later. That way we have a year together before we have to go off in different directions."

Elaine thought for a moment. "We could get married on the first of March which is a couple of months away, but there would be a lot of planning to do. Much confusion. We need to notify the Registry Office about when and where we are going to get married. If we plan it that soon I don't think we can arrange for a church wedding in Frodsham. And your parents are in Nigeria for another two years."

"Do you think your parents would be willing to arrange something less formal?" I wondered.

"I don't know, but I'll ask them when I'm up there in a couple of weeks' time. First I need to know how they feel about our getting married. In the meantime, you'd better write to your parents and see what they think. Remember, you're still dependent on them for living expenses."

I was amazed by how practical Elaine was being, while I was a bundle of nerves and anticipation.

"I do have another reason for suggesting the wedding take place right away. I have to confess, I'm not altogether happy with our arrangement here. We're all crammed in together eating, working, and sleeping in this apartment and there's minimal privacy. The walls are so thin. It's time for us to find our own place. I want us to be on our own. What day of the week is the first of March anyway?"

"I think it's a Friday. As I recall, we were half-planning on a bottle party with the Fishers on that day. If we get married here we could make that a reception. We haven't got any money for anything else. It's a thought anyway."

I wrote to my parents the next day. Mother replied immediately and was very pleased with the idea. She agreed that we shouldn't wait and was sorry that she and Father would miss the ceremony. A few days later I got a rare letter from Father who was less enthusiastic about the idea. He stressed that marriage was a big step to take and wanted to make sure I had taken everything into consideration. He mentioned the responsibilities of being a husband, the prospects of having a family which, he reminded me, was not always easy to plan, and then emphasized the point that I would then become responsible for looking after Elaine. But it was our decision and he hoped we would be happy. He also said that he would continue with my allowance until I finished Medical School, but quickly added that under no circumstances could he increase it. Then he suggested that when we got married we should take the time off for a proper honeymoon. For some reason he felt this ritual was a very important part of getting married.

Elaine visited her parents the next weekend. When she got back she was rather quiet. After supper, she confessed the atmosphere at home had not been good. "My father said that I would be on my own when I got married. He would no longer provide my allowance. He thinks I'll stop my studies once I get married and that will mean three years of tuition money and expense money wasted. Mother was also not pleased. In short, I received no help or advice."

"What do *you* think we should do?" I asked. I had half-expected them to be ambivalent about the idea, not out of any dislike for me, but for fear that marriage would end her career. Neither of us saw their concern as a problem. Quite the reverse. Dual careers in medicine was very much a part of our attraction to each other.

Elaine paused and examined her hands as if they held a record of possibilities. "My grandmother has promised me two hundred pounds when I get married. That's equivalent to eight months of Father's allowance and, as far as I know, there are no strings attached to the money. I also get a few pounds each month from my County Council grant and I don't think there's any risk of that being stopped if I get married. So we should be able to manage for a year if your parents continue with your allowance."

The idea of getting married on the first of March continued to appeal to us. We had two student friends who were married and we talked to them at some length. After more thought we decided that we would go ahead with our plans. We invited my cousin Anne, Mike Boundy and Emma, Mike Wynne and Jean, as well as Mick and Joan to the ceremony. Elaine talked to the Fishers upstairs about holding the reception party.

My sister Marjory was in Birmingham visiting our Aunt Alice while on leave from the WRAF. Unfortunately the invitation I sent her did not get to her in time for her to arrange a trip to London for the wedding. We decided not to let Elaine's parents or my aunt in Worksop know of our final decision. In hindsight this was a bit selfish and perhaps thoughtless, but we knew what their response would be and were concerned they might try to stop us. I wrote to my parents giving them the wedding date and got a nice letter back from them wishing us all the best. Elaine found a one-room flat to rent in Belsize, just south of Hampstead Heath, so we had somewhere to live once we were married.

We got married on March 1, 1957, in the Registry Office in Hampstead and had a "reception/bottle" party in the Fishers' art studio. About seventy-five medical students and some of the Fisher's art crowd came to the party. Elaine and Lillian made the cake and Mike Boundy took the photographs. We escaped for a brief weekend stay on the coast near Brighton, which was all we could afford. Nor could we afford the time away from our studies. Nonetheless, I like to think my father would have been pleased with this small gesture.

We did not keep the event a secret. We wrote to all our relatives letting them know that we were married and giving them our new address. As expected, Elaine's parents disowned us. My Aunt Ethel wrote me the most chilling letter I have ever received. I still have it as a reminder of how easy it is to upset other people, unintentionally. Never again did we raise the topic of our marriage with Grandfather, Ethel or George, but years later my Aunt Alice told me that she had not been aware of how much Ethel had been opposed to our actions.

Our one-room flat was uncomfortable and inconvenient to Guy's by train. We were able to use the shower facilities at the hospital gyms, but our room was too small for both of us to study. There was no kitchen which meant that we ended up eating at the hospital cafeteria—an added expense. Elaine started house-hunting again and found a two-room flat with kitchen and bathroom on the ground floor in Hungerford Road, about six houses up the hill from Hungerford Prison. It was within easy walking distance of the Northern Line and the price was affordable, so we took it.

Not long after we had settled into our new flat we discovered Elaine was pregnant, but since there were only a few months left before she qualified we felt we could manage. Ironically, Elaine's mother wrote to us at this time suggesting that Elaine visit home soon to "show herself." There were rumours going around the village that Elaine had had to get married. After her visit the ice was broken and the relationship with her family improved. I visited my aunt in Worksop that Christmas, but the topic of our marriage was not raised and the only comment Ethel made was that she thought Elaine was a bit of a cradle-snatcher. This observation astounded and amused me—Ethel was ten years older than George while Elaine was only one year older than me.

Our time in Hungerford Road was a happy one. Helen, our daughter, was born on August 16, 1958. My mother was in England at the time. She was with us for the birth and helped Elaine with the new baby. The only stressful occurrence was that Elaine failed one of her M.B. B.S. exams, which was a first for her—she wasn't pleased. She had to revise and rewrite the exam and this put her plans to qualify back by six months.

In our third year of clinical practice my class returned to general medicine and surgery, but we were now the senior students on the firms. We were involved in more of the day-to-day care of patients and made some decisions about ordering tests and even medications, although we were supervised very closely by the housemen and the senior nursing staff. Rounds were more nerve-wracking as the consultants would frequently ridicule us if we did not know the answers to questions they asked. This increased pressure helped to prepare us for our final exams, which were now only a few months away.

My class was expected to take the University of London's M.B.B.S. exams (Bachelor of Medicine, Bachelor of Surgery), which were held in the summer, as well as the College of Physicians and Surgeons examinations called the Conjoint Exams. These exams were held two to three months ahead of the London M.B.B.S. exams and passing them allowed one to register with the British Medical Council. Once you were registered you were able to start the required internship year. It also meant that you could do locums. These jobs were usually replacing house doctors who were on holiday or on leave. In our household, earning money was becoming a very serious consideration so I decided to take the Conjoint exams. Working locums would provide us with an income and would be good practice for the coming M.B.B.S. exams.

By this time my class was becoming quite confident about our clinical skills and we were now expected to help the junior students find their way around. This interaction was my first experience in a teaching role. Although it was a short-lived responsibility I found teaching engaging and seductive. I began to understand some of the difficulties and frustrations involved when helping others learn, remember and use taught information. Pedagogy gave me a new insight into and appreciation of what a career in medicine could achieve.

The last two units at Guy's were an elective and a revision course designed to teach us how to take exams. I chose Urology as my elective because it was supposed to be a light firm, and thus would leave me more time for studying. This was important if I were to have any hope with the Conjoint Exams. There were four main exams held every three months. I decided to take the whole lot at once in October 1958. I was successful in general medicine and surgery, but failed Obstetrics and Gynaecology and Pathology. I sat those exams again in three months and was successful. I immediately informed Elaine of my results. We had been living apart for a short time while I finished my exams and while she fulfilled her houseman duties. When

Helen was six and half months old, in March of 1959, Elaine's mother promised to help look after her granddaughter if Elaine could get a house job nearby. Elaine's parents had moved to The Wirral (an area in Cheshire quite close to Chester Hospital) from Frodsham. Luckily, Elaine managed to find a house job in Chester Hospital and she moved into her parent's house with Helen, thus saving us the expense of maintaining two residences.

As I prepared to sit my M.B.B.S. final exams, I continued to search for work. These finals were gruelling. I had to write two three-hour papers in each subject, followed by six clinical examinations, two in each speciality. I was required to see a patient for twenty minutes and then present the history to two examiners who could ask me to demonstrate my findings or spend ten minutes discussing the case. I was surprised by the depth into which the examiners went. These tests were followed by ten minute *viva voces* in each speciality. At these sessions there were two examiners who took turns asking questions and the exams went on for four to six weeks.

Once I was qualified I knew I would have to apply for locum jobs as a houseman. I felt I should try for my first locum somewhere nearby so I asked the Medical School Office for assistance. A few days later they suggested I might go to St. Mary's Paddington for a two-week medical houseman's locum. My interview was set for the following Monday. Since I was running a bit late that day I borrowed a car and parked it just outside the hospital and rushed into the interview. The interview went well and I was asked to start work in a week's time. I was elated although the glow of my success was soon removed. When I got back to the car a policeman was writing out a ticket for illegal parking—the penalty, a two-pound fine—an expensive start to paying my own way.

The locum job paid the grand sum of twenty-four pounds after taxes. Even so, my first pay cheque seemed like a "king's ransom".

* * *

After my short locum at Paddington, I was determined to find more permanent work, closer to Elaine and Helen. There were no jobs in Chester but I found a six-month position in Shrewsbury, which was only thirty-five minutes from Chester by train.

In Shrewsbury my job was as a house surgeon to Mr. Lincoln-Lewis, a consultant and well-known surgeon who had his M.S. (Master of Surgery), as well as the FRCS. He proved to be a good teacher who enjoyed mentoring new physicians. There were rumours that he had come to Shrewsbury to get away from the politics of London and to collect fine antique furniture.

My next house job was in general medicine at Chester City Hospital where Elaine was working and we were allowed to share a room. Because she was also a medical houseman, we were on call alternate nights and we did not get any time off together. Besides, Elaine was anxious to go to her mother's to see Helen whenever she could. Elaine and I would go up to "Weatherall", her parents' house, together when we were off at the same time. Nonetheless tension still remained and I never went to see Helen on my own.

When I found a placement in Chester my job was working for a consultant who specialized in heart disease while Elaine's boss specialized in respiratory diseases. Between the two of us we got a good grounding in the things that can go wrong with the heart and lungs. After three months, we had to decide what we would do next. Elaine felt that she should take a break from work to look after Helen who was now eighteen months old.

Even with two incomes and paid housing we were not saving any money. More of an issue, as far as I was concerned, was that Helen was living full-time with Elaine's parents. We didn't have any debts, but if Elaine were to quit working I could see that my houseman salary alone wouldn't be sufficient to sustain us. The other option was to find a GP's assistant position, but I wasn't sure that my obstetric and paediatric experience was enough to embark on that line of work.

A third option was to look abroad for employment. In essence, to follow in my father's footsteps. This possibility set us looking for jobs in the overseas section of the *British Medical Journal*. One morning

I found an advertisement for a job as an intern at the Grace Hospital in Winnipeg, Canada. The job description stated that the internship would rotate though general medicine, surgery, obstetrics, gynaecology and paediatrics. The salary was twice what I was getting in Chester and included married accommodation. In addition to these perks, the hospital was offering to pay for either a return airline ticket or one-way tickets for up to three family members. One of the hospital's orthopaedic surgeons was scheduled to visit London and would be available to interview any interested physicians during his stay.

This opportunity looked like an ideal way for us to gain new experience, see North America, and secure the extra training I thought I needed. The only commitment was that I would have to work there for a year and pay for our way back to England. After considerable discussion we decided that I should at least go for an interview.

Dr. Welpley, the orthopaedic surgeon from Winnipeg, was staying at the Savoy in London while he was on holiday in England. He invited me to have lunch with him one Saturday in April, 1960. Dr. Welpley had also finished his medical training in London. He had immigrated to Canada several years before so he had a good idea of the impact of the decision I was about to make. The décor of the hotel, elegant and tasteful, was intimidating, while lunch was a radical departure from the cafeteria fare to which I had become accustomed. We were seated in a quiet corner of the dining room.

"Why are you interested in coming to Winnipeg?" he asked.

"For a combination of reasons," I said. "First, I feel I need some further training. At the moment I'm uncomfortable with my knowledge of obstetrics and paediatrics. And second, my wife and I are interested in visiting North America where, from what we've been told, the training and medical practices are quite different from what we've experienced. Finally, if we stay in England, out-of-hospital accommodation is prohibitive."

I paused and studied him. "What would my job at the Grace Hospital entail?"

"It would be similar to what you're doing at the moment except the patients are admitted and looked after by general practitioners.

Your job will be to admit patients, take histories, assist at operations and generally help look after day-to-day patient care. You will get a better idea of what general practice involves. There are no consultant firms and the surgeons do not have blocks of operating time. You will not be attached to any specific surgeon or specialist as you are here. You work for the hospital to help care for inpatients who are primarily looked after by their admitting GP."

"What obstetric and paediatric experience can I expect to get?"

"The plan at the moment is that all the interns will have one month of obstetric experience and eight weeks of paediatrics at the Children's Hospital, which is part of the University. During the rest of the year you would be a rotating intern covering general medicine, surgery and orthopaedic surgery. However, if any of the interns have special interests we will attempt to accommodate them. The jobs are recognized by the Canadian College of Physicians and Surgeons for the purpose of getting registered in Canada. However, your British work and qualifications are accepted by the Manitoba College of Physicians and Surgeons.

"I've worked in both systems, the private system in Canada and under the National Health Service in England. There are, of course, some problems with both systems but I prefer the greater input that physicians have in the Canadian system. I must say that economically we are better off."

I found the last part of his answer exactly what I wanted to hear. More money coming in with accommodation included might be exactly what would convince Elaine to take the risk. It would give her valuable time with Helen, something lacking from both of our lives for far too long. We needed time together as a family.

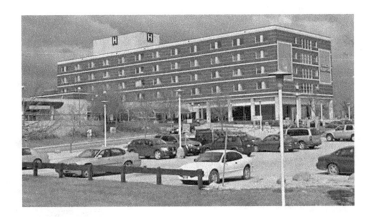

In the 1960s Bernard practiced medicine in a variety of settings, including Grace Hospital in Winnipeg, Manitoba (top), hospitals in the newly independent country of Uganda (right and bottom), as well as the United Kingdom.

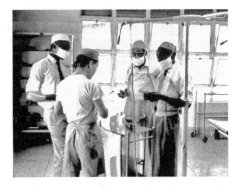

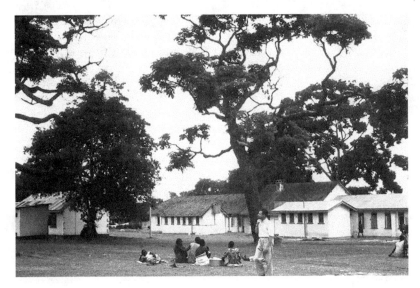

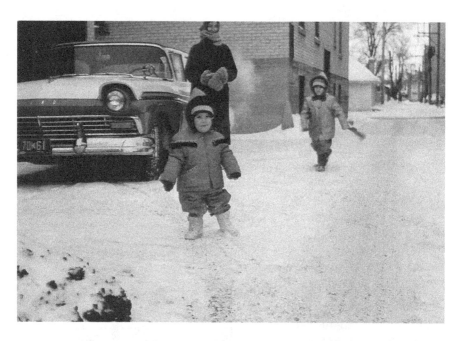

Bernard, Elaine and their young children making the most of a cold and snowy Winnipeg winter in the 1961.

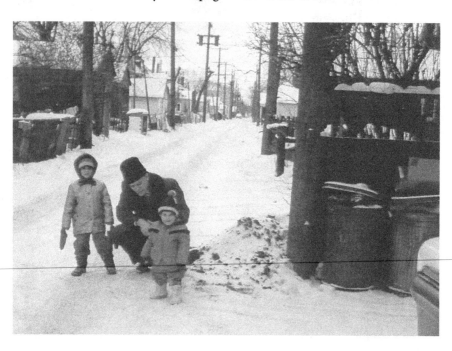

Chapter 8
Canada: The First Time

Making the decision to go to Canada was the easy part. Elaine and I soon discovered that there were several hoops to jump through before actually travelling. The most troublesome were the two interviews at Canada House in London. These were difficult to arrange because I was working full-time as a houseman in Chester.

The first interviewer was from Toronto and he was curious to know why we were planning to go to Winnipeg. He could not understand why anyone would choose that part of the country over Ontario. I explained that I had been offered a job there and we thought it would be a good starting point from which to explore Canada, especially since we didn't know anything about Winnipeg or the Prairies. He seemed satisfied with this explanation, wished me luck, and hoped we would at least have a look at Eastern Canada. In passing he mentioned that Toronto was a long way from Winnipeg, three to four hours by airplane. He also suggested we should apply for full immigration status and not for a one-year work permit. He felt that doing this would make our lives a lot easier if we decided to stay for longer than a year, which he felt was likely.

Once our application was approved the whole family had to return to Canada House for the second interview and for medical examinations, various tests, and vaccinations. This gave me the opportunity to talk to a Canadian physician about working conditions and Winnipeg. He was encouraging and felt that working in a private practice would not be a problem. By the time we had been processed for the move Elaine had finished her house jobs and was fully registered with the General Medical Council. She wanted to try General Practice and, because her mother was still willing to look after Helen, she applied for a GP locum in the Chester area. She got the job and worked for several weeks. This gave her good experience and helped a bit with our meagre bank balance. In the meantime, I finished my house job and got registered with the GMC.

After lengthy discussions we decided I should go out to Canada first to test the waters in Winnipeg and make sure we would be comfortable. Most important, we needed to make sure the married accommodation promised was suitable.

In June 1960, I boarded a plane, my two suitcases having been checked. We left Heathrow at dusk. The night flight to Winnipeg was a long journey in a turboprop aircraft. We stopped at Gander, Montreal, and Toronto, each stop giving a new dimension to distance. This was the first time I had ever seen the arc of the earth.

Gander Airport, at that time, was quite busy. It was a major fuelling stop for transatlantic flights and one of the ports of entry into Canada. I had to go through Customs and Immigration there and was able to look around the large duty-free shopping area, even though with empty pockets. We refuelled again in Montreal and arrived in Toronto just before sunrise. In Toronto, I was told, I had a three-hour wait before catching my flight to Winnipeg.

Compared to Heathrow, Toronto's airport was small. I found a seat that looked out onto the runway, but there wasn't much to see. Inside the terminal, there were a few concession stores but they hadn't opened yet.

While waiting, I began to wonder what I was doing there, thousands of miles from home, my family and friends. From everything that was familiar. In spite of its British and French heritage, this was a foreign country with different customs and philosophies. Initially the idea of coming to Canada and North America seemed like an adventure, but while sitting alone in an empty lounge in an alien airport I began to have doubts.

I was thinking that perhaps we had made a big mistake, when I noticed that the sky over the runway was brightening. Purple grey steaks changed to bright red reflecting off some high cirrus clouds. Then the horizon changed to a brilliant red-orange and the halo of the yellow sun, increasingly dazzling, edged its way up over the runway. The rest of the sky turned from black to a deep blue. Although the sunrise lasted only a few minutes it cheered me up and I began to feel more optimistic about our decision.

I noticed the smell of coffee and heard some clattering just around the corner from where I was sitting. My flight wasn't due to depart for another hour, so I stood up, stretched and walked to the small coffee bar that had just opened. Behind a counter with glass panels there were a variety of snacks with unfamiliar names. The girl behind the counter saw me looking at them. Perhaps she saw the look of puzzlement on my face.

"Can I get you something?" she asked.

"The coffee smells good and the buns look appetizing but I don't have any Canadian money on me," I replied.

"What sort of money do you have then?"

"I have a couple of English pounds."

"I think we can exchange them for you. What would you like to try?"

"A coffee with milk and sugar and one of those spiral cinnamon buns. They look awfully good. I haven't seen them before. What are they like?"

"They're quite yummy. Sweet and sticky with a cinnamon taste. You'll need a knife and a paper serviette."

Armed with a coffee, paper napkin, knife, butter, and cinnamon bun, I returned to where I'd been sitting and watched the start of the day on the runway. A plane came in and docked just outside the window where I was sitting. Two men pushed a set of stairs up to the plane and the door opened. About forty passengers spilled out and came in through the gate. Most of them were wearing light business suits, but a few, including children, were casually dressed in shorts, holiday shirts and light summer dresses.

Eventually my flight arrived and was ready for boarding. We walked out to the plane and I was amazed at how hot it was so early in the morning. The plane was a North Star—designed specifically by Douglas for Trans-Canada Air Lines—which carried about fifty passengers. The takeoff was noisy and reminiscent of my first flight to Nigeria in 1950. A breakfast consisting of waffles, crispy bacon and maple syrup was served shortly after takeoff. This North American-style breakfast was a pleasant surprise.

From my window seat I had a good view of the landscape as we flew to Winnipeg. At first we flew over farmland, the farms mostly rectangular and not very large. Most of the crops were vegetables, but many fields grew a bushy plant with dark green foliage that I didn't recognize. I later discovered it was tobacco. An hour out we passed over a huge lake which I surmised must have been one of the famous Great Lakes I had been taught about at school. I looked it up on the map in the airline magazine tucked in the seat pocket in front of me—Lake Huron. Later we flew over part of Lake Superior. The vastness of these lakes astounded me. They dwarfed the other lakes I'd seen. Next we flew over the Precambrian Shield with its thousands of smaller lakes and boundless coniferous forests. I could see the occasional road but there were very few towns or villages. The topography appeared to be rocky and relatively flat. But it was the sheer endlessness, a new form of duration, which impressed me the most.

As we drew closer to Winnipeg we crossed another lake dotted with thousands of islands of various sizes. Some of these had small buildings on them. I later discovered this was the Lake of the Woods and that I was looking at holiday cottages. Passing over the north shore of the lake, I spied clouds of white smoke and steam spewing from a pulp mill in the township of Dryden. Shortly after this, the landscape changed again, forming a giant grid map of large, strikingly square green fields and farmhouses. The fields were grain, mainly wheat, the earth powder dry as the occasional vehicle skittered along a road followed by a plume of reddish dust. We had arrived at the start of the famous Canadian Prairies. The land would be flat all the way to Winnipeg—then on for another thousand miles before rising into the Rocky Mountain foothills.

As we approached Winnipeg the pilot came on the intercom to tell us that it was a glorious summer day with a slight breeze. The temperature was ninety degrees Fahrenheit! We had to walk about a hundred yards from the airplane to a small airport; ninety degrees felt stifling after sitting in a suit in the air-conditioned plane. I could feel the hot concrete through the soles of my shoes and was relieved to get into the air-conditioned terminal.

When I got to the baggage collection area I was approached by a middle-aged gentleman, wearing a light grey suit. He was quite athletic looking with a roundish face, his blue eyes slightly hooded. "You must be Dr. Binns," he said with what I thought was a New Zealand or Australian accent.

"Yes," I replied.

"I'm Dr. McCreath, the medical superintendent at the Grace Hospital. Your bags will appear over there shortly." He pointed to a one-foot-high platform area about fifteen yards away. "Do you have much luggage?' he asked.

"No, just the two allowable suitcases. They're quite heavy, though," I said as we walked over to the platform.

"You've arrived at one of the nicest times of the year. It's not too hot yet and the trees have got their foliage. The dust isn't too bad and the mosquitoes are still tolerable. We haven't had much rain yet this year. I think you'll find Winnipeg a nice city to work in but you will also find that things are a bit different from the UK. I did my postgraduate training in London and worked there for a few years before coming here. There is plenty to do in your spare time which you'll have more of than you did during your pre-registration year."

"That'll be a nice change. Elaine, my wife," I explained, "and I didn't get much time off and we've been working in different hospitals for the past year."

When my luggage appeared, he picked up one suitcase and I took the other and we walked out to the car park. About fifty cars were parked in the lot, nearly all of them American models, mainly Fords, Chevys, Buicks and Chryslers. What struck me was the size of these vehicles. They were enormous compared to cars in England.

"Mine's the dark red Buick," he said pointing to a car ahead of us.

By the time we had walked fifty yards I felt suffocated by the heat. It reminded me of my arrival in Kano, Northern Nigeria. As we got nearer to his car I noticed there was an electrical plug in front of each parking space.

"What are all those plugs for?" I asked.

"Oh, in this heat they must seem a bit absurd if not ironic. They're the plugs for the car block heaters. It gets very cold during the winter months and if a car is left unplugged for more than three or four hours, there's a good chance it won't start, especially if it's an older model with an old battery. But don't worry about that yet. Fall doesn't arrive until the end of September and the really cold weather occurs in January."

"That's good news," I said.

"You'll find that you're a lot better off here than you were in the UK and you'll be in the market for a car within a month or so." We got to his car and he opened the very large boot—trunk, he informed me, in North America. There was more than enough room for my two bags. Automatically I walked around to the left side of the car and he said, "Sorry, Bernie, you can't drive yet. You'll probably go down the wrong side of the road, which might startle a few of the locals!"

"Right. I forgot, you drive on the other side of the road here."

Dr. McCreath laughed. "You'll soon get used to the idea."

We climbed into his Buick, which was the largest car I'd ever been in. It was even bigger than the luxury car that had picked up Elaine and me when we had been hitchhiking in France. The seats were a deep red leather and very luxurious. The engine was quiet, the interior air-conditioned, a new innovation to me.

"This is a very nice car," I said.

"These cars are very different from European models. You'll see a few English and other European cars in Winnipeg, but they don't run well in winter when it gets down into the minus thirties."

By this time we were out of the parking lot and heading south towards Winnipeg. Once again I was overwhelmed by the sheer flatness of the place. I could see the city about ten miles away and noticed there were not many multi-storey buildings. The road we were driving along was straight and the intersections were all at right angles. Major intersections were controlled by traffic lights, not roundabouts. The road, though straight, was quite rough and dusty with a lot of pot holes, some of which were quite deep. I noticed that Dr. McCreath was careful to avoid them as much as possible. The sun was glaring and the air dusty. And yet we rode in plush comfort inside the car.

"Two big rivers merge at the centre of Winnipeg," he explained as we passed over a bridge, "the Red River and the Assiniboine. The Red comes from Minnesota and the Assiniboine from Saskatchewan. By the time they get here they are big rivers and after joining they flow north to Lake Winnipeg, which is some five hundred miles long. The lake empties into the Nelson River which ends up in Hudson Bay."

"That's a big lake. How far is it from here?" I asked.

"About fifty miles. It's said that you could take England and Wales and drop them into the lake and lose them."

"What surprises me is the small population. It's much less than the UK."

"Yes, and seventy five percent of the people live within seventy-five miles of the American border," he said. "That's a pretty thin line when you consider the border is more than 5,400 miles long."

We had arrived in the city outskirts and were passing through a residential area. The houses consisted mainly of two-storey, wood frame dwellings, which stood close to each other. Most houses had lawns and small flower beds in front. There were sidewalks next to the road, lined by oak, spruce, fir, pine, silver birches, elms and willows. We arrived at Portage Avenue, a four-lane highway fronted by two- and three-storey commercial buildings.

"This is one of the two main roads in Winnipeg. It runs east-west and joins up with Main Street about three miles east of here. Main runs north-south and crosses the Red River before reaching the US border, about seventy miles south of here. The hospital is just off Portage on Arlington Street. We're almost there," he said, turning left onto Portage Avenue.

"We've placed you in a room in a house just opposite the hospital until your apartment is ready. But don't worry, it'll be ready well before your wife and daughter arrive."

After turning onto Arlington Street, a large red brick building appeared on the right. Over the entrance concrete letters identified the building as the Salvation Army Grace Hospital.

"Here we are. This is the front entrance to the Hospital. The Emergency and Ambulance entrances are at the back, which is reached by going down the parallel road, Evanson Street. Your digs are here," he said as we pulled up in front of a two-storey wood-frame house.

"Come, I'll introduce you to the Boychucks. They're an elderly Ukrainian couple. By the way, there are quite a few Ukrainians, Mennonites and Hutterites in Manitoba. There's also a whole area of Winnipeg called St. Boniface which is predominantly French Canadian. It's south and east of the Red River. They account for nearly forty percent of Winnipeg's population."

We got out of the car, fetched my luggage from the trunk, and climbed the stairs to the front door. As we stood waiting for someone to answer, Dr. McCreath took a quick, somewhat furtive look at me.

"If you're not too tired," he said finally, "you might drop by my office after you've unpacked. It's on the ground floor, beyond the foyer. You can't miss it."

After meeting the Boychucks, unpacking my few things and stowing them away in an old-fashioned wardrobe, I walked over to the hospital through a blast of heat. Entering the building I was surprised by how cool it felt. Then I heard the hum of the air-conditioning system. I was soon to learn that this was an essential piece of equipment in the heat and humidity of a Manitoba summer—neither patients nor medical staff would have survived without it.

The first thing Dr. McCreath did was introduce me to Colonel Gage, the Salvation Army hospital administrator. She was a charming person, with an expression of contentment on her face. She was interested in learning why I had decided to come to Winnipeg. She assured me that I could always come to her office at any time to discuss any problems I encountered in the hospital, but added that Dr. McCreath was the Medical Director and that medical problems were to go to him. Dr. McCreath then gave me a brief tour of the hospital before I returned to my room and collapsed on my bed in a stupor. The trip had seemed interminable; I was a long, long way from home.

* * *

Over the next few days I discovered that the Grace Hospital had two hundred and fifty beds for general medical and surgical care including elective Orthopaedics, Obstetrics and Gynaecology. There were no Neurosurgical or Paediatric patients. These were referred to the Winnipeg General or St. Boniface hospitals. There was an on-call Anaesthesia Department and a twenty-four hour Emergency Department. Bacteriology, routine chemistry and general pathology, including autopsies, were done in the hospital. X-ray and cardiac assessment departments were also on the premises. Like a lot of hospitals, there were new and old parts of the building. The new wing (about ten years old) housed the Obstetrics Department, Emergency, the operating rooms and the hospital cafeteria. The older part of the hospital accommodated the patient wards.

Unlike the hospitals I had previously worked in, the wards were divided up into rooms that contained two, four or six beds. Each ward also had a couple of single rooms. Initially I thought this would be rather inconvenient and difficult to work in, but the rooms were larger than they were at home and they were definitely more private for the patients. The corridors in the older part of the hospital were only just adequate for transporting patients on stretchers. The patients were segregated into male/female Surgical and Medical Wards.

To look after the inpatients there was a "medical staff" that consisted of specialist consultants to whom the general practitioners referred their patients directly. For elective procedures patients were seen privately outside the hospital in doctors' offices or medical clinics and only came to the hospital for the procedure to be done. Patients in the Emergency Department or obstetrics were initially seen by their family physicians.

A high proportion of the patients were admitted and looked after by their general practitioners who had varying degrees of operating or care privileges. The medical staff did not confine their activities to one hospital and most consultants saw patients at more than one. These included the larger Winnipeg General and St. Boniface hospitals, which dealt with more complicated medical and surgical problems.

The junior hospital staff, which included me, consisted of one senior resident and ten interns who came from various parts of the world and had different levels of experience. Five of us were from the UK. One was a Canadian trained in the UK. Two were from India and two from Czechoslovakia. Our senior resident was a trained surgeon who had decided to immigrate to Canada from England. The rest of us were recent graduates except for the two Czechoslovakians who were both middle-aged refugees and still had some language problems to overcome before being allowed to start private practice.

Unlike the UK hospital system there were no consultant "firms." Patients were admitted under their own family physicians, of whom there were about forty on staff. There were thirty specialists who covered surgical, orthopaedic, urological, paediatric, obstetrics/gynaecological and internal medicine consultations, as required. However, some of the specialists only attended patients at the Grace Hospital on an occasional basis.

On admission, all patients, except women in labour, were seen by one of the junior staff who completed a history and physical examination and then contacted the patient's doctor to let her or him know about the admission and get further orders for care. This gave us the opportunity to discuss patient management with the attending physicians. It meant that our responsibility for drug prescribing, investigation and planned management was much less than it had been in the UK, but the opportunity to discuss patient care with a wider group of physicians and consultants was greater. As most of the primary physicians were general practitioners this meant that we got a much better insight into what general practice was all about.

When consultants were involved we did get the opportunity to discuss cases with them on an informal basis and not as a part of the organized education of the junior staff. Our education was limited to two or three one-hour seminars per week where we received didactic lectures or had case presentations for discussion. These seminars were run by the consultant staff from the various departments. We did have to assist at surgical cases, but we were usually the second assistant. The general practitioners liked to be the first assistants.

There was an assistant's fee involved that I suspect accounted for their hands-on enthusiasm.

Once I got used to the different system I had far less responsibility for care and decision-making than I had had before. The good news was that I was only expected to work from 8 a.m. to 6 p.m. Monday to Friday; and to be on-call to cover emergency admissions twice a week and one weekend in four. Because of this system we saw a wide variety of clinical problems. I was pleasantly surprised when I got my first pay cheque after two weeks and found it was twice as much as I had been receiving in the UK. I was a bit concerned about not being involved in obstetrics and asked Dr. McCreath about it. He told me that obstetrics was not part of my rotation. He said he would look into it and discuss it with the Chief of Obstetrics.

At the same time I asked him about the married accommodation and was assured that it would be ready before Elaine and Helen arrived. This was timely news as they were booked to arrive in five weeks. I was surprised at how quickly I had become steeped in this variation on a medical theme and pleased with how quickly I had adapted. Yet I looked forward to being reunited with my family; to sharing this unfolding adventure with Elaine. Already I had much to tell her.

After the first few weeks a few of us started to explore Winnipeg. The downtown area was easily accessible by bus and had two large stores—the Hudson's Bay and Eaton's—near the junction of Portage and Main. This intersection had the reputation of being one of the coldest and windiest in the world. At the moment this notorious crossroads was benign. In a few months we would learn how ferocious the meeting of the winds could become.

Surrounding this core were several commercial buildings, including the Winnipeg Grain Exchange, banks, insurance companies, the Canadian Pacific railway station and other smaller shops and restaurants. Portage had four driving lanes with metered parking on either side of the street and an elevated dividing strip down the centre. Trolley buses with overhead power lines ran down the street. The tallest buildings, the Bay and Eaton's, dominated the south side of the street. They were seven storeys high with elevators and escalators between floors. Adjacent to these buildings were two multi-storey car parks with direct access into what were called "department stores", in which everything was sold—from clothing to hardware to furniture to paint to sporting equipment to kitchen goods.

This was totally different from shopping in England. Much of the merchandise was new to me. Refrigerators and cookers were much larger than those in England. The heavy-duty winter clothing on display, which included Russian-type fur hats, heavy coats, overshoes and parkas, seemed ridiculously inexpensive when compared to prices for these articles in the UK.

One afternoon I walked along South Main Street for about a mile. This route took me past the railway station which had an impressive gothic entrance, topped with a clock and turrets—an odd mixture of architectural designs. The station was the main loading area for grain being shipped either east or west from the Prairies. Passenger services were also available to Toronto in the east and Vancouver in the west. A branch line ran north to Churchill and another headed south to Fargo, North Dakota—Winnipeg was the hub of a transportation wheel. But the majority of trains transported freight.

Further along, the road crossed a bridge over the Assiniboine and then immediately intersected with a larger bridge which crossed the Red River. The Red River was flowing rapidly and was wider than the Thames at London Bridge. The water was muddy but I didn't see any rubbish riding its whirling current. I strolled up the sidewalk to the middle of the bridge and stopped to have a look. On the other side of the river I noticed a large building with a tower and a cross on top. A middle-aged man stopped next to me.

"The river's still high, isn't it?" he observed.

"Yes, I guess it is, although I have to confess this is the first time I've seen it. I've only been in Winnipeg for a couple of weeks."

"Where are you from?" he asked, with a trace of a European accent. "You sound English."

"Yes, that's right. I've come from the UK to work at the Grace Hospital. I'm doing a bit of exploring."

"This bridge crosses the Red River which flows north. Over there is an area called St. Boniface. That's where I live. It's predominantly French Canadian but we all speak English as well."

"What's that large building with the cross on top," I asked, pointing in the direction he was looking.

"St. Boniface, one of the two university hospitals. The other is the Winnipeg General, which is north of Portage Ave."

"Why is there a cross on top?" I asked.

"It's run by the Grey Nuns."

"That's interesting. The Grace is run by the Salvation Army. I've not come across hospitals run by religious organizations before. These are my first."

"It's quite common in Canada and the USA. They do a good job." He paused and glanced at his watch. As suddenly as he had stopped, he seemed anxious to be off. "Anyway, it's been nice talking to you. I'd better be on my way. *Bonne chance.*"

And with a slight bow at the waist and nod of his head, he continued his walk across the bridge. I wondered how many more times in my life I would have this sort of surprise encounter with complete strangers. Many, I suspected.

On my way back to the bus stop at Portage and Main I stopped at one of the car dealerships to look at some of the cars on the lot. Three of the other interns had bought cars and I knew it was not too difficult to arrange financing. I also realized it was going to be difficult living in Winnipeg without one. The city was so spread out.

The next day I was having coffee with Brian, Rodney and Goetz, three of the other interns, and I asked them what they thought I should do about a car. "You'll certainly need wheels when your family arrives," said Brian. The other two agreed.

"How long is it now before they get here?" asked Goetz.

"About five weeks. I can't in all conscience splurge on a car, especially when we're expecting another child in September. Elaine might question my priorities."

"Where are you going to be living?" asked Brian.

"They've promised us a flat in the Baldwin apartment block. I've not seen it yet. It's still occupied and they want to decorate it before we move in. What's yours like, Goetz?"

"Quite pleasant. And it's well-fitted out. We didn't have to buy any big items. It's on the third floor which is a bit inconvenient. The elevator's small and slow at times. But you can't beat the rent."

The next four weeks flew by. With Elaine's encouragement in a letter, Goetz and I went out to buy a car. We looked at some twenty models on different lots, and took several out for test drives. I took an immediate dislike to many of the aggressive salesmen. Eventually we ended up back at the lot by the bridge. Harry, the salesman, showed us a Ford with low mileage and in reasonable shape. After a bit of haggling I managed, with Goetz's help, to get him down to a thousand dollars, which I didn't feel I could afford. In the end, Goetz and Harry persuaded me to go for financing though the dealership over two years, with the option of paying off the loan any time after the first three months. There was a problem; I didn't have a credit rating. But after lengthy deliberation, the dealership decided to take a chance on me, and I purchased the car.

We found our new lives in Canada a bit topsy-turvy. So much seemed upside-down, backwards or slightly off-kilter. For example, when I told Brian that we had been allocated a flat in the Baldwin apartments he told me that he and Rodney, both bachelors, were in a flat at the top of the same block. This seemed an odd choice since the apartments also served as the Salvation Army's home for unwed mothers! Pregnant girls came to the Salvation Army for help—they came from Winnipeg, from other towns and cities in the province of Manitoba, and sometimes from remote parts of Canada. The young girls spent several weeks in the home before delivery and some lingered and spent time recovering after they had given birth. Most of these young women put their babies up for adoption; thus the place was not a nursery. All seemed so vulnerable. Brian and Rodney were decidedly out of place. Right away they discovered they had to obey the same house rules as everyone else, which included no partying and strict visiting hours for guests.

Before Elaine arrived, Brian, Rodney, and I spent many evenings out looking for good restaurants and pubs. But all we could find were barn-sized, bare-walled beer parlours, which were for "men only". We were taken aback when we were told that we could not move from one table to another with a drink in our hands. Later on we discovered that people were not allowed to have open liquor on the streets, in vehicles, or in the parks. To us these restrictions seemed uncivilized, if not punitive.

The only place where you could take a lady out for a drink was at a restaurant or cocktail lounge, for a meal or light snack. One day we went to a grocery store to buy some beer and liquor for a party but couldn't find any alcohol on the shelves. The proprietor told us that we had to go to the Liquor Commission down the road. Once we got there we found that we had to fill in a form listing what we wanted to buy and take it up to the counter. There were lists on the walls of what was available but we couldn't browse around looking at the wines before making a purchase. After shaking our heads at the "weirdness" of it all, things got even more surreal when we were asked to provide identification by the clerk, something we had never experienced in our home countries.

As we settled into our new lives, our Canadian colleagues raved about Winnipeg's lively theatre scene, its orchestra and art gallery, and the world-class ballet. None of us were prepared for the high quality and enthusiasm of the performances—the exuberance that one associates with youth. We were also told about the lakes and provincial parks that were within easy driving distance. We visited two of these lakes, the water crystal clear and warm, the beaches soft and sandy.

Family camping, swimming, fishing and boating were popular and the parks crowded at the weekends. The Manitoba mosquitoes soon found us and had a feast. The mosquitoes looked like anopheles, one of the malaria carriers. When I raised my concern I was told not to worry, there was no malaria in Manitoba. The malaria parasite needed a high temperature for at least forty-eight hours to mature. Yet western equine encephalitis did appear on a regular basis and new cases were monitored closely.

By the time Elaine and Helen arrived in July, I had adjusted to the much lighter work load and the added benefit of not having to sleep in the hospital when on call—after all, we lived right next door to the hospital. Also our responsibilities were fewer. We were not expected to prescribe any drugs or initiate any investigations without first confirming them with the patient's attending physician.

Elaine only had two months to go before our next child was due so we had to find someone to deliver the baby and decide which hospital to use. Dr. McCord suggested we approach Dr. Marty Robinson who worked at the Manitoba clinic and at the Grace Hospital. He was new to Winnipeg, having trained in London, Ontario, and Oxford, England, and was looking for patients. We were assured that since we were both physicians and I was working for the hospital there would be no charges for the services. In 1960 there were no provincial or federal health-care schemes.

If we had not been members of the medical profession these costs would have been in the region of about a thousand dollars. To cover the cost of doctors and medical treatment some people had private medical insurance. Others had medical insurance coverage with the companies they worked for, but a lot of people had no coverage whatsoever. For help and support, the latter relied on charity from organisations such as the Salvation Army and the Grey Nuns. Many physicians altered their billings to accommodate the financial status of their patients and many bills were simply written off. This was an aspect of medicine with which I was completely unfamiliar. I soon realized that as members of the profession we had certain privileges while for others getting medical attention could be more like a lottery. With no National Health Service in place, we could appreciate the serious impact that the costs of medical care might have on some families.

Having a baby meant Elaine got firsthand experience of private practice medical care as a patient. She commented on the differences in both outpatient care and hospital practice. The maternity wards were like the rest of the hospital with one, two or four beds to a room, offering more comfort and greater privacy than the single wards we had known at home. At the time there were no midwives in Canada, which meant that all maternity care was performed by physicians, in our case, by an obstetrician, and he was there to do the delivery. In the UK, maternity care was the responsibility of midwives.

In Elaine's opinion the absence of a midwife was not necessarily a good thing. She let her doubts be known and mentioned that she felt a bit cheated when for no apparent reason outlet forceps were used to shorten the second stage of labour. Later she made it clear that she was much more comfortable with the natural birth she had experienced with Helen. Another major area of concern to her was the advice she got about breast feeding, which was encouraged in the UK but discouraged in Canada.

My professional experience in this area at the time was very limited and it was many years before I could analyze the situation and contribute meaningfully to the debate between bottle and breast. Because I was working in the operating room when Elaine went into labour, I was not at the delivery of our second child. A theatre nurse rushed in to tell me that we had another daughter and that all was well.

Kathryn was born on the morning of the 30th of September, 1960. When Elaine went into the hospital the trees on Arlington Street and Vimy Park, located next to our apartment block, were green with foliage. That night I had to get out of bed to close the windows. The weather had suddenly turned cold and the wind blustery. When I went across to the hospital the next day the cold penetrated my light jacket and the sky filled with low, dark clouds rolling in from the north. When Elaine came out of hospital five days later, there were no leaves on the trees and a sprinkling of snow covered the ground. I asked about this sudden change at coffee in the operating room lounge and Dr. Waugh, one of the senior surgeons, said, "That's why we call it 'fall' and not autumn. Welcome to your first Winnipeg winter. It's a little early this year."

"It came on rather quickly, didn't it?" I asked.

"No. This is quite common. The wind comes in from the north and the temperature drops rapidly. You may have noticed geese flying over us for the past few days. That's a sure sign that winter is on the way. Many of the other waterfowl have been migrating south for the past few weeks, but most people don't notice them. Don't be surprised if the temperature drops to ten or fifteen degrees below zero in the next week. We'll probably get our first proper snowfall soon. Once it arrives winter is truly here, and the snow could stay with us until April. You'll be wearing a hat, gloves and overshoes for the next five to six months."

"That seems a bit extreme," I commented.

"It's the Prairies. It gives us a chance to get down to some real work. There's little else to do," someone else piped in.

"That's not entirely fair," said Trevor Kent, one of the family practitioners, who was well known for his outdoor pursuits. "You can go hunting for the next five to six weeks. You have a choice of ducks and geese, or deer and moose. Some people go after bear, which seems a waste of time to me. Not really very sporting. Then there's ice fishing, once the ice is thick enough. Cross-country skiing is popular. And skiing. But you have to go a hundred miles or so to La Riviere or the Lake of the Woods to find any downhill slopes and they're not very good. The runs are too short. If you're interested, theatre, ballet and opera seasons start soon. We have an ice hockey team and the Canadian Football League goes on until the end of November. So there's quite a lot to do."

"What Trevor says is true. There's plenty to do during the winter, but one has to be proactive. Several social clubs offer indoor sports—badminton, squash and curling come to mind—as well as other activities," said one of the other doctors.

Dr. Waugh's forecast proved accurate. By the middle of October the weather turned frigid and we bought some warm outdoor clothes. For the children we found full-body parkas with hoods and a long zip down the front. I was surprised by how easy they were to put on and take off. Watching Helen and, the next year, Kathryn trying to move in their new outfits was hilarious. They looked like tiny robots lurching about and falling into snow banks. Happily the suits were well padded.

The heavy woollen suits I'd brought with me from the UK were far too hot to wear indoors. They were perfect for poorly heated English houses and buildings but in the balmy seventy-degree heat maintained by the central heating systems in Winnipeg, I was continually stripping down to my shirtsleeves. In the end I had to buy lighter suits in order to be comfortable at work.

When Winnipeg received its annual forty-inch snowfall, it remained all winter. The snow ploughs piled the snow on the sidewalks, where it stayed until the spring melt. Learning to get the car out of snow drifts and manoeuvring on icy rutted roads was an adventure. I was surprised at how few accidents there were considering the conditions. Most of the time the sun shone, but when it got cold, Portage Avenue disappeared in a fog from the clouds of steam condensing from car exhausts.

The cold had its own beauty. On calm days ice crystals hung in the air. When the sun shone on them they refracted the colours of the rainbow. At temperatures below minus thirty, two sun dogs appeared, either as bright spots on each side of the sun or as partial halos around the sun. They were caused by atmospheric ice crystals and often heralded a change in the weather. Winnipeggers took some pride in the fact that their temperatures usually ranged between –40 degrees F. (–40 degrees C.) in winter and +40 degrees C. (+110 degrees F.) in the summer. I found both extremes hard to tolerate. The saving grace was that it was very dry.

Within a few weeks the two rivers had frozen over and people were able to walk across the ice safely. Our first blizzard arrived just before Christmas. Fortunately the central heating was reliable and efficient as the temperature plummeted precipitously and the wind howled past our double windows. At these low temperatures many of our windows iced up on the inside and we saw ice crystals in the apartment. Outside I could see the snow driving past but it was not until I crossed the street to the hospital that I faced the full force of the cold. In spite of my heavy coat, mitts and fur hat, crossing the street was a struggle I didn't think I'd survive. I felt as though I was on an arctic expedition. I turned my back to the wind and, when I entered the hospital, I had ice crystals in my nose and outside the corners of my eyes. There were no other people out and no cars to be seen. Although the storm had only been raging for a few hours there were high snow drifts on the sidewalk and road.

Later, looking out of one of the fifth-storey windows, I could see the wind and driving snow cover and swirl over the whole of Winnipeg.

This was a scene I could never have imagined when I visited Canada House to arrange my family's migration to the middle of Canada. Nor could I have envisioned wrestling with the elements as a part of my medical education and training. Anticipating my career now included measures beyond those encountered on a ward or in a classroom or with a firm.

Most of Winnipeg came to a standstill during blizzards. The hospital remained open but elective surgical cases were cancelled because the patients or surgeons could not get to the hospital. Emergencies and labouring mothers, who managed to get to the hospital, were looked after by the staff who happened to be there when the blizzard started. They remained on duty until it was over. What surprised me was how the electrical power and water supply remained in place. The facilities had backup generators available, but to my amazement they were not needed very often.

The high winds and snow lasted thirty-six hours and then stopped as quickly as they had started. The sky cleared and the sun came out, but the temperature remained very low, between minus twenty-five and thirty degrees. This weather did not stop the city from coming to life again, albeit in slow motion. People shovelled their driveways and their sections of sidewalks. Snow ploughs arrived and cleared the main streets. Cars crawled around mountains of snow.

As soon as she saw others moving about the city, Elaine suggested we do some grocery shopping. We were low on supplies of just about everything. We were not used to the idea of stockpiling in case of a blizzard. Our car was parked in the street and I had forgotten to plug in the block heater. There was a snowdrift at the front and the windshield was covered with several inches of snow. I took my mitts off to open the door and when I grasped the door handle my hand stuck to it. Fortunately, I remembered my experience in Kashgar and waited a minute or so for the metal to warm up before pulling my hand away so as not to pull off a layer of skin.

When I got in and turned on the ignition all the lights lit up but the starter motor wouldn't turn over the engine. I plugged the block heater in and retreated back into the apartment for lunch. I asked Goetz how long I should wait before trying to start the car and he said four hours. In the meantime I cleared the ice and snow from around the car.

After four hours the engine turned over slowly with a lot of grinding noises I didn't like. Eventually I heard a thud and the engine fired up with an enormous cloud of black smoke. Although the engine was running, it sounded rough as if it were firing on three or four of its six cylinders. To my relief, eventually the engine warmed up and ran smoothly. I turned the heater on and a cloud of snow blew into my face. When the snow had cleared from the vents the heater came on. Then the windows immediately fogged up and frosted over. I couldn't see out at all. I was sitting inside an igloo of my own making.

As the defroster laboured to clear the frost, I scraped the inside of the windows so I could see out. I then put the car into gear but it wouldn't move. Even though it was in gear the engine continued to strain. I put the car back into neutral and got out to see if there was anything preventing it from moving. Nothing. I got back in, put the car in gear, and revved the engine. The car lurched forward with a loud clunk and stopped. When I tried again to inch forward, it moved, but the steering felt heavy. At the same time, the whole car bounced up and down. I got out to have another look at the wheels and road. Everything appeared normal enough so I had another go at getting it to move forward. This time I kept the car moving but it felt as though I were driving over a giant washboard. I kept going and things gradually smoothed out. As I was walking back to the apartment I ran into Goetz and I told him about this strange experience.

"Square tires," he said, laughing and shaking his head. At that moment I didn't see the humour. "Tires flatten when the temperature drops below minus twenty-five, especially if the car has been standing outside for a few days. Then you get a bumpy ride. Welcome to the Prairies."

Once we adapted to the winter conditions, Elaine and I found living in Winnipeg not that different from living anywhere else. When we went out for walks with the children, we put Kathryn in her carry-cot on a sledge, which one of us would pull, and Helen would bundle up in multiple layers and trot along beside. We ventured out to several nearby parks and the zoo where Helen took great delight in talking to and teasing the animals. Elaine, who had learned to skate when she was at school, loved watching the skaters on the outdoor pond at Assiniboine Park. She especially loved to see them jump and spin and couples dance. Young boys stick handled after hockey pucks and dodged around other skaters.

For the most part we stayed in Winnipeg, happily occupied with the children and work. Some nurses and doctors headed to their cottages at La Riviere to ski and party, a common pastime during the winter months. Our group of twelve interns in the Baldwin Apartments often socialized on the weekends. Keeping the beer cold was easy. All we had to do was put it outside a window for a few minutes.

Shortly after the Christmas festivities ended, the temperature began to drop. I watched in awe as the mercury dipped down to minus thirty and stayed there. The dangers of this hit me one day when I heard on the news that a young person had frozen to death in town while trying to walk home from a party. The news item said that he only had on a light coat and that he had tried to walk about a mile. The night wind had driven the wind chill factor down to the minus sixties. This sort of accident, I was told at coffee in the doctor's lounge the next day, was not uncommon on the Prairies. Such accidents also happened when a car broke down and the occupants were not prepared for the cold.

Towards the end of February we experienced one of nature's quirks. As I walked over to the hospital on a brilliant sunny morning, the snow began to melt. I thought this must be the beginning of spring and mentioned it at coffee.

"Don't you believe it. This is the Bonspiel thaw. It will only last a few days and then the cold will be back with a vengeance and we'll probably get another dump of snow. The annual Winnipeg Curling Bonspiel is planned for this time of year and this unpredictable weather is very annoying for the organisers. The ice on the outdoor rinks melts and makes curling difficult if not impossible. Warmer weather at this time is quite common, but unlike the Chinooks— warm to hot winds that come up from the deserts in the States that hit places like Calgary—this sudden change in temperature doesn't wake up the trees in Manitoba. Chinooks cause a lot of problems with tree growth in southern Alberta and many species that we have in Winnipeg wouldn't survive there. Not to worry, though, it will only be balmy for a couple of days and then the temperature will drop down again," said Dr. McCord.

McCord was right. It turned cold again and more snow arrived. It was not until March that the temperature started to warm up a bit, almost reaching 32 degrees Fahrenheit during the daytime, but dropping well below freezing at night. Later, in March, I heard the geese; I looked up and saw the first of many flocks of Canada geese flying north over the city. The occasional flock of snow geese also appeared. Then, within a week, the temperature climbed into the seventies and stayed above zero at night. This increase in temperature caused the snow drifts piled on the sides of roads, laden with their reddish dust and other rubbish, to melt quickly. Large puddles of muddy water formed everywhere.

Walking became hazardous. Passing cars threw up large waves of water when they drove through puddles. When the roads flooded the works department sent out the "steam enema" team, as the doctors used to refer to them, to unblock the storm drains. This problem only lasted about a week. Then the city dried out. Dust and sand from the streets blew around, getting in everything.

The deciduous trees turned green with new leaf buds and spring officially arrived. Fruit trees blossomed as well as the lilac bushes, with their fragrant purple flowers. Colour returned to the city after six months of snow.

One morning in the operating room I was told I should walk down to the river to have a look at the "break up." The best place to see it was on the bridge over the Assiniboine River, which was not far from the hospital. As I neared the bridge I could hear a low-pitched crunching noise coming from the river. It was caused by ice that was flowing down the river, grinding and breaking up. The river moved fast—in chunks—the pieces of ice, massive. When they collided with the bridge supports the whole concrete structure vibrated creating even more noise. Intermingled with the ice blocks were other bits of debris—tree branches, old doors, window frames, sofas, chairs, mattresses, garden refuse and other rubbish that had been thrown onto the river during the past six months. Although I didn't see any on this occasion, at other times when I visited this spot, I was surprised by the number of dead animals caught up in the rush of ice and water.

Both the Assiniboine and Red Rivers overflowed their banks frequently at this time of year. Winnipeg had been so badly damaged by flooding in 1950 that the provincial government had built a ten-mile floodway around the city to protect it. At the time it was the second-largest earth-moving project in the world, bigger than the Suez Canal but smaller than the Panama Canal. Named after the premier of the day, it was affectionately known as Duff's Ditch. In the winter months, parts of the canal were used to dump snow collected from the city streets, which in turn were used as toboggan runs.

I had been working as an intern for about three months when I was asked to call in at Dr. McCreath's office.

"I've asked you in today to let you know we've arranged for you to go to the Children's Hospital early next month. You will be there for eight weeks and will be expected to live in for part of the time, depending on how many interns they have on their rotation. It shouldn't be too heavy a commitment.

"As far as obstetrics is concerned, the rotating internship here does not usually include that experience. However, our obstetric resident will be finishing shortly and we don't have a replacement. I've discussed the problem with administration and the University Department of Obstetrics and we would like to offer you the post, but you would have to make a one-year commitment. The pay would be better than what you're getting now and we would continue to give you the apartment on the same terms. The position would be recognised by the College of Physicians and Surgeons as part of the Fellowship training, so if you decided to pursue a specialist training program in the future, you would not be wasting your time."

I was pleased. To have this verbal affirmation of my work was encouraging, but more to the point it confirmed many of the thoughts I had had about the future. There was so much more that I wanted to know about medicine, especially about how it was taught.

"I'm glad about the paediatrics. I was beginning to wonder if that was going to happen. I had not really planned on spending a whole year in obstetrics, but I would certainly consider it. I'll have to discuss it with my wife before saying yes, though."

"Can you let me know in a day or so? There's another advantage. You would be entitled to an extra two weeks' holiday if you decided to do the whole year."

When I discussed the position with Elaine, she thought it was a good idea and felt that staying one more year would give us a chance to see what career opportunities Canada and Manitoba had to offer us. We had certainly enjoyed our stay so far.

The Winnipeg Children's Hospital was administratively part of the General Hospital, but it was a separate physical entity which had been established in 1909 and rebuilt in 1958. It had four storeys and 127 beds to service the needs of Manitoba, eastern Saskatchewan, northwestern Ontario, the Keewatin area of the North West Territories and North Dakota. There was an emergency department and facilities for looking after burns, neonatology, paediatric oncology, neurosurgery, plastic surgery, medical and other surgical specialties.

As an intern I had the unique privilege of being taught by Jack Bowman, a paediatrician, and Rinehart Friesen, an obstetrician. These two men had pioneered the research into the problems of blood type incompatibility and newborn mortality. Their research was done in conjunction with the Red Cross blood transfusion services in Winnipeg and they developed a vaccine for Rh disease, a potentially deadly disorder for fetuses and newborns. Since the 1960s the vaccine has benefitted Rh negative women worldwide and allowed them to have healthy Rh positive children. This vaccine is often cited as the single most important medical research discovery in Manitoba's history. Working with them for eight weeks sparked my own curiosity about the wide-ranging possibilities of research.

On the wards of the Children's Hospital I was intrigued by the effectiveness of the steam room, which was used for the treatment of children with life-threatening croup, a relatively common respiratory problem in young children in the dry, cold winters of Manitoba. While there I also saw patients with convulsions related to high fevers and severe drug overdoses. I worked for short periods of time in all the departments and the experience filled in gaps in my understanding of paediatrics. Some areas were depressing; the outlook for curing children with leukaemia and brain tumours was poor.

Over time I realized that Canadian-trained residents and interns were more academically orientated than I was. They tended to rely on laboratory investigations more than the actual hands-on physical examinations of patients to make decisions about treatment. While their undergraduate training was much less practical than mine, their theoretical teaching was more extensive. Our respective programs were the same length in time, but patient contact and responsibility for patient care was much less in Canadian medical schools. Their internships covered a broader range of medical disciplines than mine had in the UK—for example, everyone spent time doing maternity and paediatrics. I wondered if these differences had any long-term consequences in our roles as family practitioners.

My Canadian colleagues were also much more outgoing than I remembered my British colleagues being. Partying was an important part of their lives when they were off call. Like their UK counterparts many were unmarried and the nurses they worked with were often their partners for social events. I was a bit taken aback one morning when I arrived in the on-call room to find two interns lying on beds hooked up to intravenouses. When I asked why they were taking intravenous fluids I was told that it was the best way to get rid of a hangover. They were especially proud of themselves—they had added vitamins to the IV fluids. The idea of rehydrating using hospital equipment struck me as mischievous, but I had to concede that I might just be naive and a bit old-fashioned.

When I finished at the Children's Hospital, I became the new obstetric resident at the Grace Hospital and was no longer expected to do general duties. The chief of Obstetrics, Dr. W.J. McCord, was a tall, bespectacled, stylish Manitoban, who had spent time in Sheffield, England during his training years. He took me under his wing and helped me gain some self-assurance. My duties were primarily to the labour suite and on the maternity ward, but I was also called to maternity and gynaecology patients in Emergency, and I was responsible for admitting them to the hospital. I was also expected to assist at gynaecological cases in the operating rooms. There were about 1,400 deliveries a year so it was a busy place to be.

The delivery suite, in the newest part of the hospital, was spacious and air-conditioned, with four delivery rooms, one of which was equipped to act as an operating room for emergency forceps and caesarean sections. There were two special-care rooms. The postpartum rooms had two or four beds. There was twenty-four-hour anaesthesia coverage and simple laboratory investigations. An X-ray technician was on call twenty-four hours a day. The deliveries were all conducted by a physician, which was a new concept for me; I was used to normal deliveries being conducted by midwives.

If a physician was not able to get to the hospital in time for a delivery, I would be called to attend and manage the delivery. My most memorable delivery was a breech. Fortunately all went well except when the nurse mistakenly gave me a pair of artery forceps when I asked for the obstetric forceps to help with the delivery of the head after the feet and body appeared.

The unmarried mothers' home that the Salvation Army ran, mostly housed in the Baldwin Apartments, had its own clinic in the hospital. It was my job to look after these patients under the supervision of the "staff man" of the month. The number of patients I saw varied, but averaged fifteen per clinic, comprised of prenatal and postnatal patients. Some of the patients were divorced or separated and a small percentage of these patients were having their second or third babies. Not all of them stayed in the Baldwin Apartments, but they were all being assisted by the Salvation Army and were not charged for the services provided unless they could afford to pay.

I was surprised to learn that these patients came from all strata of society and that there was a high percentage of Indian, Métis and Inuit women. Some of the social problems they presented included parental violence, rape, incest and literally being thrown out of their own homes. Many had just been abandoned by their spouses and families. These circumstances were completely beyond my experience. Not only was I outraged by what I witnessed but the emotional toll was sobering and exhausting. I felt both anger and sorrow. I began to appreciate how lucky I had been as a child. The nurses and caregivers were surprised by my naivety, and put me in the picture when they thought it appropriate. At that time abortion was a criminal offence, but it was discussed occasionally and I was shocked to think about the problems some of these patients had to face. During that year I did not see any patients who had had a criminal abortion but I learned that criminal abortions could be obtained and that serious medical, social and legal problems occurred as a result of this activity. Most of these women were seen at the Winnipeg General Hospital.

By the time I had spent a year as a resident at Grace Hospital I could see that the specialty of obstetrics and gynaecology had much to teach me. The work was predominantly with younger people who were relatively healthy. The care of pregnant patients most often had happy outcomes, although there were some dramatic and stressful times.

The classic situation was when both the mother and unborn child were at risk of dying. Obstetric care required a good in-depth knowledge of general medical and surgical conditions. The impact of pregnancy on these conditions could be considerable. For example, if a pregnant patient had a cardiovascular or respiratory disease, the expanding uterus compressed the chest and caused more stress on these already struggling systems. Added to this problem was the impact of a forty percent increase in cardiac output, increased blood volume and weight gain. Such a situation could rapidly become life-threatening. Similar problems could be encountered with other general medical, surgical, orthopaedic and psychiatric conditions. Care of these women required the close co-operation of the different specialists and a mutual understanding of each other's area of expertise.

The volume of hands-on practical obstetrics during my year on the ward was limited to only one caesarean section, twenty low-forceps deliveries, four mid-cavity rotations and deliveries, two manual removals of the placenta, a breech delivery and two sets of twins. After a year I felt this was not a lot of experience. On the other hand, I was involved in the care of several patients with severe toxaemia. One woman had convulsions, which was extremely distressing. Two patients had severe haemolytic disease where the newborn babies required exchange transfusions. Yet I felt that since the specialty was a practical one, another year would not be adequate preparation for the position of a consultant obstetrician. By this time, O & G was a specialization I was seriously considering.

The residency programs for specialists in Canada were four years long. In Obstetrics and Gynaecology, two years had to be spent in these disciplines, eighteen months had to be spent in general surgery, basic science or research, and six months as an elective where one could choose from a number of options or, alternatively, do more obstetrics and gynaecology. At the end of this four-year training program, the candidate qualified to sit the certification or fellowship examinations in the specialty. If successful, one obtained a licence to practice as a specialist.

The gynaecological experience I gained during the year was also limited to a few minor procedures—miscarriages, ectopic pregnancies, ovarian cysts and assisting at hysterectomies. As a "bonus" I was taught how to perform neonatal circumcisions, which was a routine procedure at the time. I had some misgivings about this operation, but it was part of medical practice and expected. Being an "assistant" at surgical procedures, which meant I was a spectator rather than a practitioner, was useful but did not help me actually learn the surgical techniques involved; this omission was of major concern to me. As my current job was only recognized as an obstetric residency, the gynaecologic experience was just an add-on, at least as far as the College was concerned.

One of the highlights of my job was presenting cases at the Hospital Grand Rounds once a month and teaching other interns some obstetric principles. I was expected to attend Grand Rounds at the Winnipeg General on Friday mornings. There I had the opportunity to meet and discuss various topics with Professor Raulston and members of the Department. These sessions gave me another opportunity to taste the thrill and satisfaction that accompanied teaching.

Many of the senior staff had spent time in the UK or the USA gaining additional practical training. By the end of the year I had decided that I would like to become an obstetrician and I asked the College what further training I needed. They told me that I required one further year of gynaecology and a year of basic sciences. If the college would accept my general surgical and medical internship work in the UK, I would only have to do two more years before sitting the exams.

After lengthy discussions with Elaine, Professor Raulston, Dr. McCord and Dr. M.L. Robinson, I finally decided I would go for more training. Dr. McCreath suggested I should do six months of pathology to fulfil my basic science training, since there was a recognized pathology resident at the Grace Hospital. This meant that we could continue to stay in the accommodation the hospital had provided. There was one added benefit. By this time, Elaine was anxious to get back to work. She had made some enquiries about positions at the Misericordia Hospital, a short walk away, where they were looking for interns.

In May 1961 I was told I had two weeks of holiday and that I should take the time off in late June. So far, we had made limited excursions in Manitoba; now we decided a camping trip to Yellowstone

Park, south of the border, might expose us to a different way of life. I'm not sure what we expected. On the way we would pass through North and South Dakota and get some sense of how the USA differed from Canada.

On a glorious summer day in late June 1961, we loaded the car with camping equipment and the two children. We got away at ten o'clock in the morning. The drive south on Highway 75, to the American border, was along a straight two-lane highway with the typical squared farmland on either side. The fields of wheat, barley and, from time to time, sunflowers were well established and green. The farms varied in size and state of repair. Some were being painted while others looked derelict. Everywhere we glanced we saw windmill water pumps, which Helen began to count, dilapidated sheds and outhouses. Elaine and I agreed that the places looked quite primitive and that life as a homesteader must be tough, a mere scratch on the earth, especially during the dead of winter. Most of the farms were surrounded by windbreaks of scrub oaks, willows and thorn bushes. We saw little in the way of livestock, but most farm yards had a few chickens and two or three dogs. We passed several small townships some of which had towering grain elevators over-shadowing them, a sure sign a railway line passed though the town.

Once across the border, Highway 75 changed to the I-29 and the road quickly became a smooth four-lane highway. As the highway improved we saw a big notice warning drivers that the speed limit would be patrolled by radar, police on foot, motorcycles, and in police vehicles, both marked and unmarked; and just to make the threat palpable, also by aeroplanes. While the latter possibility seemed a bit extreme to me, I decided I best not speed.

For the first few hours the countryside was much the same as in Manitoba but the farm houses were larger and better kept. Like a piece of taut string the road was straight and seemed to go on forever, as if out of what I remembered of Hitchcock's film *North by Northwest*.

It was not until we got into South Dakota that I noticed the topography had changed to undulating hills. The elms, poplars, and willows had become much larger than those in Manitoba. As planned,

303

we turned onto I-90 at Sioux Falls and headed towards the famous attractions of Rapid City, the Badlands National Park, and Mount Rushmore. The next day we intended to drive to the Badlands—a "must-see" according to our friends in Winnipeg.

The next morning we drove west for three hours before we came to the turnoff to the Badlands National Park. The terrain was more barren and less populated than the undulating prairie we had been travelling through. Quite suddenly, after driving over a slight rise, a spectacular if not dramatic view of the Badlands spread out before us.

They consisted of multiple razor-sharp hills with very steep sides rising several hundred feet towards the intense blue sky. They looked like giant figures grasping for the clouds. The colours of the rocks— red, brown and orange—were vibrant in the clear air and full sun. Adding to the drama, the sharp pinnacles gave us the sense that we had arrived on another planet. Scattered about were a few thorn bushes and some sage. Large trees could not survive here. The soil was too poor and water scarce, except during flash floods. A dry river bed, filled with boulders, wound into the hills.

At the national park information kiosk, we learned that the hills had been carved by water and wind erosion over several million years. Wildlife could still be found in these hills in which indigenous peoples had once lived. From a map of the area we got directions to the campsite where we planned to stay the night—down a steep road, about a mile away from the viewing point, beside the river bed, close to the beginning of the Badlands. Here the topography of the rock formations became even more wistful.

Forty-five campsites formed a circle around a central building. Each had room for a tent and a standard camp table. I always made a point of boiling the water we drank when camping, but it was re- assuring to read a sign stating that the tap water was drinkable. As we unloaded the car we noticed that there were only half a dozen other campers.

Multiple deep cracks in the ground suggested to me that perhaps there had been water in the area recently. Because of this I chose a site that was elevated a few inches above the others and we set up our tent.

After supper we took the girls for a short walk to the dry river-bed. I was struck by its deep crevasses, which were two to five inches across, carved in the dry clay soil. On the walk a few lizards scuttled away to hide in sage bushes. I kept my eyes open for snakes because we had seen a notice warning of rattlers. On the way back to the camp the sun started to set and the magnificent colours of the hills contrasted impressively with the areas that were now in shade. Several other campers had now arrived.

We retired to bed early.

Except for the distant sound of the wind circling the pinnacles, a hush fell over the campsite.

Sometime in the early hours I was woken by a flash of lightning and a boom of thunder. Then the wind keened and I thought the whole tent was going to blow over. I sat up and held onto the centre pole to keep it in place.

"What was that?" Elaine asked, sitting up.

"A storm brewing, I think."

"Should we get into the car?" Elaine asked, as the tent whipped in the wind and threatened to tear.

"Let's give it a few minutes. It may be just a sudden gust and a bit of lightning. Getting everyone into the car in the dark might be a bit tricky," I said.

Immediately the rain hit. It came down in large drops with such force they caused a fine spray of water to come though the tent wall. When I played the flashlight against the wall I could see that water was streaming off the canvas. But there were no more flashes of lightning so I felt it was going to be easier to stay where we were than move to the car. After half an hour the deluge subsided. During this time I heard a number of car doors bang shut, but we were still reasonably dry. When the rain stopped I unzipped the tent fly and had a look around with the flashlight. We were perched on a tiny island in a sea of water. Our neighbour's tent, only feet away, had collapsed and was covered with water.

As the storm receded I got back into my sleeping bag. I woke up a few hours later as the tent walls flapped wildly in another strong gust of wind. I noticed that the temperature in the tent had gone up noticeably. When I opened the zip I could see that dawn was breaking and the sky was clear. We were still surrounded by water, but it was not as deep as it had been the last time I looked. There was no point in doing anything as Elaine and the children were still sleeping, so I closed my eyes and drifted back to sleep. When I next woke up Elaine and Helen were chatting.

When we finally climbed out of the tent we could see how the small mound on which we had pitched the tent had saved us from getting swamped by the torrential rain. Several of the other campers were busy sorting through the shambles left by the storm.

When we broke camp the ground was almost dry and there was no sign of the water that had poured down during the night. We were awed by the power of the rain and gained some insight into how the Badlands had been formed

Our original plan was to go directly on to Yellowstone National Park. However, after looking at the map we realized we had five hundred miles to go. We decided to break the journey and took the road going southwest, out of Rapid City, into the Black Hills, heading towards the famous sculptures at Mount Rushmore. The road wound around, up and down, as if we were on a roller-coaster.

We came round a corner onto an unexpected view of the Mount Rushmore presidents. Nothing can prepare you for the suddenness of this view, or for those stone faces out there in the wilderness. Although I had read several articles about these giant sculptures I had no idea how large they were or how accurately they portrayed the four men. And why those four? We did not spend much time in the Mount Rushmore area but I had a chance to reflect on the improbable tasks some men set for themselves and complete. Sometimes to an unknown end.

Our route took us through Sheridan and Cody, and past Buffalo Bill State Park. We had heard these famous names, so much a part of America western lore. As we drove further and further into Yellowstone Park and came upon volcanic remains we had the sensation we were travelling back through time. Where the hillsides were not covered by trees one could see the red and yellow colours of the volcanic soil. Near the lake we passed through extensive grasslands and saw a small herd of shaggy bison. Not that long ago, they would have looked at us as the oddity in this setting. Now they were the exhibit. Next we saw two moose standing in marshlands. They merely lifted their heads and sniffed as we passed.

In total, we stayed in Yellowstone Park for five days. During that time we had a good view of the Yellowstone "Grand Canyon" from our campsite. We drove to the mudflats and saw the geysers and Old Faithful. As neither Elaine nor I had ever seen anything like it, we began to understand why Yellowstone Park was a mecca for American campers, some from as far away as Alaska, Florida and Texas.

After five days we moved on to Waterton Lakes Park in Canada. To get there we had to drive north for two days. En route we visited the south end of Glacier National Park. When we got to the top of Logan Pass, on the "Going-to-the-Sun" route, we drove through ploughed snowdrifts that were five to six feet high. I was surprised by the height of the snow even though it was warm and the snow was melting. This drive took us through the eastern side of the Rockies with their soaring, craggy peaks. Towns were few and far between.

Waterton Lakes Park was not nearly as well groomed as the American parks we had visited. By then we were preoccupied with getting back to Winnipeg. Our return trip home was via Lethbridge, Alberta, and the Trans-Canada Highway through Saskatchewan, which at that time was only two lanes wide and, for long stretches, had yet to be paved.

When we got back to Winnipeg I started my new job as the Resident in Pathology at the Grace Hospital. This experience was a complete change from what I had been doing for the last two years—for the first time in my career I wasn't expected to see any "live" patients. The majority of the work involved doing autopsies, and then looking at the pathological slides and coming to a conclusive diagnosis. I also had to look at the slides from surgical specimens taken in the hospital. This experience was invaluable because it meant that I was finally able to talk intelligently to pathologists about the results of biopsies. It was not uncommon for surgeons to come to the department to discuss slides with the pathologists.

One of the senior pathologists had been taught to do autopsies with his bare hands. He said that the rationale for this was that by using bare hands one was less cavalier about how one handled the sharp instruments. The logic of this escaped me and I felt he was taking unnecessary risks. However, he said that in all the years he had been doing autopsies he had never managed to hurt himself or get an infection.

The other big advantage of my new job was that I was encouraged to attend as many of the educational sessions at the university hospitals as I could get to. I did not have to confine this to pathology sessions and therefore was able to pursue my interest in obstetrics and gynaecology. Pathology did not have on call responsibilities or include evening hours so I helped out with the children and had a little family time. Elaine found some part-time intern work at the Misericordia hospital. She liked working again and the girls enjoyed their time in nursery school.

As our evenings and weekends were free we were able do things outside of the hospital. With the encouragement of friends I took up the game of golf, which at first I thought was a stupid game but soon came to enjoy. In the fall of 1961 I was introduced to hunting upland game, ducks and geese. On one of these hunting trips I learned the hard way how easy it was to get lost in the bush. All I did was step off the footpath and walk ten or fifteen yards off course. When I turned round to get back to the path I misjudged the angle and spent the next four hours trying to find my way out. I didn't have a compass with me and had to rely on some of the skills I had been taught in high school with the Army cadets. I was able to identify where north was and walk east in a relatively straight line. Eventually I found a wire fence and followed this back to the road.

While stumbling through the bush I spotted what I thought was a large dog coming towards me, but it wasn't until the animal was fifteen yards away that I realised it was a timber wolf. I think we were both equally surprised to see each other because the wolf just walked on by without acknowledging my presence while I trudged on avoiding eye contact. My hunting colleagues were getting worried by the time I got back to them because they realised that if I had gone north there was nothing but bush for three hundred miles. I learned my lesson and since then have never been hunting, fishing, or tramping through the woods without a compass and, at the very least, a knife and matches.

Although life in Winnipeg and working as a pathology resident was instructive I felt that to become an obstetrician and gynaecologist I needed some in-depth practical training. I could see that the training program in Winnipeg was not going to give me the experience I felt was necessary to be competent. In fact, most of the obstetricians and gynaecologists I met in Winnipeg had spent a year or more working in either the UK or at one of the large public hospitals in the United States. I also wanted to take the London M.B. B.S. exams again. Failure had not gone down well. I also felt that I should have the London University degree; after all that was where I had studied. In addition, I was homesick and wanted to see my parents again.

Elaine and I discussed the idea of moving back to England and we agreed that it might be a good move at this point in our careers. Dr. Robinson had spent time in Oxford and offered to write to them to see if they could find a place for me in their training program. This resulted in my being offered a position as a house surgeon in Oxford starting in July 1962. Oxford was a well-known and respected teaching hospital where I would be working for the highly respected gynaecologists, Mr. Stallworthy and Mr. Hawksworth—an opportunity I could not afford to miss.

We left Winnipeg on January 20, 1962. We well remember the day because it was 25 degrees below zero, beautifully clear, with a gentle breeze. On the way out to the plane, Helen, who was wearing a heavy coat, mitts and a woollen hat, said that she was too hot. When we got off the plane in London it was well above freezing, but with a fine drizzle, and she complained bitterly that she felt cold.

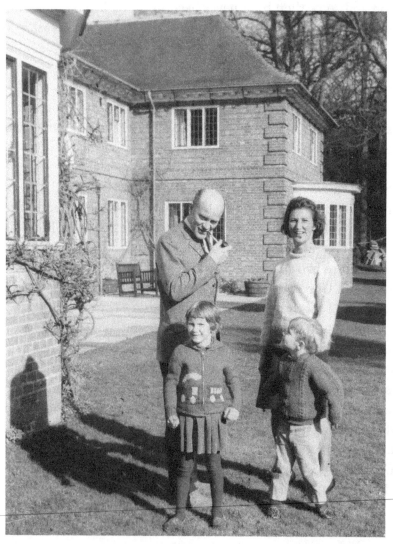

The family while we were staying at Sir John Stallworthy's mansion in Oxford.

Chapter 9
Return to the UK: Learning to be an Obstetrician/Gynaecologist

Once back in England, we stayed for a few days in London and visited with old friends we hadn't seen for two years. We had a lot of catching up to do, especially about the ways in which our careers had taken different directions. Once again I appreciated how much teaching methods differed on either side of the Atlantic. It was fun comparing stories, although I was already beginning to wonder how I would fit back into a system I thought I knew so well. Observations and expectations were clearly at odds in the two systems.

Then we picked up our new car and drove to my parents in North Yorkshire. At first we didn't realize how well off we were after only two years in Canada. We had easily saved enough money to fly back to England, as well as pay for a new car before returning home.

My parents were now living in Eston, a dreary suburb of Middlesbrough, which was notable, from what I could see, for being close to several pollution-producing commercial enterprises—a steel works, Dorman Longs, a Palmolive soap factory, and two oil refineries. It was January. Damp and dull. But what struck and bothered us was the constant fog. I found the place depressing and wondered why my father had decided to work here. His explanation was straightforward: he had returned directly from his Colonial Service job in Nigeria when that country gained its independence, he didn't have a job in the UK, and the one in Middlesbrough was the first that came up. It was that simple!

In Middlesbrough he was the medical officer in the Department of Health, a position he held for two years. At the end of that time he found a job as a school's medical officer in Saltburn-by-the-Sea, a town about forty-five miles South of Middlesbrough. He and my mother spent the rest of their lives there and never traveled internationally again. My mother died when she reached seventy and Father continued on until he was almost ninety. He enjoyed his work as the school's medical officer and continued on well past retirement age. In his spare time and as a pastime he also found that he could teach children how to play the flute. He gave free lessons until he died. He was also active in the musical community of Saltburn and Whitby and travelled to London at least once a year to see musicals.

My parents had rented a modern four-bedroom house in Eston with a tiny garden in the front and a slightly larger one at the back. It was comfortable, although a bit boxy, but had ample space for us all. After the initial few days and the excitement of seeing my parents again, I set off to find work.

My first concern was to find a six-month job in gynaecology that would be recognised by the College, before taking up my position in Oxford in July. This did not give me much time. Fortunately, Father subscribed to the *British Medical Journal* and had saved the recent editions. Several jobs interested me but the most attractive post was one advertised at Grimsby General Hospital—it came with married accommodation. When I phoned the hospital they said that the job was still available and that I should come for an interview the next day. I drove the hundred and twenty miles and was interviewed by Mr. C.R.M MacDonald, the consultant gynaecologist and a hospital superintendent. The interview went smoothly and he offered me the job starting the next week.

To my surprise Grimsby General Hospital was a busy place. Housed in a grey stone building were departments of General Medicine, Surgery, Gynaecology, Paediatrics, an emergency area, and two operating theatres. The maternity unit was housed in Nunsthorp Hospital, just up the road. As the Senior Medical Officer in Gynaecology, I had twenty beds to look after with the help of a registrar, Ms. Billy Greening, a gynaecologist in training from Australia. She had to cover the maternity unit up the road as well. On my half-day a week and one weekend in three off, Dr. Greening covered any problems in the Gynaecological Ward. Most of the junior staff members were from India or Pakistan.

After two weeks Elaine and the girls joined me. Our housing was close to the hospital and I was able to walk there when emergencies came in. A short time later Elaine found someone to look after the children while she did some locum work for a local general practitioner.

Sister Cuthbert, an attractive, middle-aged lady, had been running the Gynaecology Ward at Grimsby for ten years. Silence surrounded her. After my first week at the hospital she took it upon herself to make sure that I understood the nature of my job. One morning, at coffee time, she invited me into her office, a small room partitioned off from the rest of the ward. The office walls didn't reach the ceiling and we were privy to the patients' conversations. She said she thought I might be interested in what I heard.

The patients hadn't noticed I was in the office and they spoke freely about their sex lives, giving some intimate and detailed descriptions. Everything they said was undisguised. I was taken aback by the crude language some of them used. Sister had obviously spotted that I was still somewhat naive and needed to be "put in the picture". One patient referred to me as that innocent young doctor from Canada, who was going to learn a few things about life in a small fishing village in the north of England. Sister told me that these patients were very careful about how they spoke around me. They didn't want me to form "bad" opinions of them or brand them as lower class.

My job was to admit patients to the Gynaecology Ward, arrange for any investigations that were necessary, and confirm that the surgical plans were correct. There were two operating sessions a week and on most of these days we would do two or three major and several minor procedures. Thanks to my experience in Canada, I soon demonstrated that I could assist at both minor and major surgical procedures. I often became the first assistant to Mr. MacDonald when Dr. Greening was busy or at the maternity hospital. Towards the end of the six months I was allowed to perform minor procedures on my own and, after discussion with the registrar, I was allowed to care for emergencies including operative procedures.

Mr. MacDonald had one gynaecological outpatient session a

week which I had to attend. At these he would see patients referred to him by the general practitioners in the area and from Louth. At these outpatient sessions I had to see the post-operative patients and discuss with him any complications of which I had become aware. I was also expected to see some new patients and discuss them with him or Dr. Greening. The result of this arrangement was that I saw a lot of new and post-operative patients and learned a lot about the complications of gynaecological surgery. While in Grimsby I performed abdominal hysterectomies, pelvic floor repairs, treated ovarian cysts, ectopic pregnancies, incomplete abortions, septic abortions and some less common gynaecological problems. Birth control problems were not looked after in these clinics; there was a National Service in place for this purpose, and their clinics were held in a separate area.

One Friday, about six weeks after I'd taken up my post, Sister Cuthbert approached me. "I hope you have a good weekend but be warned, the abortionist is in town and you may be seeing a few septic abortions."

I was not sure how she knew about the abortionist and asked, "Are there any legal implications I should be aware of with respect to these patients?" Abortion was illegal in England at this time.

"It's very unlikely you'll get any information out of the patients. In fact, they rarely admit they're pregnant and will tell you all sorts of stories about why they're 'ill'. If there is any reliable information you feel could be used in the courts, please let Mr. MacDonald know as soon as possible. However, the chances of this happening are exceedingly remote."

Since I had no experience whatsoever with botched illegal abortions, I read as much as I could in the library, but the information available was limited. The most important clinical aspect I needed to be aware of was that the uterus could be perforated, resulting in an abdominal infection, internal bleeding, chemical irritation, air in the abdomen causing shock, and sometimes death. The other major complication that could develop was a massive infection of the womb and lower genital tract, which usually took a day or so to develop. If I had good evidence that a criminal act had occurred then I had to inform

Mr. MacDonald who in turn had to notify the police.

At 10:30 Friday night I was called to the Casualty Department to see a young lady of sixteen complaining bitterly of abdominal pain. The casualty officer did not think she had acute appendicitis and wondered if there was a gynaecological cause for her pain. She looked a little flushed, was obviously in pain but was otherwise well. Her temperature was 99 degrees F., her pulse was slightly raised, but her blood pressure was normal. I went through the usual list of questions and established that the pain had been there for a few hours and was "crampy" in nature. She had not vomited but had felt a bit nauseated since the pain started. I explained that I was the gynaecological house man. I would have to ask her some rather personal questions and it was very important that she answer them accurately. She seemed to understand, and agreed.

"How old were you when your periods started?"

"Twelve."

"Are they regular," I asked, "and when was your last period?"

"They are very regular. The last one was two weeks ago."

"Was it normal and was there any pain associated with it?"

"It was perfectly normal with the usual few cramps."

"Are you sexually active?" I asked as discreetly as I could.

"No. I've never had sex," she replied.

I then asked her about her family history and what she was doing. She was living at home, attending school and hoped to go to university. Apparently she was a good student. She had never had any serious illnesses or been admitted to hospital. She was not taking any drugs or medications. I explained that I would have to do a full physical and pelvic examination, which she agreed to, although with some reluctance. When I examined her chest she was obviously embarrassed and it was difficult to recognise any breast changes. Her abdomen was moving normally and there were no obvious scars or other abnormalities. On palpation I noticed some tenderness but no guarding. The tenderness was most pronounced over her lower abdomen. The pelvic examination was not easy because of her embarrassment and unwillingness. The small speculum went in easily but visualization of the cervix was difficult. Bimanual examination was exceedingly difficult because she would not relax. I noted that her cervix was a little soft but I couldn't feel the uterus. She was excessively tender over both ovaries but I couldn't feel any masses.

This young woman presented me with a very difficult clinical problem. I suspected that she was not telling the whole truth about her sexual activity. I asked her again, explaining that it was extremely important that we know. She still refused to admit she had been sexually active. The possibilities that went through my mind were that she might have a mid-cycle ovarian bleed, a ruptured ovarian cyst, pelvic inflammatory disease, or a ruptured ectopic pregnancy. I tried to explain this to her and told her that she would have to be admitted to the Gynaecology Ward for observation and further investigations. These included routine blood work, a urine analysis and culture, a urinary pregnancy test (at this time it took 48 hours to get a result), and a chest X-ray.

When I came to see her in the morning she looked ill and had a temperature of a hundred. Her pulse rate was one hundred and ten and her blood pressure was one hundred over sixty. The staff nurse on duty said she was not happy about the patient. The results of the blood test showed that she was anaemic. She had a slightly raised white cell count, her urine analysis was essentially negative, and the X-ray of her chest was normal. Her abdominal signs were more marked but there was no localisation. I, too, was uncomfortable with her progress and phoned Mr. MacDonald. He instructed me to arrange for an abdominal X-ray with the patient standing, and suggested that I put up an intravenous drip with saline. He said that he would be in within the hour. When the X-ray was taken I had a look at it and could not see anything unusual. Once Mr. MacDonald had seen the patient and examined her we went back to Sister's office.

"I don't really like the look of this young lady. I think she's a lot sicker than she seems. I agree with you Mr. Binns, I don't think she's telling us the whole truth. Let's go and look at that X-ray."

"I looked at it, sir," I said, "and couldn't see anything unusual about it."

When he got the film up on the viewer he looked at it for a few moments. "Yes, as I suspected, we have a problem. This is why I asked for a standing X-ray of the abdomen. If you look carefully at the left diaphragm you can see a dark shadow below it. That's air and should not be there. We're going to have to open her up and have a look to see what's going on. You better get some blood cross-matched and some intravenous saline running through a large gauge needle. I'll talk to her parents and explain what we have to do and get their consent. She's under age. We won't know until we have her abdomen open exactly what has happened but I suspect it's going to be a bit of a mess. Staff Nurse, can you get hold of the parents for me?"

"They're in the waiting room and are very worried. I'll tell them that you want to see them."

We took the girl to the theatre that afternoon by which time her temperature had gone up to one hundred and one and her pulse was running at one hundred and twenty. She looked sick, was flushed and sweating. Mr. Macdonald had talked to her again, but still couldn't get any further information out of her. He told her that he would have to make a vertical incision in her abdomen because we weren't sure what the problem was. Under anaesthesia I catheterized her to empty her bladder and Mr. MacDonald suggested that I do a gentle pelvic examination. I found that her vagina and cervix were soft. Her uterus was difficult to feel. I could not detect any masses, but after the examination I noted that there was some blood in the vagina. When I told Mr. Macdonald this he instructed me to wash out the vagina with an antiseptic solution. After the usual abdominal prep and draping Mr. MacDonald opened the abdomen through a lower para-medians incision.

"Well, she certainly has some bleeding in here. We'll soon find out what the cause is. Mr. Binns do you notice anything else unusual?"

"Not really, sir."

"I think I can smell Detol," he said. "I think we better get blood into the operating room. We may need it before we're done, Sister."

"It's already here, sir."

By this time we could see that there was a considerable amount of blood in the pelvic cavity. Once the small bowel was moved out of the way it was easy to see the pelvic contents and uterus. We could see that there was a tear in the top of the uterus and that there was some placental tissue protruding through the tear. The ragged edges of the tear were black and looked very unhealthy.

"We do have a mess here. I don't think we can safely save this uterus so we'll have to do a hysterectomy," said Mr. MacDonald. "You'd better start running that blood in," he said to the anaesthetist.

The actual hysterectomy was uncomplicated. At the end of the procedure all the blood and other fluids in the pelvis and the rest of the abdomen were sucked out. Then Mr. MacDonald washed the peritoneal cavity out with saline.

"How's the patient making out?" he asked the anaesthetist.

"Very well, considering I've given her one bottle of blood. I think she'll certainly need another. Her temperature is not too high and she's stable."

"Well, she's a healthy young woman and will almost certainly survive this operation. That this is the result of a criminal procedure I have no question. However, I doubt if we will get any history or evidence to present to the coroner or police. These patients and their relatives are very loyal to the abortionists. We never have enough evidence to proceed to criminal charges. We know that an abortionist visits this area every six to eight weeks. We think she comes from Sheffield but we don't have any other details. Over the years I've seen several criminal abortions and occasionally one of these patients dies, usually because of sepsis or uncontrollable bleeding. Mr. Binns, you will probably find this a rather sobering experience, but there is a lot to learn from this case. Thank you, Sister, and everybody else concerned. Keep a close eye on her for the next twenty-four hours and put her on penicillin for five days. Leave the drain in for forty-eight hours. I'll be in to see her in the morning. Let me know if there are any more problems. I'll go and talk to the parents."

Mr. Macdonald was right. Our young patient was much better the next day and we were able to send her home a week later. In spite of a lot of pressure from both Mr. Macdonald and the Nursing Sister we were not able to get any information about where or by whom the abortion had been performed. The police were notified but after a brief interview they decided there was nothing further they could do.

This patient raised many serious medical, legal, and moral questions for me. As students, we had been taught about illegal abortionists and there were some examples of damaged uteri in the Gordon Museum, which I remembered well. However, this was my first experience as a clinician. The situation of a sixteen-year-old being subjected to a procedure that rendered her sterile and which could easily have ended in her death distressed me. And I wondered how the young woman's parents would cope with the knowledge that their daughter would never have children of her own.

Prevention is always better than the cure, which raised the question of birth control and sex education for teenagers. In 1962 this subject was taboo. Sex education was not taught in schools; the subject was left to parents to discuss with their young adolescents. Family planning clinics were only available to married women or those about to get married. The birth control pill was just coming onto the market and yet sexual activity in teenagers was fairly common. The only methods of birth control were *coitus interruptus*, the so-called "safe time", condoms, spermicidal agents, diaphragms, cervical caps, and intrauterine Graphenberg rings. In order for a teenage girl to receive birth control advice from her doctor or a clinic, she had to get permission from her parents. Most parents were not approachable and, consequently, their teenage daughters took risks. Since I didn't have any religious or moral beliefs that prevented me from dealing with these problems, I decided that I would always help out in any way I could.

The other area of Gynaecology that I was introduced to graphically and personally at Grimsby was the management of cancers. During my six months there I saw several different cancers. These included disease of the cervix, uterus, the ovaries and one case of a vulvar cancer. After discussions with Dr. Greening and Mr. MacDonald, it became apparent to me that the management of genital cancers differed in different regions of the UK, Australia, Canada and the USA.

In the Sheffield region early cancers of the cervix were treated by surgery. I was privileged to assist at three Wertheim hysterectomies. This procedure was the most complicated surgical procedure that a gynaecologist was expected to do, and involved the removal of the uterus tubes, sometimes the ovaries, the upper third of the vagina, adjacent tissues, plus dissection and removal of the lymphatic drainage of the cervix. The operation was extensive and could take up to four hours. Patient selection was important; preoperative assessment, vital. Mr. MacDonald only performed this procedure when he felt it was important to preserve ovarian function and a normal sex life. The alternative was heavy irradiation with a combination of intrauterine and external X-ray treatment which did not preserve the remaining ovaries' ability to make estrogen.

The different approaches to treatment were widely discussed. The idea that there were different ways of treating the same medical condition was new to me and somewhat disconcerting, especially since practitioners of each theory thought their particular practice was the correct one. Mr. MacDonald, who was an experienced man, was pragmatic; he maintained that one had to know what the options were and then individualise before making the final decision on management.

In Grimsby I received a comprehensive introduction to gynaecological practice in the UK. My daily encounters provided limitless lessons on the relationship of medicine to life, perhaps because I worked with two exceptional people. The consultant, Mr. MacDonald, was thoughtful; he was both a good surgeon and a wonderful teacher— the perfect combination at that stage in my career. Billy Greening, the Australian registrar, had first trained as a nurse midwife and had spent time in the Australian Army. She had taken up medicine late in life. Like Mr. MacDonald, she had a wide range of practical experiences, which when coupled with maturity added balance and perspective to my youthful exuberance.

Elaine also benefitted from her general practice locum work, but we had little social life. We certainly didn't form lasting friendships with any local people. We soon discovered a seaside resort town close by in Lincolnshire. Fresh fish from Cleesthorpe became a legendary culinary delight, one of those memories we have shared on a regular basis down the years.

After six months we moved south to my position as a lowly houseman in Oxford. There were two Departments in Obstetrics and Gynaecology. One was the University Teaching Unit which was run by the well-known Professor Chasseur Moir and his staff. He was world-famous for his work on blood transfusions in maternity care and repairing vesico-vaginal fistulas. Patients were referred to his centre from all over England and from abroad. The other unit was the National Health Regional Department, run by Mr. Stallworthy (known as "JS") and Mr. Hawksworth, both of whom were New Zealanders. Their unit worked out of both the Churchill Hospital in Headington and the Radcliffe Infirmary in the centre of Oxford. It was a very busy unit.

I was based at the Churchill Hospital. Built in 1940 and named after Clementine Churchill, Prime Minister Winston Churchill's wife, it was constructed to look after the wounded from the London Blitz in World War II. There were never enough of these patients to use it to full capacity, and so the hospital was leased to the American Army and reverted to the local Oxfordshire Council at the end of the war when it was operated as a conventional general hospital, minus an emergency department.

Like the resident staff-nurse and junior medical staff accommodation, our housing was in army Nissen huts, which had been put up during the war. The Nursing Sisters resided in part of the main hospital complex, which formed a square, housing the administrative offices and the hospital cafeteria along one side. The four operating rooms were at one corner of this section and the maternity unit was opposite. The patients were lodged in eight twenty- to thirty-bed wards down the next two sides of the square, with an extra ward in the middle. The third side was where the newborn nurseries were and where the Nissen huts started. All the wards and departments were connected by an open, rectangular walkway. Going from one area to another meant the staff stayed fit.

My primary responsibility was to the maternity unit, but twice a week I had to assist at gynaecological operations and cover the gynae-cology ward when the other houseman had his day off. There were two senior registrars, six registrars and eight housemen covering the two hospitals. We all had to attend the consultants' rounds and the "tea party" which was held once a week, on Thursday evenings, at the Churchill. The tea party was an educational session where interesting cases from the week were presented, discussed in detail, and their management decided upon.

The maternity unit was a self-contained unit with four delivery rooms, one of which was an operating theatre where caesarean sec-tions were performed. There was a small ante-partum ward and a twenty-bed post-partum ward. The newborn nursery had a special section for premature and other sick babies. These special care facili-ties were required because Churchill Hospital was the referral hos-pital for the region, which extended from Banbury in the north to Swindon in the south and halfway to Wales on the west. Many of the patients were referred from other hospitals, family practice units, and family practitioners who ran district midwifery practices.

My responsibilities were to the labour floor, and to the ante-partum and the post-partum patients. Labouring patients were in-itially looked after by the midwives who were responsible for normal deliveries. When problems arose with labouring patients the mid-wives referred them to me. During the six months at Oxford I man-aged to gain a considerable amount of experience with difficult deliv-eries and the care of abnormal obstetrics. I also became practiced at doing caesarean sections.

Much of my maternity teaching and advice came from the midwif-ery staff, led by Peggy—an attractive, hard-working, auburn-haired Sister. She ran the unit with military precision. It was a brave indi-vidual who dared to disagree with her. Even Mr. Stallworthy thought twice before offering a criticism.

Peggy first introduced me to clinical research. I was sitting in the doctor's office in the maternity ward when she came in. "Mr. Binns, I have a job for you. You see the charts stacked on the shelf just above your head. They need to be completed before they can be sent back to medical records for filing. There is a white sheet attached to the front of each chart and your job is to fill them in and then return them to my office. I'm sorry there are so many of them, but your predecessor did not do them before he left."

I looked up at the shelf and estimated that there were more than two hundred charts! "What are the forms all about?" I asked.

"Oh, it's some research project of JS's. The information that you put on the forms is entered onto computer cards and then analysed by the university computer department. The information they want is quite detailed but once you get the hang of going through the charts you'll find it quite easy. Here, I'll show you." She leaned over me and pulled out one of the charts.

The form on the chart was very busy, with code letters and numbers around the edge and questions about the patient, her admission details, progress, treatment, method of delivery, and discharge in blocks on the inside. There were coded answers to the questions and a tick had to be placed against this code on the margin of the form. There was a space for comments when the proper code was not to be found. Peggy showed me how to go through the chart and fill in the form.

"It's not that difficult but it's time consuming. JS is insistent that we get them done. He was not very pleased last week when I told him that your predecessor had not done them. It's a medical project, so you will be responsible for them."

"It looks like a big job. Will there be more charts coming?" I asked.

"Yes. It's an ongoing project for the next year."

"Okay, I'll see what I can do to catch up."

Getting caught up took me four weeks and I never heard what the outcome of the research project was. I suspect that one of the registrars got a couple of papers published out of the information. The activity introduced me to simple clinical research and the collection of data. That so much could be mined from so little fascinated me and I began to realize how much information there is on medical charts, some of which is very private.

Oxford was a schizophrenic city with a large academic population and with an even larger population manufacturing Morris cars at the Cowley works. It was a city of both divergence and convergence. Being in labour and having a baby reminded everyone of their common humanity. The response to pain and the emotions involved with childbirth were the same.

Peggy and her midwives taught me much about people and their response to pain and how to handle these problems. For women in labour we initially used mild analgesics and then progressed to nitrous oxide. This was often all that was required for a normal labour and delivery. But some patients required stronger sedation. For these we had Pethidine (Demerol), morphine, and even heroin, which was a very effective and useful drug. When these became inadequate we resorted to caudal anaesthesia, which is very similar to the modern day use of epidurals.

These anaesthetic techniques first came into vogue during the 1940s in the United States, but were not used in the UK until after World War II. Oxford was one of the first centres to use this method of pain relief in childbirth. It was an excellent procedure and allowed the obstetrician to do operative deliveries without general anaesthesia. The dangers of general anaesthetics in maternity care were well documented. Occasionally caudal anaesthetic was even sufficient to do a caesarean section.

Sir John Stallworthy was a remarkable man who took on the responsibility of running the unit just before the Second World War started. He had just completed his specialist training under Chasseur Moir and was ready to move back to New Zealand. He was actually packed up and prepared to move with his wife and young family when the Oxford Region decided they needed a new department in addition to the Nuffield Department run by Professor Moir. They offered the position to Mr. Stallworthy.

In New Zealand, JS had been a good rugby player and was an All-Black trialist when at medical school. He was very strict about how the unit was run and developed what came to be called the Oxford method. His mentor was the famous Victor Bonny of Queen Charlotte's and the Middlesex Hospital, London. Many of the surgical techniques that we learned in Oxford came from him. JS was a dedicated teacher and was interested in how his juniors were progressing. He was often hypercritical of individual performances and was feared by his staff, but he never let us lose sight of our primary purpose—to care for the patient. JS was a superb technician himself and would not allow his junior staff to perform procedures until he was convinced they were both capable and reliable. Safety always came first.

He was keen on research and was always open to new ideas and ways in which to find answers to problems. And yet before presenting anything new to him we had to have a very good understanding of what the issues were and be confident that our personal solution might be an improvement over existing practice or theory. He could be very set in his ways, if not stubborn, especially in defence of theories and practices that were proven. He wouldn't accept change for its own sake. Although he sometimes rebuked me, largely for what I felt was my lack of experience, I never thought he was being unfairly critical. I knew he was only interested in making sure I learned from my mistakes. While some of his subordinates felt abused by his apparent intolerance, I was fine with his judgements. His approach was similar to what I had known as a medical student at Guy's.

The other consultant, Mr. Hawksworth, was a different proposition; a different sort of master. He was always a complete gentleman, with the emphasis on gentle—soft-spoken and empathetic with both patients and staff. While an excellent obstetrician and a good gynaecological surgeon, he took comfort from the familiar rather than experiment with new techniques. He simply didn't like risk in medicine.

Yet both of these consultants used the same patient management principles, so there were no major differences to be learned in this regard, unlike in Winnipeg where, within reason, different treatments and patient strategies were encouraged. This did mean that we learned a singular way to practice, but we were told that it was not necessarily the only way to do things and that our options would broaden when we became consultants. During my six months in Oxford I discovered that there was a lot more to obstetric care than I had known and understood to be the case while working in Winnipeg. My vision of the field expanded and deepened.

Unfortunately there was no married accommodation available for junior staff in Oxford. This meant that Elaine and the girls had to stay with my parents in Saltburn-by-the-Sea. There was a short period of six weeks when they were able to come and live in Oxford. One of the anaesthetists was away on holiday and wanted somebody to look after his house in Banbury Road, close to the Radcliffe Infirmary and downtown Oxford. House sitting gave us the opportunity to explore the beautiful old city and visit some of the colleges. Since it was during the summer months, at the height of the tourist season, most of the colleges and churches were open to the public. We spent many hours investigating ancient stone buildings, walking along the canal, and visiting famous pubs we'd read about in novels and histories or we'd heard associated with famous Oxford residents.

I was sorry when my six-month contract came to an end. I had applied for and got a gynaecological senior medical officer's job in Manchester. This position would complete the gynaecological requirements for the Royal College of Obstetricians and Gynaecologists (MRCOG) exams. These exams were the next step towards becoming a specialist in the field. Besides, I was lucky to get this job as it was also a university-affiliated post.

Shortly after I arrived at St. Mary's Hospital, Manchester, Elaine decided that she and the girls had spent enough time living with my parents. Our next child was expected in May and she wanted to be in a place of our own before she had the baby. She visited her parents on the Wirral, a peninsula bounded by the River Dee, the River Mersey and the Irish Sea, just north of Chester. She found a small furnished cottage to rent in Lymm, which was on the outskirts of Manchester. This location was a convenient distance from the hospital and close to Elaine's parents.

During our move to Lymm, in early February, 1963, I learned one of my most important medical lessons. While moving our things to the cottage, I suffered my first serious physical injury. I was dragging a sea-trunk of packed goods that was too heavy to lift. There was snow and ice on the path and I thought it would be easier to drag the trunk along the path instead of end over ending it. I was on my own and had just got to the door of the cottage when I felt some severe pain in my lower back. When I tried to straighten, I found I could only get three-quarters of the way up. With great difficulty, I managed to get the door open and roll the trunk into the house. When I tried to find relief from the pain I realized I had probably prolapsed a vertebral disc. I found a door, and after putting a small book under the open end, so as not to pull the door off its hinges, I hung there for as long as I could. This gave me some relief and I managed to get back into the car and drive to the hospital.

By this time it was ten o'clock at night. I was on duty the next day. I decided that if I could get up to my room, I would see how things felt in the morning. When I tried to get out of the car I found the only way that I could do it was to roll out and crawl the few yards to the doctor's entrance and pull myself upright using the door handle. With considerable effort I found the lift and got to my room, where I had some painkillers. After swallowing a couple of pills and lying very still I was reasonably comfortable and fell asleep.

When I tried to get up in the morning the pain returned with a vengeance, so I phoned my registrar who came up and agreed that I had "slipped a disc". He gave me some more painkillers and suggested I rest for the day. Things were a bit better the next day, but the consultant who came to see me insisted that I have some back X-rays. When they came back normal he sent me to the physiotherapy department for stretching and heat treatment. This went on for several days. My first experience as a patient was humbling.

At the time I assumed I would get better, but I have to admit there were moments of doubt and I did wonder what I would do if I did not recover completely. What impressed me most was the attitude of the caregivers and their genuine concerns about my progress. Fortunately, I was back at work within a few days, but it was a significant new experience. Since that episode I have always felt that all doctors should spend a few days of their lives as patients.

* * *

February was not the best time of year to acclimate to a large northern English city like Manchester—a cold, dull, often foggy, damp, and rainy place.

St. Mary's Hospital on Whitworth Park was established in 1790 as a hospital for women and was relocated in 1903 to its present location. Built out of local stone, it had wide corridors and windows that looked out onto a dreary view of grey buildings, a few trees, and a scruffy lawn. The corridors had concrete floors; the walls were painted with a heavy-duty paint, medium green for the first four feet and then cream to the ceilings. The corridors were noisy and echoed. There was a constant sense of playback.

The wards were open, with sixteen beds down each wall, and a Sister's office at the entrance. The utility rooms and bathrooms were at the far end of the wards. The beds were the typical white cast-iron hospital issue on wheels. Each patient had a chair and small cabinet for personal items. The portable screens, also on wheels, were stacked near Sister's office. Surprisingly, most of the patients were cheerful and appreciative.

The operating theatres were spacious, well-lit, but windowless. The Outpatients Department had a large waiting room and six examining rooms. Each consultant had one day a week for his clinics. There was no emergency department, so patients who came in as emergencies were transferred to the General Hospital, which was not far away, or would be admitted directly to the wards.

The housemen had rooms on the fourth floor which were adequate, plus a common room with an attached dining room. One feature of the common room was a small medical library. However, I only used these facilities one night in four and one weekend in four. The rest of the time I joined Elaine at our cottage in Lymm.

I had been appointed as Senior Medical Officer to Dr. A.H.C. Walker, who was one of the four gynaecologists working in the hospital. A university professorial unit also worked there. As most of the junior staff were preparing for the MRCOG exams, we attended all the teaching rounds that we could. The general gynaecology work was similar to the work in Grimsby, but there were a few philosophical differences in the management of uterine prolepses, genital cancers, and urinary incontinence. The management of uterine cancer was more conservative with much greater reliance on radioactive radium insertions and deep X-ray therapy. Even so, there was considerable debate about the best way to treat these patients. We did learn how to interpret the research work that was being published with a critical lens. Screening for cancer of the cervix with Ayer's and Papanicolaou smears (now simply called cervical smears) was still in its infancy, but was available, and we were taught these techniques.

Before I qualified to sit the MRCOG exams I had to prepare and submit the "Book"—a collection of twenty obstetric and twenty gynaecologic case histories of patients I had managed. The cases selected had to be representative of the speciality and illustrate that I had a broad experience of it. The case histories had to be detailed and I had to make appropriate commentaries after each case. There were also two long commentaries of about five hundred words each to do, about cases that I felt were particularly interesting. The "Book" was a sort of thesis, in length and detail.

I included cases from Canada and the UK and was able to discuss some of the philosophical differences in the practice of the specialty on either side of the Atlantic. The final hurdle was finding someone to type my "Book". The manuscript was 255 pages long with some photos and graphs. Getting it typed professionally would have been expensive, so Elaine took on the job, much to her consternation, which kept her occupied for a month or so. After I had completed my time in Manchester, the "Book" was finished and accepted in November 1963.

Elaine and I had our third child while I was working in Manchester. My mother was able to come and stay with us when the baby was due. Patrick, named after my father, was born on the seventeenth of May. Once again I was working at the hospital when I received news of the happy event. Husbands being present for the delivery was not an accepted practice at that time, unless it was a home birth. Our first child was born in a London maternity hospital, the second in a hospital in Winnipeg and the last in a hospital in Manchester. Helen was delivered by a midwife and Kathryn and Patrick by physicians, although the doctor barely got there on time for Patrick. Elaine felt that the English approach with midwives in control was the most satisfying for mothers because midwives were more patient—they weren't in a big hurry to get it all over and done with. As an obstetrician who spent most of his time trying to sort out problems in the delivery room, I had to admit I saw things differently. When something went wrong at home the stress on everyone could be enormous, as I was to find out years later in my own practice.

The summer months in Lymm and Manchester were spent with family, with frequent visits to Elaine's parents on the Wirral, and the occasional excursion to Saltburn-by-the-Sea. Towards the end of my six months in Manchester I faced the perennial problem of finding another job.

Positions in England were scarce. There were no registrar jobs in Manchester or the greater region. I would have liked to have gone back to Oxford but there were no jobs there, either. The next best area for us would have been the South Birmingham region and I searched the journals for jobs there. Again, nothing.

Eventually a middle-grade registrar job was advertised in Swindon, which was in the Oxford region. Although I was not really senior enough to be a middle-grade registrar I applied for the job giving Mr. Hawksworth and Mr. Stallworthy as my references. The interview was held in the Oxford Hospital Board room at the Radcliffe Infirmary. The interview was not until midday so I drove to London and spent the night at Mike Boundy's house. About 9:30 p.m. the phone rang. It was Elaine. She told me that Mr. Hawksworth wanted to talk to me before the interview. I was to meet him in the operating room at the Churchill hospital in the morning. This surprising request made me wonder if I had done something I shouldn't have.

When I got to the operating room Mr. Hawksworth was in the middle of a hysterectomy so I had to change before going in. As I came through the door he looked up: "Ah, Binns, nice to see you. How are things going in Manchester?"

"Very well, sir. But as you know the job comes to an end in a few weeks and I'm looking for work. I've applied for the Swindon job but I may not be senior enough to be eligible."

"That's why I asked you to come in this morning. We are giving you our complete support and I think you will get the job, but we have a vacancy here that has come up rather suddenly and we wondered if you'd like to come back to Oxford instead."

I could hardly believe my ears.

"I'd be delighted to come to Oxford, sir. How soon would you want me? I have a couple of weeks leave due at the end of my present job so could be here in four weeks."

"Hmmm. We were hoping that you might be able to get here sooner, but I think we can manage that long. One of our registrars has had to go back to Australia for a family bereavement and is not planning on coming back."

"Thank you very much, sir. What shall I do about the interview?" I asked.

"Oh. Don't worry about that. I've spoken to Mr. Kent, the consultant, who said something about us stealing his candidates. He was quite understanding." And he chuckled. "We look forward to seeing you as soon as you can make it. You'll get a written offer in the mail in a day or so. When do you plan on taking the exams?"

"Next year, sir. I have all the cases I need for the 'Book' and I should have it finished in a couple of months."

"That's good. Let me know if I can be of any help. It's quite a test and difficult to put together."

"Thank you, sir. Yes, difficult indeed, but I'm actually enjoying the challenge. It's an excellent test of what I've learned in my career to date." At that moment I felt as though I were going to explode with joy. Restraining myself was difficult. I wanted to leap about the room, but I stood there, transfixed. "And thank you for the job. I'm really looking forward to being back in Oxford and feel very privileged. Is there anything else today or can I get back to Manchester?"

He smiled. I was certain in that instant he knew how I felt. "No. Have a good trip back and we'll see you soon."

I returned to Oxford as a middle-grade registrar based at the Churchill Hospital. I was now responsible for patient care in the maternity unit, where I had worked as a houseman, as well as for the twenty-bed gynaecology ward, which included two fully dedicated operation days a week. As a registrar I had to cover emergencies in two hospitals when on call. Outpatients were all seen at the Radcliffe Infirmary. This gave me the opportunity to attend the excellent teaching rounds that were put on by Professor Chasser-Moir's department. As a registrar I had teaching responsibilities to the housemen and the midwifery school at the Churchill Hospital.

There were three outpatients clinics a week at the Radcliffe. These looked after both ante-natal and gynaecologic referrals from general practitioners. The ante-natal patients were first screened by the midwives and the registrars saw the gynaecology patients in preparation for presentation to the consultants who made the final decision on management and dictated the letters to the practitioners.

The maternity patients were all high risk, referred by their practitioners for hospital delivery. The reasons for such referrals were laid out quite clearly for some situations such as primi-gravida (first baby) or grand multiparity (over five children), previous caesarean section, breeches, previous mid-cavity forceps delivery, post-partum haemorrhages, etc., but others were less clear and included socio-economic situations. This screening procedure was helpful to us and clarified in advance many of the problems the midwives might otherwise face.

In order to provide as safe a district service as possible, the concept of a flying squad was developed in several regions of the UK. The first was set up in 1933 by Dr. H.J. Thomson in Bellshill, Lanarkshire, Scotland, and the concept of sending help out to labouring mothers in the district spread from there. A team was on call twenty-four hours a day that could go out to patient's homes to help in emergencies. Our Oxford team consisted of the on-call registrar, with a houseman, and a senior midwife. If a general anaesthetic was needed, then the on-call anaesthetist was brought on board. Emergency problems in the district had been studied and the conclusion reached was that it was safer to deal with an emergency at home and stabilize the patient before transferring them to the hospital. Since the problems could range from acute foetal distress to life-threatening bleeding, we had to be prepared for almost any eventuality.

Anaesthesia was a major concern. The registrar had to inform the on-call anaesthetist when he felt their attendance was needed. The registrar's car served as transport for all the equipment required whether for a forceps delivery, repairing a genital tract laceration, or manually removing the placenta. We carried separate packs for baby resuscitation, giving open anaesthesia and setting up drips for shocked mothers. We also took two bottles of Rh O negative blood with us.

We were drilled on flying squad call procedures. The most important was being sure to get the patient's address written down carefully, so that we knew where to go. Directions could be confusing. Very few patients had phones in their homes and the calls we received often came from public phone booths. A detailed map of the Oxford district was always a part of our pack, but, fortunately for us, most of the midwives knew the area well and we managed to find the patients.

When it was foggy and difficult to see where we were going, I instructed the husband to stand on a street corner waving a torch to guide us. There was an emergency ambulance service which we called if we felt the patient would have to be moved to the hospital. The drivers and assistants of the ambulance service were not trained in resuscitation procedures as they are today; their main purpose was to provide a comfortable transport to the hospital.

These call-outs were stressful but they proved to be a valuable part of the maternity service in the region. They brought us face-to-face with some of the problems that doctors and midwives had to face when delivering babies at home. The occasional tragedies that happened usually resulted in the death of the baby, but during the years I was in Oxford I never knew of a maternal death in the district.

Except in emergencies, as a registrar I was always supervised directly by a Senior Registrar or Consultant. I was also constantly under the watchful eye of Peggy and her staff. They consulted us when there were obstetric problems and did not hesitate to let us know when they thought we were mistaken in our assessments. I could get things under way if we were unable to contact a superior. In dire emergencies we did go ahead while waiting for the call back but this was only done if the whole team—surgeon, midwife and anaesthesiologist—all agreed.

Early on I learned the value of being efficient when running a department. In 1963 money was scarce, but it was not until I became responsible for organizing the operation lists that the seriousness of our lack of funds came to my notice. One day I submitted a list to the Theatre Sister that included two consecutive vaginal hysterectomies.

"You cannot do that, Mr. Binns. Mr. Stallworthy will not wait for the instruments to be sterilized between cases."

"I didn't know there would be a problem."

"We only have one full vaginal and one full abdominal set of instruments to work with so you cannot do two vaginal or two abdominal majors in a row. We have to sterilize the instruments between the cases and that takes twenty minutes or so. Neither Mr. Stallworthy nor Mr. Hawksworth would be happy with that as it is not an efficient use of their time. I did ask Mr. Stallworthy about getting some more instruments, but he told me that if we alternated cases we could save the money and spend it on something more critical. This does make life difficult at times, but we manage. Perhaps one day we will have the luxury of more instruments. You can put in a minor between cases if you like, but both consultants prefer to get the majors out of the way first, if they can."

"Thanks for the advice, Sister. I didn't realize that money in a teaching hospital like this was that tight."

"It's been like this since the war. We're still struggling. It's only because of the efficient way we run this hospital that we stay well within our budget most of the time. The services of consultants like Mr. Stallworthy and Mr. Hawksworth allow the hospital to survive."

"I see." To be honest, I was shocked. That there might be limits to what we did had never occurred to me. None of the senior staff let on that finances were a problem. I think if this had been common knowledge, the reputation of the hospital might have suffered.

"You've just returned from Canada," she said, "I don't suppose you had this sort of problem there."

"Not that I was aware of, but I was only a junior intern and was not privy to the budgeting and running of the hospital."

Following this conversation I began to notice how well the whole unit was run and became aware of the importance of efficiency and reducing waste at all levels of patient care. This applied to obstetrics and percolated into the intensive care nursery which was run by a senior Sister who was totally dedicated to looking after sick neonates. She would spend hours personally looking after sick babies and this showed in the results that came out of the unit. The survival of premature babies was better in her unit than in most reported studies and it was probably a result of the personal attention these babies received.

The importance of inter-departmental communication was another aspect of patient care that came to my notice. There was a very good relationship between our department, internal medicine, surgery, anaesthesia and paediatrics. I was involved with a very complex case of severe systemic lupus erythamatosis (one of the collagen diseases) during pregnancy. Very little was known about the impact of lupus on pregnancy and the unborn baby. My patient became quite ill during her pregnancy and during the last few weeks I observed that the foetal heart rate was very slow (forty-fifty beats per minute), which indicated a complete heart block.

Her overall care involved three departments with careful monitoring. She went into premature labour at thirty-seven weeks and we used experimental heart rate monitoring equipment (electro-cardiography) on both her and her baby during labour. The equipment came from the paediatric department and the mother's care was the concern of the internal medicine department. All I had to do was oversee the labour and delivery of the baby. The significant thing was that we all worked together. We were able to monitor both heart rates during labour and delivery. The baby was delivered alive with his complete heart block. Unfortunately, he was also found to have systemic lupus and did not survive more than a few days.

I was surprised by how low I felt after this loss. I wasn't at fault for anything that had happened and yet I took it personally. In medicine we always want to win even though we know this is impossible. Intellectually I understood what had happened, but emotionally I felt gutted. Perhaps it was the irony that struck me—that with so much cooperation could come such loss.

When I presented the case to the Tea Party, Mr. Stallworthy said that in view of the unusual nature and rarity of this case, he thought that I should present it to the Royal Society of Medicine meeting in London the following month. He also suggested that Dr. Hull and I should write the case up for publication. Although terrified, I agreed.

The pressure of presenting material to the Royal Society of Medicine was soon apparent. I was allowed only fifteen minutes to put this complex case and its significance before the august group of senior members of the medical profession. It was a daunting task. Fortunately, David Hull (paediatrics) was a great help putting things together. I don't think I have ever been so nervous as I was that night. I managed to stay within the time limit and then was asked a few polite questions which I managed to answer reasonably well. The whole episode was a major learning experience.

The next hurdle I had to overcome was the MRCOG exams, which were regarded as the Obstetrics and Gynaecology equivalent to the FRCS or MRCS examinations in Surgery and Internal Medicine. The examination dates came quickly and I did not have much time to prepare. The whole process was long. Each paper in each division was three hours long. Then there were long case presentations where we had to take histories, and examine and discuss those with the examiners. Following this there were the notorious *vivas* where the examiners could ask us questions about anything in the field. And sometimes outside it!

Amazingly I did not feel worried going into these exams, probably because I did not expect to pass them on the first occasion given their terrifying reputation. I wasn't as intimidated by the examiners as I had been during my previous clinical exams. The examiners certainly were very detailed and went on for a long time. A few days after my final exam, Mr. Hawksworth met me in the corridor and congratulated me on my performance. He told me not to worry about my results and said I would get official confirmation soon. I was both surprised and pleased with the news.

Some months after this Elaine and I discussed what the next step in my career should be. We considered our financial position, which was a lot worse than it had been in Canada, even though my job there had been a junior one. We couldn't keep our bank balance out of the red each month, in spite of Elaine's excellent money management. We were going broke.

We were in rented accommodation and liked living in Oxford. Helen had started school, but there was no work available for Elaine, probably due to the fact that many of the professors at Oxford universities were married to physicians. These spouses were doing any part-time work that became available and they got preferential treatment when jobs came up.

We thought that if I could get a senior registrar's post we could manage with the increased salary, but the three senior registrars in the Oxford region were all recently appointed and there was no prospect of a job coming up for another two years. I had not got round to discussing the topic with Mr. Hawksworth or Mr. Stallworthy but I was considering returning to Canada where I felt my job prospects might be better, even if it meant working as a general practitioner and not as a specialist. I was still registered to practice medicine in Manitoba and had reciprocal privileges in Alberta, Saskatchewan and the Maritime provinces. After over four years of training it seemed bizarre not to continue with the specialty.

One night, at one in the morning, I was called to deliver one of Mr. Stallworthy's private patients. He was on the way into the hospital, but he was not going to get there in time. He had just spent several weeks touring East and South Africa as a visiting Sims Black Profes-

the delivery, out of the blue, over a cup of coffee, he asked: have you ever considered working in Africa?"

I said. "My father spent twelve years working in Northern Nigeria and I visited him and my mother several times. When I think about it, watching him work there was probably one of the reasons I took up medicine. Why do you ask?"

"As you know, I've just got back from visiting there and they really could use our help. The staffing conditions in Mulago University Hospital, Uganda, are very limited, and they're doing a lot of very good work. They only graduate sixty doctors a year from their medical school, which is the only one in the whole of East Africa. The county needs trained doctors and the teaching and clinical experience of working there would be invaluable to a young person like you."

"I agree. But what concerns me is that I've not finished my training and really should be looking for a senior registrar job. I was hoping there might be one coming up in the Oxford region, but that won't happen for at least two years and our finances are looking a bit grim these days. Elaine and I were talking about this recently and wondered about going back to Canada. But that would probably mean going into general practice which is not what I really want to do."

"Yes, I'm aware of your problem. Perhaps if you would consider going to Africa for a year or so, I think I could guarantee you a senior registrar job in this Region when you get back."

"I'll consider it, but I'll have to see what Elaine thinks about the idea. The whole family would have to go and there are health hazards associated with going to places like Uganda and Nigeria. My other concern is that once I step off the ladder of promotion here I would lose my seniority," I said.

"Well, think about it, and, as I said, I will find a job for you when you return, if you decide to go. Thank you for looking after Mrs. Castle for me. She's a nice lady and she also asked me to thank you."

The next day I discussed the prospects of going to Africa with Elaine and, to my surprise, she thought it was a good idea, especially when she heard that Mr. Stallworthy had promised to look after me when we came back. I remained apprehensive and told Elaine that

that might not happen. Two years was a long time and I was not sure he was really in a position to make such a promise. And yet I was interested in going to Africa and felt that we could always return to Canada if things did not work out when we got back to England.

The next day I told Mr. Stallworthy that Elaine was agreeable and he suggested I start looking for a suitable posting that would be financially viable. So it was back to the BMJ job section once more where the Ministry of Overseas Development was advertising for an Obstetrician and Gynaecologist in Uganda but not at Mulago Hospital. It was a government job which was two-thirds funded by the British government and one third by the Ugandan government. It was described as a consultant posting in Obstetrics and Gynaecology and the salary was reasonable. The contract was for two years and included all travel and accommodation expenses. I wrote to the Ministry and they invited me to an interview.

The interview was conducted by two physicians and a representative from the Ugandan government who asked all manner of questions about my background and why I was interested in the job. At the end they told me that they were hoping for someone with more experience than I had. The job was a consultant post, but they would get back to me after talking to my references. I did not really expect to get the job after what they had said and was surprised three weeks later when Mr. Stallworthy told me they would employ me, but only as a special-grade medical officer. He told me they would still pay me the same salary and expenses, but that they might ask me to do some general medical duties. This did not concern me too much when I considered what my father had done most of his life.

Everything was finalized a few weeks later with a contract signed with the Ministry of Overseas Development and the Ugandan government. We were to fly to Uganda as a family in a few weeks. Our scant belongings would follow us by sea. My parents thought that our going overseas was a good idea. Father said that I would enjoy myself, but warned me that there would be a lot of frustrations along the way. Elaine's parents were not so enthusiastic, especially as it meant we would not be seeing them for a couple of years. They also had some concerns about the health of the children, in particular from tropical diseases. We flew from London's Heathrow Airport to Entebbe, first class, on the second of February, 1965. The next phase of my medical education was about to begin.

Chapter 10
Uganda

On the long flight from London to Entebbe, Patrick attracted all the attention, from crew and passengers alike. He was only eighteen months old at the time and didn't have a seat of his own. The stewardess offered him a baby cot but he was too large for it and spent most of his time crawling and bunny hopping up and down the aisles between the seats. Fortunately his behaviour was more of an amusement to the other passengers than an annoyance. In those days "buckling in" was less of a concern than it is now, although if there had been an emergency, one of us, Elaine or I, would have scooped him up. The girls settled in, each with a picture book. At some point we all managed to sleep.

We cleared customs and immigration, which reminded me of my trips to Kano, Nigeria, when I had visited my parents. As we moved out of the baggage area I was once again struck by the bright, colourful dress of the locals. It was like walking through a field of exotic flowers.

We had arrived first thing in the morning, but it was midday when we got through the paperwork. I was expecting to be met by somebody from the Medical Services Department. This had always occurred when my father had arrived at his new postings and whenever he travelled out of Nigeria. I enquired at the desk if there were any messages for us but, no, there were none. When I phoned their offices they informed me that they had been expecting me a month earlier and had assumed I was not coming. Thus they had not made any arrangements to meet us or arranged any hotel accommodation. When I asked the gentleman who had answered the phone what I was supposed to do with my wife and children, all of whom were sitting in the airport, he was obviously a little flustered. He had no idea what he should do about us. When I suggested that I might just get on the next plane back to London, he got rather excited and told me there would be transport arriving at the airport in the next half-hour to take us to a hotel.

Three-quarters of an hour later a bus arrived to pick us up. When we got to the hotel, the receptionist said she had no idea we were coming and that there were no rooms available. By this time I realized I needed to be more forceful, although I felt uncomfortable behaving like an entitled colonial. The posturing worked, though, and she managed to find a room. But, she told me, she could not guarantee we would have a room the next day. This would be a little embarrassing and awkward, I said; the next day was Sunday and we had no idea where we might find another hotel. I explained to her that we were concerned about the way we were being treated. She told me the only other option would be to go into Kampala, which was thirty-five miles down the road, by taxi. Luckily this didn't happen. Once matters were sorted, we found the airport hotel in Entebbe comfortable and the food tasty.

At ten o'clock on Monday morning a white Land Rover with "Given to the Uganda Government by UNICEF" written in bold letters down both sides arrived to take me to Medical Headquarters. There I was to be interviewed by the Deputy Minister of Health, whose office was situated in a compound of several buildings surrounded by palm and tropical fruit trees. I noticed that the road into the compound was a reddish *murrum*—another reminder of Nigeria. It was warm, and I saw the odd lizard scuttling away as I walked over to the main building. The Deputy's office was located in a large bungalow. I climbed the four steps that led up to a wooden veranda where the doorkeeper sat in a hand-carved chair next to the main entrance. He greeted me and asked who I was. I told him and he instructed me to go through to the office at the end of the corridor.

I knocked on the door and a deep voice instructed me to "Come in". A slim, middle-aged Ugandan, dressed in a suit and tie, rose from his desk and greeted me. When we shook hands his grip was firm but not challenging, and his eyes quickly assessed me.

"Dr. Binns, I am Francis, the Deputy Minister of Health of Uganda. For some reason we thought you were coming a month ago. I'm sorry about the confusion on Saturday. I hope you had an enjoyable weekend at the hotel and that the accommodation was not too uncomfortable. How did you and your family find the trip?" he asked with a friendly smile.

"I'm not sure why the confusion arose. I received the tickets for the trip three weeks ago and I have a letter from your department giving details of the flight and travel arrangements. Everything seemed organized from my end. Perhaps the confusion originated at the Ministry of Overseas Development."

He nodded.

"I see from your file that you have been appointed as a Special Grade Medical Officer in obstetrics and gynaecology. Since your appointment has not been designated as a consultant we will be expecting you to do some general duties while you are here. We have planned to send you to Gulu, which is two hundred miles away, in the Northern region. The hospital you'll be working at is the regional hospital for the area and is quite busy. The medical personnel consists of a general surgeon and his wife who is a general practitioner, a Russian paediatrician, a North Korean eye specialist, and two Polish doctors, one of whom is an internist and the other a trained surgeon. There is a medical superintendent, Dr. Edyago, whose duties are purely administrative.

"You'll be the only doctor there who has been trained as an obstetrician and gynaecologist. You'll be expected to see patients referred to you from four other centres, Kitgum, Mayo, Lira and the furthest away, Arua, which is one hundred and fifty miles on the other side of the Nile, on the Congo border. A house with hard furnishings is provided. You will be able to arrange for servants when you get there. I think you and your family will find the weather quite pleasant. Not too hot. You must remember to take your anti-malarial pills. Malaria is very common in this area." He paused. "Do you have any questions?"

"As I mentioned at my interview, I'm happy to take on some general duties but you need to be aware of my limitations. From what you've just said I'll be the only obstetrician and gynaecologist in the area and presumably be on-call all the time for emergencies. This means I'll not have any time off. Frankly, that seems unfair."

The Deputy Minister leaned forward and looked at the stack of files on his desk.

"The problem is that there isn't enough staff at the hospital and we were hoping that you would be prepared to do some general duties to help the other doctors who work there. The other specialists at the hospital are already doing this. Dr. Edyago asked us if you would cover one night a week on call and we agreed on your behalf. My apologies for being so presumptuous. But the extra duties should not be that difficult for you with your training. And it will spread out the workload."

"If everybody else is doing it I wouldn't want to be the only one who refuses." Realizing there was no way I could avoid extra duties, I changed the subject.

"How am I supposed to get to Gulu?" I asked.

"You will go up by car. It takes about five hours to get there."

"As you must know, I don't have a car," I said.

"Of course. Forgive me. We'll need to do something about that. Usually we arrange for new doctors to buy a car with an advance on their pay, at minimal interest. You'll be able to claim travelling expenses and we guarantee you'll have paid off the car by the time you leave here in two years. We'll arrange for you to go to Kampala tomorrow to buy the car. Since you have a family I suggest you buy a Peugeot 304. They are quite roomy, reliable and economical."

This was a surprise. I had assumed a vehicle would be provided. I also wondered what sort of arrangement he had with the Peugeot dealership in Kampala.

"Is there anything else I should know about Gulu?"

The Deputy Minister shook his head. "Not that comes to mind."

"What time will the driver arrive tomorrow morning to collect me?" I asked.

"He should be there at about ten o'clock." He turned his head and looked away from me for a moment, as if he were doing a complicated computation. "We'll expect to see you back here in a few weeks' time to report on how things are going. At our next meeting you can

344

request any extra equipment you require to do your job at the Gulu hospital."

Then abruptly he stood up and walked around his desk. "It's been a pleasure meeting you. We're glad you decided to come to Uganda. I hope you enjoy your time here." We shook hands, he summoned the driver, and I was taken back to the hotel.

After lunch the children, Elaine and I went for a walk around the hotel grounds. The airport hotel in Entebbe stood in an expansive and lush compound. Cars drove up a circular driveway, two to three hundred yards in length, to a covered front entrance. Guests would then climb a flight of stairs and enter the lobby through two heavy glass-filled wooden doors. Simple but elegant. The driveway was lined by an oleander hedge that had a few white and pink flowers poking through. Fragrant jacaranda and flame trees spread their limbs over areas of scant coarse grass. Two garden boys cut the grass with curved, two-foot long knives, like scythes. At the back of the hotel we discovered a swimming pool surrounded by deck chairs, tables and umbrellas. Although it was still early in the day a few people had beer or long drinks at their sides. We were weary from our journey and retired early after supper.

The next morning, after breakfast, the receptionist told me the driver had arrived. Elaine decided she would stay at the hotel with the children while I went to buy the car. As I walked out into the bright sunny morning I saw the same UNICEF Land Rover, which I now realized was an ambulance, waiting for me. A cheerful middle-aged Ugandan, dressed in a light grey suit with a floral, open-necked shirt, greeted me.

"Are you Dr. Binns?" he asked, blinking several times. "Please call me Charles. I have come to take you to Kampala to help you buy your new car."

On the drive to Kampala we passed through several small villages filled with people, children, stray dogs, and chickens. The trees and cooking aromas again reminded me of Nigeria. I was surprised by these similarities. The main difference here was that the road was paved and people drove faster. Like Rome, Kampala was originally a large city situated on seven hills. And never dull. It was a busy place with people walking and cycling down streets in all directions. It had the feeling of a market town on a large scale.

"First I will take you to the Mercedes dealership where you can look at the luxurious cars though I doubt if you will be buying one, sir. But it's fun to look at them," said Charles.

"It might 'be fun' to look at them but I'm sure they'll know I can't afford one."

"Next I'll take you to the Volkswagen dealer. They are very popular but I hear you have a wife and family with you and the Beetles are not very big. They are the cheapest cars to buy in Uganda. Volkswagen also makes a wagon but it is expensive. After that we will go to the Peugeot dealer."

When I explained to the Mercedes dealer that I would have to borrow the money from the government, they agreed I wouldn't be able to afford one. The Volkswagen dealer, on the other hand, was very keen to sell me a car. He had several Beetles in the shop and one Karmann Ghia sports car. Although I was tempted to buy the sports car I knew what Elaine would say. It was hardly suitable for a family of five. The Peugeot dealer had two main models. One was a 403, a comfortable large car but outside my price range, and there were some 304's.

When I explained that the government was going to be lending me the money for the purchase, the dealer seemed pleased and said that he could have a car ready for me, fully licensed and insured, in an hour's time. It was obvious to me that my earlier suspicions were correct. This sort of transaction was common; all the paperwork was in place.

Charles took me for lunch at a Chinese restaurant and after lunch we returned to the dealership. As promised the car was ready. And so I purchased my first French-made vehicle, a comfortable car suitable for the rough back roads of Uganda.

The next day, after an early breakfast, Elaine and I loaded children and luggage into the Peugeot and we drove into Kampala to buy food and basic supplies before heading off into the wilds of northern

Uganda. White cumulus clouds punctuated a blue sky. It was hot. The car didn't have any air conditioning so we opened the windows to the sounds and smells of an African city, all of us chattering away about the new things we were seeing. After leaving the downtown area of Kampala we drove past a large seven-storey building with lots of windows, a large car park, and a surrounding area with several trees, bushes and patchy grass. As we went past the gate I noticed that it was the Mulago University Hospital, which had been built about two years earlier. It was impressive but it would be some months before I actually visited there.

The road out of Kampala was winding and paved and busy with traffic of all descriptions—carts, trucks, motorcycles, bicycles, cars and swarms of pedestrians. Chickens and stray dogs, wary of cars, ran along the shoulders of the road. Once we were out of the city the traffic decreased and we found ourselves driving through typical African bush land. Fifty miles out of Kampala we passed through a small village and, on the other side of the village, the road changed to a graded reddish gravel road—more *murrum.*

Ten miles further down the road a truck going the other way threw up a large stone which hit the windshield of our brand-new car. The impact broke it into small pieces. Unable to see through the shattered glass I promptly punched a hole through it with my fist, cutting my knuckles in the process. Once I stopped the car I realised that I'd have to knock out the entire windshield if I were to see where I was going. Elaine and I discussed going back to Kampala to get a new one installed, but we agreed that since we were about half way to our destination we should carry on to Gulu.

Fortunately I had a pair of sunglasses with me, which I put on and was not troubled by the insects, dust, leaves and other bits of debris that flew into the car when we passed vehicles going the other way. In the back seat the children had to duck down when they saw cars coming. By the time we got to Gulu, the inside of the car was covered in fine red dust and we looked like a bedraggled tribe.

It was approaching four o'clock in the afternoon and we were not certain where we were supposed to spend the night, so I decided to drive to the hospital. Luckily the route was well signed. When we reached the entrance a man in a khaki uniform waved at us to stop.

"Where are you going, sir?"

"I'm the new doctor. We've had trouble with a broken windshield and I'm not sure where we're supposed to spend the night. I thought I'd come to the hospital to find out."

"Oh dear, that's why you look such a mess. I think all the doctors have gone home. You'd better go to the Acholi Inn just up the road on the left, past the magistrate's building on the other side of the road," he said, pointing towards some white buildings.

Just then a stocky white man in an open neck shirt, shorts and sandals came out of the main hospital entrance and walked over to see what was going on at the gate. "Can I help? I'm Dr. Zamorski, one of the doctors here. Have you had an accident?" he asked, speaking with a pronounced mid-European accent.

"Thank you. We're merely dusty, but fine. We've come from Kampala. On the way a stone shattered the windscreen. I'm Dr. Binns, the new gynaecologist, and was wondering where we're supposed to stay tonight."

"I think the best thing is go to the hotel which is just up the road on the left. They should be expecting you. I'm sure the Hospital Superintendent has booked you in. We heard that you were coming, but we didn't know for certain when you would be arriving. I look forward to seeing you in the morning. I'm sure you're wanting a good bath and meal."

At the hotel, the front desk was not expecting us, but fortunately they had plenty of rooms available. We dusted off, bathed, changed clothes and went to the dining room for a much needed meal.

"This has been an interesting introduction to Uganda," Elaine reflected at dinner. "I get the impression that the left hand doesn't know what the right hand is doing. I was rather surprised they weren't expecting us. That's a bit worrying; they should have known."

"To be honest, I was not entirely surprised about them not knowing when we were arriving. My father said it was a common occurrence in Nigeria when he was working there. It seems they have a way of looking at time and events that's different from ours. Things will probably improve when we get into the house and I start work. I will go and see the Medical Superintendent after breakfast tomorrow. In the meantime, we might as well enjoy the luxury of the hotel."

Uganda had obtained independence from Britain on the ninth of October, 1962, just over two years before we arrived. The country had been administered as a British protectorate since 1894. Consequently there were many functional government departments and systems in place. At the time, the transition of power to a self-governing Ugandan republic was probably going better than similar transitions in Kenya and Tanzania. That being said, as a general rule, communications between governmental departments were not smooth; many of the expatriate administrators had abandoned the country shortly after independence. Some had stayed on for personal reasons, but they had to contend with the general policy of "Africanizing" senior positions and often found themselves replaced by Ugandan nationals.

Administrative departments that continued to use the structures put in place by the British included medical, educational, legal, and district administrative services, plus the police and army. Due to the lack of trained or experienced Ugandans a lot of work done in these departments was provided by individuals from various volunteer aid organisations. The main contributors of trained specialists were America, Sweden, Finland, Germany and Britain. Within the medical field there were individuals from many other countries. We were a very multicultural group.

Dr. Edyago, a British-trained Ugandan, had been appointed as the senior medical administrator of the northern region, which had a population of several million people. He was in charge of running five hospitals as well as the district medical and nursing services. His job was administratively and politically complicated. He openly supported the government of the time, while others supported Idi Amin. Dr. Edyago kept to himself and didn't mix with the hospital staff. He was very dictatorial and never asked for advice even when he was dealing with issues about which he had little knowledge.

When I first went to see him he took me round the hospital and showed me the delivery unit, the maternity wards and the gynaecology ward which was part of the general surgery wards. He told me that I would have ten beds available for gynaecological work and that the maternity department had a twenty-bed ward for pre-and post-natal patients, separate from the general wards. Forceps deliveries could be done in the delivery rooms of which there were three. All caesarean sections had to be done in the operating room. He explained there were no medical anaesthetists but there were two nurse anaesthetists who provided this service.

The hospital had two general surgical wards and two general medical wards. These housed forty beds each, but, he explained, there were always more than forty patients in each ward. As in Nigeria, many patients slept between the beds or even under them. Most of the patients brought their own bed linen, but in emergencies the hospital did supply bedding. The beds were the typical black-painted metal frames on wheels. There was a separate children's ward, and an isolation ward for seriously ill patients with smallpox and other infectious diseases. There was also a small ward for leprosy patients. On the hospital grounds there was a kitchen, a laundry, an outpatients department, a Grade "A" outpatient clinic (where some private patients and other special patients were seen) and Dr. Edyago's administrative offices.

As I looked around I could see that all the buildings were single storey, had corrugated iron roofs, and open windows without any mosquito netting. The walls were white-washed and the floors were concrete. Concrete-covered walkways connected the surgical ward, the delivery suite, the maternity ward and the operating theatres, providing shade as well as cover during the rainy season. The various buildings were about fifty to sixty yards apart, surrounded by *murrum* and scanty grass. Flame, jacaranda and other tropical trees provided shade for patients waiting to be seen in the outpatient department. There was some running tap water and electrical power, which went on and off unpredictably. The whole compound was surrounded by a six-foot barbed wire fence and there was a uniformed guard at the gate at all times.

After Dr. Edyago had shown me round the hospital and answered a few of my questions, we went to his office. Once seated, he said, "Now you've seen the hospital. I expect it's a little different from what you're accustomed to. However, we do a lot of good work here. We are the main referral centre for the whole of the northern region and patients are sent here from quite long distances. There is a network of nurse practitioners and midwives who work in the district and refer patients to us when necessary. Four smaller hospitals exist in the region, which have one, two or four physicians running them, but they will also be referring patients to you. I've taken the liberty of telling them that you'll be joining us."

He then outlined my job responsibilities. "You will have two days a week for gynaecological operations and you will be on-call for the maternity unit emergencies all the time. We have nobody else here who can handle them. You will also be on-call on Wednesday nights to cover general emergencies—we simply don't have enough staff."

I was still concerned about his last comment. "They told me at Medical Headquarters in Kampala that this would be the case and I have agreed. But I did mention to them I was not very comfortable with the idea."

"I don't think you'll find it too difficult," he said. "Most of the emergencies are either surgical trauma or severely ill patients with general medical conditions. Your training is such that you can probably manage these and you can always phone up and ask for help from the internist or our Russian paediatrician. She is a bit of a headache for me because she refuses to see any adult patients. Her rationale is that because she specialised very early on in her training, she is not qualified to treat adult patients, only children."

I wondered if this remark was directed at my reluctance to perform general duties. But his facial expression gave no hint that this was the case.

"The other physicians," he continued, "are all generalists and will be more than happy to help out. Your other responsibility will be teaching in the midwifery school. We graduate sixty midwives a year from the school and they come from all over the country. We have a Nursing Sister who oversees the school's curriculum and instruction. She has one assistant who helps with teaching and has requested that you help her teach the students about medical problems in midwifery."

"I'd be delighted," I said. This was an area in which I felt I had something to contribute and in which I felt I could make a difference in patients' lives.

There was a lull in the conversation and I got to ask the question that most concerned me at that moment.

"When will we be able to move into our house?"

"It's ready for you. I'll get the clerk with the keys to show you around when you're finished here. Then you can plan on moving out of the hotel in the next day or so. I'm sure you'll have to buy a few things but the essentials are there."

"Some of our things are being shipped by boat and they may not arrive for a few weeks, but I'm sure we'll manage."

After a short silence we both stood up, neither of us certain of what to say next. Then it dawned on me: "When do you expect me to start working?"

"Come round tomorrow morning and I will introduce you to the others. After that you can start work. They'll be delighted to see you." We shook hands.

My first impression, based on my initial tour and job description, was that things were going to be difficult to start with and that I wasn't going to get much support from Dr. Edyago. Yet despite my misgivings, work and life in Uganda turned out to be most agreeable.

After three weeks in Gulu we became acclimatized to the high temperatures and bright sun. I marvelled at how quickly we started to enjoy ourselves. Our new home, large and spacious with high ceilings, turned out to be the typical expatriate house commonly found in the British colonies. It was built of grey stone bricks and had a corrugated iron roof that sounded like someone was doing drum rolls when it rained. There were three bedrooms, a sitting room, dining room, kitchen and bathroom. Electrical power had arrived three years before so there was a modern refrigerator, running water, as well as a telephone. The hard furnishings, supplied by the government, were satisfactory and they kindly loaned us some linen until our belongings arrived from England.

Within a few days of our moving in, several house boys, ayahs, garden boys and cooks came looking for work. As Europeans, we were expected to have servants, so we hired a houseboy, ayah and garden boy. The applicants were all Sudanese with different levels of spoken English. Lem was the successful house boy/cook. Kamysa looked after the children when Elaine was busy, and Euruneo was the new gardener. Their wages were miniscule by European standards, but high compared to the local rates. Elaine had brought an electric iron from England but Lem had no experience with electric irons. After burning a few things Elaine told him to use the charcoal one he was familiar with and there were no more issues with ironing after that.

The garden around the house was filled with tropical fruit trees, including some mango trees, a few straggly banana trees and one avocado tree. There were several oleander and other decorative tropical bushes, some small jacaranda trees and two or three larger flame trees. A small circular driveway with a shade tree in the middle of it fronted the entrance. Behind the house there was a vegetable garden which had very little in it when we arrived. It promptly became a project for Elaine. She increased its size substantially and planted vegetables that supplied us with fresh food all year round. One of the most popular foods was peanuts. Using two grinding stones, Kamysa quickly turned the crop into peanut butter. The children watched on, eagerly awaiting their first sticky spoonful.

There was a lawn, if one could call it that, made of coarse Kikuyu grass, typical of the tropics. The reddish-brown soil turned to red mud when it rained and became a dusty, crumbly hardpan when dry. Poisonous snakes were reputed to live in the area but we never saw any during our time there. Two or three small termite hills rose like miniature mountains in the compound. Frogs, toads and chameleons had lots of insects to feast on.

Fifteen expatriate houses had been built around the last two holes of a nine-hole golf course. The golf course acted as a mosquito barrier as well as a recreational area. The Gulu Golf Clubhouse was situated just past the ninth hole and it was here that the expat community congregated. The club had two tennis courts, a bar, a full-size snooker table, and a large room that could be used to dine in or to view movies. There was a kitchen but it was only used on special occasions. Members of the club included thirty to forty residents of Gulu who were responsible for a lot of the administrative duties of the northern region—physicians, nurses, teachers, bankers, engineers, game wardens, district administrators, members of parliament, and a vet. There were another fifteen people who worked outside of Gulu and who kept vacation houses there. Many of these were volunteers from various parts of the world who typically spent one or two years in Uganda before moving to another country.

It was in Gulu that Elaine and I learned to play golf, a game that has both fascinated and frustrated us ever since. After work we often played nine holes of golf. During the monthly "mug" tournaments up to eighty people in the club would enter the competition. People came from as far away as Kampala to participate. Elaine took it upon herself to organize the meals for everyone. This presented quite a challenge as there were Hindus and Muslims to feed. Curried goat was one dish she cooked frequently. Luckily fish was acceptable to everybody. The fish was supplied by the game wardens and other fishermen who brought in some large Nile perch. These fish had big heads and a firm flesh that curried well. Occasionally the game wardens would bring in other wild game animals (small antelope and wild pig) for us to cook.

In the first seven months of our stay in Gulu, all three children stayed home with Elaine and Kamysa. Elaine started teaching the girls to read and write as well as take a close look at the animal life living within our compound. Watching tadpoles in the bird bath grow legs and transform into frogs was a wonder they got to witness firsthand. Despite the initial protests of Helen and Kathryn, chickens and ducks, hatched and raised in the back of the compound and treated as pets, eventually made their way to our table. Elaine taught arithmetic using a math rods set and the girls spent hours building structures and counting the number of blocks.

To commemorate the visit of Princess Margaret and Lord Snowdon in March of 1965, Elaine had the children make little books to help develop their writing and drawing skills. This visit was a national event. Our family and most of Gulu went to see the pair. Everyone enjoyed the dancing and local shows organized to entertain the couple.

In September Helen and Kathryn attended the local school to get a more structured education. This small school serviced about thirty to forty expatriate students and the language of instruction was English. There were two English teachers. The girls were placed in different classes. School ran from Monday to Friday in the mornings only because the temperature in the afternoon rose too high. Elaine continued to look after Patrick at home while getting more involved with gardening, cooking and organizing club events. She spent her free time visiting other expatriate wives, as well as reading, golfing, and playing tennis and bridge. The life of an expatriate wife in the British Colonial Service did not leave much in the way of spare time.

The multicultural township of Gulu was situated on a small hill, a mile past the hospital. At the time, it was the largest township in the northern region and one of the largest in Uganda. People came from all over to shop for supplies and do business. Most of the shops were run by East African Asians. Trade between the west coast of India (Gujarat) and Africa had been going on for centuries. Craftsmen and merchants had settled in Uganda in the 1920s to help the British transfer cash crops out of the country and consumer goods in. Africans were not very efficient at trading goods and Europeans did not like the heat and hardship outside of Entebbe and Kampala. East Indians were happy to fill these positions. There were a few African shop owners, mostly from the Buganda tribe, while a few were Lebanese or European from Mediterranean countries.

There was one main road that was paved and lined on either side by small shops, typical of Africa and other tropical countries. The shops were usually wood and mud-brick structures, with a covered area in the front for the display of goods. Behind this was another area for storing articles for sale, a few seats or benches for customers to sit on, and a place where the owner could do the bookwork and stay out of the sun. The shop owner and his family usually lived in some rooms at the back of their shop.

Gulu had a Shell petrol station with a mechanic. The standing joke was that he had only three tools: pliers, a screwdriver, and a hammer. However, he was quite competent and managed to keep most of the cars, trucks, motorcycles and bicycles in the area on the road. He certainly had no trouble replacing my broken windshield.

Off the main road there was a small bazaar where we could purchase local produce including ducks, milk, and chickens, and once a week or so freshly killed beef. To get the beef one had to be there at the kill and wait for the vet to inspect the animal to make sure it was fit for human consumption. Elaine went to this market when she needed more than two pounds of meat for an upcoming event. She would arrive at 9:15 when the beast was slaughtered and would be walking home by 9:30. The meat was usually tough and needed to be stewed with pawpaw leaves to tenderise it before it could be made into a curry.

The town had decreed that people had to wear western clothes, but the state of the shirts and pants they wore was best described as rag-tag. Age and multiple washings kept them clean but full of holes, often revealing more than they hid. On one of her trips to the meat market Elaine came face to face with a warrior in full regalia—head dress, spear and shield—with only a bunch of feathers worn over his back side. Obviously he had not heard of the clothing decree and strode along upright and proud towards his destination.

The town was like a cauldron, hot and bubbly, alive with voices of women and children. The women usually carried the wares they were bringing to market or had purchased on their heads. In spite of the clothing decree, men were often dressed in white flowing garments and diverse head gear. Some sported European suits with jackets and ties in spite of the heat. The local vegetables that we bought from the market were good but seasonal. Aromatic cooking smells filled the air. Stray dogs and chickens were everywhere under foot. There were few set prices—haggling was expected, dickering a matter of pride.

A truck service came up from Kampala once a week with fresh foods and vegetables for the expatriates, but the prices were high and the produce was often "going off" by the time it arrived, especially butter and milk. Elaine soon gave up relying on this service except for some special items. She arranged to buy milk from a local Fulani family who delivered it to our house in a churn on the back of a bicycle. We pasteurized it ourselves to ensure that we did not get any nasty bacteria.

Gulu was located in a part of Uganda that had a very high incidence of malaria. On routine examination, seventy-five percent of the population had parasites. This meant that we had to take our anti-malarial pills regularly and we tried to avoid mosquito bites. The house had wire netting over the windows and we had mosquito nets over all the beds. Other tropical diseases, such as hookworm and dysentery, were common. We constantly reminded the children to be certain to wear their shoes and to avoid eating anything that had not been cooked well. One of Kathryn's memories of our time in Gulu was being told not to walk in puddles barefoot. With these simple precautions our family managed to survive two years in Uganda without catching any serious illnesses.

Our Sudanese gardener was rich by local standards and he could afford several wives. On one occasion he took us to his home and showed us the rondavels he had built, one for each wife, plus one for cooking. These round houses were built with mud and wattle walls and thatched roofs supported by eucalyptus poles, which were the most expensive construction material. At the top of the wall was a twelve-inch space, left open for ventilation. This gap was overhung by the roof. The only other opening was a wide door. The dwellings were very cool inside. To avoid being robbed, he hid his riches, and by wearing clothes with holes in them, he looked like everyone else and didn't stand out as being particularly wealthy. I often suspected people must have wondered how he could support his many wives.

Life in Uganda was very basic. We had lots of fun creating our own entertainment. Because there was no TV or good radio we were forced to socialize and as a consequence made good friends. The children thrived playing inside and outside with few toys but inventive games. Although we had little opportunity to see other parts of Uganda, Murchison National Park was only an hour and a half's drive away. We made several outings to see the wild animals in the Park, and on two occasions we stayed overnight at the lodge.

On one visit we took the boat trip from the lodge up to Murchison Falls. The falls are not very wide but the water drops several hundred feet creating a constant spray filled with rainbow colours. The river was full of hippopotami and crocodiles and the banks were lined by all sorts of birds. At the top of the falls lived a family of baboons that entertained the visitors with their incessant antics. They chased each other over the rocks and looked like they were taking death-defying tumbles. Others sat on shore grooming a companion. The park was always full of animals and we saw many elephants, buffalo, giraffes and antelopes, but the wild cats eluded us. We were disappointed not to see the cat that had been so much a part of our dream of Africa.

On our many day trips we saw assorted birds with brilliant coloured plumage. Some of the marsh birds, such as the shoebill stork and the pink backed pelican, were large and had enormous bills.

During a two-day road trip to Mombasa, Kenya, via Nairobi, we drove down the Rift Valley, stopping at Lake Nakuru, which is famous for its pink flamingos. The sight of thousands of birds wading back and forth feeding was spectacular.

The hotel we stayed in south of Mombasa was unique in our experience. The "rooms" consisted of individual, round, well-furnished huts topped with coconut palm thatched roofs. All were within one hundred yards of the high-tide mark so it was easy to go down to the brilliant blue sea to splash in the waves. Unfortunately the sun reflected off the dazzling, white-coral sand and the three children and I ended up with painful sunburns. Elaine, on the other hand, tanned a dark brown. She got so dark that on our return to Gulu one of our

East Indian friends asked who the new *ayah* was.

We returned through Tanzania and drove past Mount Kilimanjaro. The grasslands, scattered trees, and wildlife of the East African savannah—antelopes, giraffes, and elephants—spread out before us. At one of the parks we stopped to visit a Masai tribe, a nomadic people who live off their cattle herds. Exceptionally tall people, they are different from all other East African tribes.

Having survived the savannah during the dry season, we were relieved to get home and wash off the dust from our travels.

Theoretically I was responsible for the obstetric and gynaecological services for about four million people. The four other hospitals in the region were situated fifty, eighty, and one hundred and fifty miles away. Kitgum, Moya and Lira had one doctor each in charge and a supporting staff of nurse practitioners and nurses. Arua sat on the Congolese border, on the other side of the Blue Nile River. It had three Russian doctors and one East Indian doctor. Arua was an odd situation. Across its main street was its sister township of Aru, which was officially in the Congo, and therefore had a strong French influence.

To supplement the small number of government physicians in Uganda there was a network of nurses, nurse practitioners, and midwives. These individuals worked deep in the bush where they ran clinics. The patients came to these clinics from many miles out. The only form of transport from the smaller villages was by walking or on bicycle along rough tracks that turned to mud when it rained. Patients who were too sick to walk or ride a bicycle had to be carried on stretchers by their relatives, sometimes with the aid of a trolley pulled behind a bicycle. There were very few horses or donkeys in the area and I have always assumed that this was because of sleeping sickness which was endemic in the area. Horses and donkeys are particularly susceptible to this disease.

Most of the clinics were held in the larger villages, which were fairly close to roads that linked up with the main road network of the northern region. Many of the patients that I saw in the Gulu hospital maternity unit had taken several days to arrive. The midwives told me that often patients died on the way to the hospital but there was no record of their actual numbers. Many of these patients had already been seen by the local witch doctor and given native medicines, some of which caused severe uterine contractions and other problems.

In Gulu there were three general practitioners working outside the government medical services as private practitioners who referred patients to me. Approximately ten kilometres from Gulu there was a mission hospital established by the famous Canadian surgeon, Dr. Lucille Teasedale, and her husband, Dr. Corti. At that time they only had a small hospital but they did an immense amount of work. Since 1961 this small hospital had been expanded to be part of the university hospital in Kampala. I had the privilege of visiting and working with them during my two years in Uganda.

There were at least three major tribes in the region: the Acholi, Lango and West Nile, which was Idi Amin's tribe. Each group spoke different languages and had different customs. There was also a population of Sudanese refugees who had fled to Uganda in 1955. They were quite easy to recognise because they were physically taller, darker and had classic scars on their faces. The other minority group was the East Indians who had been part of the East African community for several hundred years.

Although there were many languages spoken in the region, the men used a common official language, Swahili, while the women often spoke only their own dialects. The nurses, midwives, and nurse practitioners came from all over Uganda and were often unfamiliar with the local dialects and languages. This gave rise to considerable difficulties in communicating with the patients. However, there were several local nurses who could speak up to seven different languages and they acted as interpreters. I sometimes wondered how accurate they were. After a few months I was able to understand much of what the ladies were saying, sometimes with a better understanding than the interpreters. This was probably because I had already learned two other languages as a child. However, I was never fluent enough to barter over the price of a piece of meat in the market.

The Gulu hospital provided an absolute bare minimum of medical equipment and technical support. We had access to simple X-rays, some basic laboratory testing, but no bacteriology. It was possible to send surgical specimens to Kampala for diagnostic purposes, but it took two to three weeks to get results. The equipment in the operating room and the maternity delivery suite was limited. There was no blood bank, and the facilities for giving general anaesthesia were basic. There was no Boyles machine for giving modern anaesthetics but there was a portable EMO machine for giving closed-circuit ether anaesthetics. The two nurse anaesthetists were very competent, but one of them liked her alcohol a bit too much so she was not always available.

Although we had the Russian paediatrician on hand, there was no equipment for looking after small babies, apart from a laryngoscope and tubes for intubation. She spent most of her time looking after young children. Apparently her services were a free donation to Uganda from the USSR. She stayed in Uganda for two years. The two Polish doctors were also on an aid program; one of them had been in the army and trained as a thoracic surgeon, the other trained as an internist. There was a North Korean eye specialist, representing another aid program. He, too, had spent time in the army and was quite competent in all areas of medicine. A surgeon from Goa had been appointed as a consultant and refused to do general duties. Obviously he had more gumption than I did. Luckily he would do caesarean sections when I was away. His wife had the DRCOG (the diploma of obstetrics) and helped out when I was not there. They all tried their hands at obstetric problems but their skills were limited so I was always called in for serious complications.

The medical team also included four senior English-trained nurses, one of whom was in charge of the midwifery school. The others were in charge of the wards. The rest of the staff were Uganda-trained nurses and nurse assistants. The outpatient area was staffed by nurse practitioners who had an additional eighteen months of training beyond their nurse training.

Before leaving England I had discussed with my father what to expect when I arrived in Uganda. On his advice I had purchased some basic obstetrical and gynaecological surgical instruments, which included some forceps for doing hysterectomies, a pair of obstetric forceps, and a Blond-Heidler saw used to decapitate the fetus in obstructed labour. Once I had established what the major problems were in Gulu I went to see Dr. Edyago with requests for some special surgical instruments.

One common problem, the most troublesome to patients, was a vesico-vaginal fistula. This condition was associated with prolonged obstructed labour and resulted in a passage developing between the bladder and the vagina. Urine leaked out of the bladder into the vagina and the patient became constantly wet and smelly. This fact resulted in their being ostracised by their community. The operative procedure to treat the problem required extra-long-handled delicate surgical instruments which were not available in Gulu. I ordered some to be delivered as soon as possible.

At the same time I asked Dr. Edyago about a blood bank and he told me that this equipment was not available in Gulu but that they did transfuse some patients after simple cross matching with blood from their relatives. When I asked if there was a suitable refrigerator for storing blood he told me there was one in the laboratory. He also informed me that the lab technician, Odongo, had been trained to run a blood transfusion bank. When I asked Dr. Edyago if I could talk to Odongo about using his services he told me to go ahead and see what could be done. He seemed enthusiastic about the idea as long as he did not have to get too involved with the process.

I found Odongo in his laboratory with his two assistants looking at urine samples, faecal material, and blood smears for various abnormalities and parasites. When I asked him about setting up a blood bank he was enthusiastic. He was quite confident about his ability to cross-match and test blood that we collected and he said that the fridge they had was perfectly adequate to store blood.

When I asked him where we would get the blood his answer came as a surprise. "We can get the blood from the schools and the prisons," he said, adding a big smile when he saw my doubtful expression.

"But we can't take blood from children. They're far too young," I said.

"*Bwana*, the boys and girls in the upper classes are all over twenty years old and would be very happy to give blood if we give them a bottle of Coke and a packet of cigarettes. The prisoners are the same but much older and we will have to talk to the prison chief. I have done this in other cities and there is no problem. We will need some transport but I think we have the bottles and intravenous tubes for collecting the blood."

"We could use my car if you think it's big enough."

"Oh, your car will be fine. It has a big boot and we can put everything into it."

"Do you think we can get Dr. Edyago to pay for the Coke and cigarettes?"

"Probably not. I will put them into my budget, and we'll see what happens."

True to his word, the following week Odongo and I visited one school and the men's prison to collect blood. I had some doubts about how old the boys at the school were, but they were physically much bigger than me and certainly looked like adults. They were enthusiastic about giving blood and were curious about what we were going to do with it. The prisoners, however, were not so enthusiastic. They were suspicious until we explained that we would give them a bottle of Coke and cigarettes for their contribution. The cigarettes were called Bicycles, a local product, and very cheap. I tried one once and found it stronger than the *Gauloises* I had smoked in France.

Once our blood bank was organized we used to go out and collect blood every week or so depending on how much was used by the hospital. We were very lucky with Odongo as he was a local and did not want to move. He was a competent and hard-working lab technician. When I showed an interest in seeing some of the parasites he observed in his lab he used to call me to show them to me. There were some very strange ones in East Africa. Malaria and hook worms were the most common but I saw examples of spirochetes, micro fillaria, common round worms, Guinea worms, loa-loa, and schistosomiasis (sleeping sickness parasites), to mention a few.

Given the medical, surgical and nursing help available to me I decided that I needed two outpatient clinic days a week. My biggest nightmare was the patients, already in labour, who came into the hospital from the bush. They were often seriously ill, frequently had a dead baby, and were invariably both anaemic and infected. Many had been labouring for many hours, if not days, before eventually arriving at the hospital.

Many of the obstetrical problems that these women presented can only be read about in classic works on obstetrics dating back over hundreds of years. The actual number of deliveries at the hospital was relatively small considering the population we were covering. The actual number of admissions to the maternity ward during my first twelve months was 1,696 and there were 1,175 deliveries. However, the obstetrical problems they presented can be gauged by the following complications and tragedies. I was involved in eleven maternal deaths and there were thirty-four neonatal deaths. By comparison I was aware of, but not involved in the care of, only two maternal deaths in the next thirty years of obstetric practice in the UK, Canada, and New Zealand.

Often the patients arrived at the hospital in dire straits, not only with problems related to their labour, but with other complicating factors such as severe anaemia, infections, malnutrition, and treatment by some very potent noxious agents given to them by witch doctors. I didn't doubt that many witch doctors were very knowledgeable and helped a lot of patients in the bush. Yet their remedies were doomed when it came to obstructed labours and did more harm than good. Many of these patients had been in strong labour for several days with obstructions due to mal-presentations such as shoulders and hands, small or deformed pelvises, and other abnormalities. The babies were often dead. Therefore, I tried to deliver these patients vaginally, if at all possible, because the risk of performing a caesarean section was considerable. This decision meant resorting to several decapitations, skull perforations and the use of the archaic cranio-clast. This was an instrument that was designed to crush the skull so that the baby could be delivered vaginally.

Obstructed labour, where the baby does not descend into the pelvis properly, was often catastrophic, with a rupture of the uterus, massive haemorrhage and a baby dead in the abdominal cavity. I was involved with seven of these cases of which two were the result of previous classical Caesarean sections. What always surprised me was that some of these patients survived. The women showed remarkable resilience and were able to recover from severe trauma, anaemia and infections. Depending on their circumstances, they were treated either by a hysterectomy or a repair of the uterus. These patients often refused to have a tubal ligation done at the time of surgery which made any future childbearing hazardous.

Twins were relatively common in this population and I saw several complications of these labours. Retention of the second twin for hours or even days was one such mal-presentation. Again, I was often surprised when the second twin survived. General medical complications of pregnancy included smallpox, severe anaemia, TB, and leprosy.

Because I was on call all the time, we had a direct telephone line installed from the hospital maternity unit to our house. When I was not at home, I was sent for by one of the orderlies who rode a brilliant yellow bicycle. He could be seen coming from a long way off, carrying the dreaded ledger from the labour floor. In this ledger there would be brief messages to me:

"We have a prolapsed cord and we can still hear the baby's heart. Please come."

"We have a patient who has been in labour for two days and is very sick."

"We have a hand presenting at the vulva. Please come."

"Dr. Stefan cannot deliver the baby. Please come."

"We have a patient who is having fits. Please come."

Under such circumstances I had no choice but to go to the hospital immediately. Sometimes the messages were about patients whose history I knew and if there was no urgency I was able to write orders in the ledger. The man on the yellow bicycle was remarkably good at finding me and I suspect that most of Gulu knew what the maternity doctor was up to most of the time.

When it came to gynaecology the situation was slightly different because the only real emergencies were heavy bleeding during miscarriages and ruptured ectopic pregnancies, which for some reason were common. The frequency was almost certainly related to the high incidence of gonorrhoea and other untreated sexually transmitted diseases in the region. Other patients presented the usual gamut of well-recognised gynaecological conditions, but had often tolerated them for longer than a patient would in either the UK or Canada. These were, therefore, more difficult to treat and included heavy menstrual bleeding, fibroids, which were often very large or degenerating, ovarian cysts, and abdominal pain associated with chronic pelvic inflammatory disease.

Unfortunately there was very little we could do for patients with cancers of the cervix, ovaries, uterus, and vulva. There were two reasons for this; the first was that the patients rarely came to see us during the early stages of these diseases and the second was that there was no radiotherapy available in Uganda. Added to this, extensive surgical procedures were not feasible in Gulu. All I could give was palliative care, and this was often limited. I got the impression that many of these patients were aware of their problems but didn't choose to come to the hospital.

Before going to Uganda I had observed Professor Chasseur Moir in Oxford operate on vaginal fistulas. When the instruments I ordered arrived, I started to perform the same surgery using the same technique. I vividly remember the first patient on whom I performed this procedure. She was middle-aged, had white hair, and had had her fistula for a considerable length of time. Probably more by luck than expertise I was successful in repairing her fistula and she was so grateful that she used to come to the hospital and wait at the gate at least once a month to thank me. She did this for the rest of my stay in Uganda. Following this initial success I operated on one or two of these patients a month. It was a very satisfying procedure when successful and very frustrating when failures occurred. But, considering the operating conditions under which I worked, I felt that my success rate of seventy to eighty percent was gratifying.

The second common gynaecological problem I saw was uterine fibroids. Some of these were very large. The largest one I removed from a patient was over twenty pounds. The usual approach to fibroids in western society is to do a hysterectomy but the Ugandan patients were very reluctant to have a hysterectomy performed. Therefore, I became quite skilled at doing myomectomies to remove these benign growths. Many of the patients only came when their fibroids started to degenerate and became painful. This could cause some technical difficulties during the surgery.

Some of the other gynaecological conditions I saw were both extraordinary and unique. I looked after two abdominal pregnancies where the baby grew in the abdominal cavity and not the uterus. There were some major problems with handling the placenta at the time of the surgeries but they had successful outcomes. Childbirth could be fatal and I witnessed two catastrophic ruptured corneal pregnancies, when the placenta implanted in the wall of the uterus where the tube entered. I also saw one patient with choriocarcinoma, which was quite rare.

People can have unique internal physiologies. I came across a patient with her spleen located in her pelvis and not beside her stomach. It was causing her pain and everyone thought she had an ovarian cyst which was why I was consulted. The most extraordinary patient I saw had a fibroma of the vulva which weighed twenty-six pounds. It had obviously been there for many years, but by the time I saw her, the patient was unable to walk because of the mass. As it was a benign condition, surgical removal cured her. I also saw one patient with elephantiasis of the vulva.

Because I was on call for general duties once a week, I ran into some other interesting medical problems. As sanitation and disease prevention did not exist, severe diarrhea and vomiting in babies and toddlers was common and often fatal. All we could do when these children came to the hospital was hydrate them with intravenous or subcutaneous fluids. The adult population also suffered the usual general medical and surgical problems. Even so, there was a percentage of interesting and, to me, unusual situations. For example, patients who had been gored by elephants and hippopotamuses. These patients were in severe shock with multiple injuries and fractures. Poisonous snake bites were frequent and sometimes fatal. We did not have any anti-venom.

Many injuries were caused by arrows and knives. Some were hunting accidents and others followed fights. Arrowheads were particularly difficult because they were quite long, up to nine inches, with spiral barbs on them. One patient managed to get one of these arrowheads into his chest by way of his neck when he tripped and fell while running after a wounded antelope. The tip of the arrow was up against the base of his heart. When the general surgeon saw him he said he would have to split the sternum to get the arrow out. He said he couldn't do anything for the man because we didn't have any bone wax.

Fortunately for the patient, our Polish doctor, who had been in the army and had had some thoracic surgical experience, felt that we could get the arrow out without splitting the sternum. Our next problem was how to put the patient to sleep. Our only anaesthetist was sick in bed. My anaesthetic experience went back to my medical school days, but I felt something had to be done. Therefore, I volunteered to give the anaesthetic. As the thorax was going to be opened, we had to give the patient some form of positive-pressure gases. I discovered it was possible to do this using the EMO machine while Doctor Zamorski proceeded to open the chest and remove the arrow, albeit with some difficulty. The patient withstood the procedure remarkably well and went home two weeks later.

One of my most worrying challenges was a twelve-year-old boy who had been wounded in his right eye. It had become badly infected and the eye was damaged beyond all hope of being saved. The risk was that he would lose the sight in his other eye if the damaged one was not removed promptly. Unfortunately the Korean eye specialist was on leave and the general surgeon was not prepared to do anything. On this occasion Dr. Zamorski and I decided that it was my turn to step outside the box, so I consulted the surgical textbooks and removed the eye. Again I was lucky and the patient went home a few days later.

Acute retention of urine in men caused by a narrowing of the urethra was common. The nurse practitioners were very skilled at inserting catheters and dilating these patients. The cause of the narrowing was strictures caused by gonorrhoeal infections. Occasionally the nurses could not get a catheter in and it became my responsibility to insert catheters in through the abdomen and then do the dilatations under general anaesthesia. The other doctors felt that as a gynaecologist this procedure was closer to my field of expertise than theirs and, much to my chagrin, I was always called in when it was necessary to perform this operation.

My other responsibility as the on-duty physician was to perform autopsies on medical-legal cases. The autopsies were done on people who had been murdered and it was our job to ascertain the exact cause of death. Some of these autopsies were exceedingly difficult because the bodies had been out in the bush for a day or so and were already decomposing. Fortunately, I had had some experience doing autopsies in Winnipeg and in most cases the cause of death was quite easy to determine. After performing an autopsy, we would make a report and this would then go to the courts. When the case came up we would be sent a subpoena a day or so beforehand in order to be ready to give evidence. Usually there was no problem with this notification. I would dress for court in a full suit, jacket and tie; the judges expected formal attire. The court would phone the hospital when it was time to give the doctor's evidence and off I would go to the court house.

On one occasion this practice got me into some political problems with one of the magistrates. I was subpoenaed to attend court but was not called during the day, probably because they had run overtime. The other doctors told me that this was a common occurrence and not to worry as a new subpoena and date would be set for my appearance. A few days later I was in the middle of my afternoon operating session when the court phoned and asked me to go over to give evidence for the case. Because I had not been given a new notification I did not have my court clothes with me. I was wearing shorts, shirt and sandals. It was also quite late in the afternoon. I phoned the court clerk to explain that I was not dressed appropriately. The clerk went to the magistrate and asked him if I could attend dressed as I was. He came back and said, yes, he had asked the magistrate, and I could give my evidence in the clothes I was wearing.

When I entered the courtroom the magistrate looked up at me and said, "Doctor, you are not dressed for the court."

"I did ask for permission to attend the court dressed as I am, Your Honour. I did not have time to go home and change into a suit to attend," I explained politely.

"I did not give you permission."

"Sir, I did ask specifically for permission to come as I am, and was told it was fine for this occasion. I apologise if I've offended you."

"I regard this as a contempt of court," he said, and turned to the policeman who was standing next to me. "Go, lock the doctor up in the cell."

I decided there was no point in arguing and was conducted to the back of the court where they had a cell into which the policeman guided me. Once I was in, he locked the door and left. When I looked across the cell I found that I was not alone. There was a very large Ugandan standing in the other corner. I realized this man was probably the person who had been accused of murder and I was the one giving evidence that a murder had occurred. I felt extremely uncomfortable and did not say a word for the next three hours. We both sat on the floor eyeing each other. I became particularly concerned when I realized that nobody knew where I was. I should have been home by this time. Elaine would have thought I had been held up with some emergency in the hospital and, therefore, would not make any enquiries about my whereabouts until well into the evening. Luckily the policeman soon opened the door, let me out, and told me I could go home.

I was troubled by this episode and went to see Dr. Edyago the next day. When I explained to him what had happened he said he did not think it was serious and that I was not to do anything about it. I told him I thought it was inappropriate that this should have happened to me and that I would write a full report to him for the records. When I talked to my friends in the station about this event they told me the magistrate concerned was very anti-European, particularly against the English. This was probably why he had been so inflexible, they suggested. Consequently, I sent a copy of my report to the chief magistrate's office in Kampala and a copy to the Ministry of Overseas Development in London. I didn't think any more about the episode until, a few weeks later, the man with the yellow bicycle arrived with a message for me to go to the Acholi Inn as soon as I'd finished my golf game.

When I got to the inn the receptionist said there was a gentleman waiting for me at the bar who would like to buy me a drink.

As I approached him, he said, "Ah, you must be Dr. Binns. I'm Chief Justice Brown. I've just come up from Kampala for some cases and I have been asked to talk to you about what happened a few weeks ago when you were asked to give evidence. What would you like to drink?"

"A beer, please," I replied.

He ordered the beer and suggested we find a table away from the bar. Once seated he said, "Our Department would like to hear the full story from you. We got your report, but we would like to talk to you about it."

I gave him the details of what had happened, starting with the autopsy several months earlier. He asked several questions about what had transpired and about the usual procedures in the Gulu courts with reference to doctors' giving evidence.

"On behalf of the Department of Justice, I would like to apologise for the way you were treated. However, as you probably appreciate, this is an awkward time for Uganda. There are some individuals who feel quite strongly that we expats have no place here. I hope you are not too upset by this episode. I can assure you that it is not usual. I hope you're enjoying your stay here. I'll make a full report to our Department."

Getting the humiliation of the courtroom out of my mind had been difficult. And the thought that there was a real possibility I might have been attacked and that my family was at risk had often worried me in the middle of the night.

I didn't think any more of this event until two weeks later when I heard via the grapevine that the magistrate concerned had been transferred to Kampala, presumably so they could keep an eye on him.

When I made trips to the smaller regional hospitals I discovered how difficult it was for a family physician to assume responsibility for administering these stations while trying to practice medicine in terribly constrained conditions. Lira and Kitgum were small stations with one doctor who looked after a hospital of fifty to sixty beds. The doctor was assisted by three or four nurse practitioners and a few midwives. He would look after what he could in the way of emergencies and, when he couldn't handle them, refer them to Gulu, which was two or three hours' drive away. The patient might survive the journey.

The number of expatriates in these stations was usually five or six, so it was a lonely existence. The other problem was that they were often moved from station to station, as had been the case in Nigeria with my parents. Arua, on the other side of the Nile, was slightly larger and a good five-hour drive. The hospital there had over one hundred beds and there were five physicians looking after it, four of them Russians.

On an early trip to Arua I realised how vulnerable one could be while driving on one's own in rural Uganda. A couple of hours out of Gulu, a motorcyclist came round a corner towards me, riding down the middle of the road. I swerved to avoid him and lost control of my car on the gravel surface. The car made a complete revolution and came to a stop, still on the road. When I recovered from the initial shock, I felt some discomfort in my right hand. When I looked down I saw that my thumb was completely displaced. I took a deep breath, mustered my courage, and manipulated my thumb back into a normal position. Fortunately I had some painkillers in the car with me. After taking a couple of these, the throbbing in my thumb lessened.

Since I had already crossed the Nile on the ferry, and was closer to Arua than Gulu, I decided it was wisest to continue on. When I arrived in Arua the Russian surgeon took some X-rays of my hand and told me that I had a fracture dislocation of my right thumb. I had got it back into a good position, but he advised putting it into a plaster. He did this and I spent the next two days in Arua discussing and treating some of the interesting patients he had for me to see. I also took the opportunity to walk across the non-existent border, the main road in both towns, to Aru.

I ended up with a cast on my right hand for six weeks, during which time all I could do was assist with operations using one hand and examine patients with my left hand. Fortunately, the number of serious obstetric emergencies was small and I was able to help the other doctors by giving them advice.

During our time in Uganda I seldom felt unsafe. However, Elaine and I heard stories that did worry us. One story concerned a Member of Parliament who was driving through his hometown. A child ran out into the road in front of his car and was killed. Deeply distressed, he got out of the car to see if he could be of any assistance. The local community was so angry and became so frenzied, they stoned the MP to death. After this incident we were warned not to stop if we injured somebody while driving and were told to go straight to the nearest police station in the *next* township to report any accident.

We did feel uneasy when political events and protests threatened to become violent. During our second year the road to Kampala was blocked for several weeks because of "bandits". We never found out exactly who they were but we were not allowed to travel outside Gulu. Elaine and I realized how fortunate we were to have freedom of movement and speech, and how fragile these rights can be. Because of increasing tensions I always kept an eight-gallon drum of petrol in the garage for use in case of an emergency. With this amount of petrol my family and I would have been able to get to the Congolese border at Arua or to the Sudanese border. However, where we would have gone after that was another question, which fortunately we never had to answer.

As time went by, the political importance of Gulu as the main centre in the northern region became apparent. One day, when I was at the bar in the club, a European stranger came up to me. "My name is Forbes and I'm with Mollems. We're here to build your new airstrip. We'll be here for several weeks and I was wondering if we could join your club."

"I can't see why that would be a problem," I said.

"We would, of course, pay whatever your dues are and if there is anything we can do to help, we would do so with pleasure."

"I'm not sure what the dues would be for a few weeks and I don't think you need worry too much about that. However, if you are laying bitumen surfaces, our tennis courts are in poor shape. If you could help with them we would be grateful."

"I think we could arrange that," he said.

"Why are they building an airport up here?"

"Haven't you been told? Gulu is going to become the centre for the army. They want us to build an airport up here so they can get troops in and out quickly. I gather the Chief of Staff, Idi Amin, will be coming up to open it when we have finished in a few weeks' time."

"No, I wasn't aware of this. I suppose it means that Gulu is going to become quite important in the future. Having a large army base up here will increase the population of the area and probably bring all sorts of other problems with it."

"Yes, you're probably right."

Over the next few weeks the club grew to include engineers, architects, draftsmen, military personnel of every rank, machine operators, material suppliers and so on. We were all invited to the ceremonial opening of the new airport, which included several parties and an exhibition of Acholi dancing. The guest of honour was Idi Amin. Gulu put on a big party for his entourage, the local administrators, and government officials. The invitations included all the local expatriates and their partners. At this party I had the dubious pleasure of being introduced to the infamous dictator. I remember him as a very large, ugly man, decked out in his uniform, who looked down on me from a great height. Although this occurred before he took over the country, I could sense his impatience, intolerance, power and dominance.

"You must be one of the foreign doctors. There will be a lot of changes here in the next few years. We will become one of the strongest countries in East Africa." We shook hands, mine disappearing into his enormous hand before he moved on to another guest. I was relieved when I felt I could politely leave the party.

Another of my major responsibilities in Gulu was teaching at the midwifery school. The class was composed of seventy students and the course took eighteen months to complete. I taught the students about medical problems which affected pregnancy, labour, delivery and the postpartum period, which included the recognition of severe anaemia, heart failure (rheumatic heart disease was quite common in Uganda), high blood pressure (with associated convulsions), gastrointestinal infections, hepatitis B, sleeping sickness, and smallpox, which was endemic, to mention a few. The students already had a school certificate, and were trained nurses. They could speak and understand English but their native languages were as different as the different parts of Uganda and East Africa from which they came. The tutor and her assistants taught them the principles and practicalities of midwifery—antenatal care, delivering babies, and postpartum care.

The practical experience they received on the labour floor was considerable. But when it came to my lectures on infections I soon realized they were unable to understand what I was saying. I could see them looking into the distance with blank faces. When I talked to them about prevention and the use of gloves, masks, gowns, drapes, and preparing the abdomen or vulva with antiseptic solutions, the message was not getting through. When I asked what they knew about bacteria and viruses I realised they really had no idea what bacteria or viruses were because they couldn't see them.

I went to Mr. Odongo in his lab and asked if he could prepare some sterile culture plates for me. He said this would be easy. A few days later he had four culture plates for me. I took these to the class-room and showed them to the girls. Then I put them in a locked cab-inet and gave them the keys. The next day we looked at the plates and they were still clean. Then I took some swabs from their hands and from between their teeth, and spread these specimens on three of the four plates. We then returned the plates to the locker and locked it up. I gave the keys back to them with instructions that no one was to go anywhere near the plates until the next day.

When we looked at the plates one was still clean but the others had colonies of bacteria on them. We took the plates to the laboratory where Mr. Odongo took some specimens off the plates, put them on slides, stained them and showed the girls the bacteria through the microscope. The girls were impressed with this demonstration of bac-teria growth and surprised at how many colonies we had obtained from their hands and mouths.

This learning experience was a good lesson for me as well. It made me aware that learning and understanding complex concepts was never easy and that different people had different ways of learning new things.

I only managed to go to Kampala three times. The first time was shortly after I arrived in Gulu when I was asked to visit the Deputy Minister to tell him how things were going and to request some extra equipment for the hospital. The second visit was a social occasion when I went to see David Norrie whom I had met in Manchester and who was now working with the Department of Obstetrics and Gynae-cology in Mulago Hospital under Professor Trussell. I got to see the beautiful tropical city and David showed me around the hospital and the department, which was well equipped and very active.

The Medical School had only been open for two years, yet had already attracted some strong department heads. The building was fresh and clean; the staff enthusiastic and hard-working. I was a little envious of their situation and wondered how I had missed the op-portunity of being involved with the school's teaching staff. The Med-ical School's goal was to produce sixty to seventy doctors a year with full training and practical experience. It was the only medical school in East Africa and supplied doctors for Uganda and neighbouring countries. I met some of their graduates many years later and was impressed by their competence. No one predicted the tragedy that was to befall this excellent centre of learning.

On my second visit to the Medical School, I spoke at a conference in obstetrics and gynaecology. My presentation was on the practicalities of trying to run an obstetrics and gynaecology service in the northern region. Dr. Rendall Short, who was working in Somalia, gave a talk on her experiences with fistulas. After the presentation I met with her and learned her experience was different from that of Professor Chasseur Moir. She was dealing with post-delivery fistulas. However, she stressed that the principles and techniques were very similar.

She also observed that while we all faced similar medical problems, there were both racial and geographic differences with which to contend. For example, the Buganda tribes had a high incidence of ruptured uteruses and a low incidence of fistulas. Elsewhere the situation could be reversed. The meeting lasted three days and gave me an opportunity to discuss some of the problems of obstetrics and gynaecology in East Africa. It was also my first presentation of a paper at a major medical conference outside of the UK.

By the time I had spent two years in Gulu, I felt I was quite efficient at handling the day-to-day problems of the hospital. However, I could see it would be impossible to upgrade the services in the region to anything approaching what I was used to. I was unhappy with my growing sense of futility and frustrated by my lack of accomplishment. Perhaps I wanted things to improve too quickly. I was impatient. When I enquired about who would be taking over from me when I left, I was told that there were no candidates and that it was unlikely I would be replaced by anybody with similar training. I realized the only lasting contribution I might make was teaching the midwives. Therefore, I decided to spend as much time as I could with them. This way I hoped that at least the quality of obstetric care would improve throughout the country.

I had kept in touch with Mr. Stallworthy in Oxford, giving him reports on how things were going and how I was enjoying the work. However, I was shocked to hear that Mr. Hawksworth had died, apparently from lung cancer. I wondered whether Mr. Stallworthy would be able to keep his promise of a post in Oxford. When I wrote to tell him I had just about completed my time in Uganda and gave him the date of my probable arrival in the UK, he wrote back to say that he could not offer me a job for six weeks. He said that if I wanted to work as a volunteer I was welcome to do so. In view of the delicate political situation in Uganda—Idi Amin was on the rise—I knew I shouldn't pass on such an opportunity back home.

One last attempt was made by the Ugandan authorities to entice me to stay on for a second tour. Although I was tempted by the money and benefits, the children would soon be going to school and Elaine wanted to get back into practicing medicine. And there were no opportunities for her in Uganda. Another dilemma was whether or not to return to England or Canada. In England I would have to do two to four more years as a senior registrar on my way to becoming a consultant. Although we decided to give the UK a go, in retrospect I find it interesting that I ordered a Volvo from Uganda for the UK—with left-hand drive!

When we left Uganda we were financially solvent. We took a train down to Mombasa where we boarded the SS *Kenya* and returned to England via the Suez Canal, which had recently reopened.

On the way past Egypt I was able to take Helen, who was eight, to see the pyramids and visit Cairo. Kathryn and Patrick were too young to appreciate a trip to the pyramids, so Elaine stayed with them on the ship as it travelled through the Suez Canal. Most of the time, she said, all they could see was sand dunes.

On our way through the Mediterranean, the SS *Kenya* stopped at Barcelona to off-load copper. In Barcelona we had one day on shore to do some shopping. We were returning to England at the beginning of winter and needed to buy some warm clothes. In her quest to buy Helen and Kathryn warm leggings, Elaine had a particularly hard time because none of us could speak Spanish. After numerous attempts at pantomime she eventually discovered that the Spanish word for leggings was *leotardos*. Upon chancing on the correct word we were immediately directed to the appropriate shop. The palaces, grand boulevards, shops, five-storey residences, cobbled streets, all contrasted starkly with Gulu and its *murrum* roads.

When we arrived in Britain the temperature dropped and rain squalls blew in off the channel. We docked in Tilbury and spent a couple of nights in London while we waited to pick up our new Volvo. As soon as we got the keys to the car we headed north to stay with my parents in Saltburn-by-the Sea.

I left for Oxford two weeks after returning. Once again leaving the family behind in Saltburn and moving into a Nissen hut in Oxford was not easy. I was now working as a Senior Registrar and on call alternate nights, covering two hospitals. When I was on call, one of the consultants (Mr. Stallworthy or, now, Mr. Arthur Williams) was always available for advice, but generally speaking I was left with the responsibilities of a consultant, which included treating outpatients and doing routine surgical procedures. During the next few months these responsibilities were expanded to my looking after the unit when one or the other consultant was away. My surgical skills were honed further and I learned how to perform a Wertheim's hysterectomy.

One day, over coffee, Mr. Stallworthy asked, "Bernie, where are your family staying at the moment?"

"In Saltburn."

"That's a long way away."

"Yes, it takes me four hours to drive, and I only get up there every other weekend. I leave on Friday, after the clinic, and get back late on Sundays."

"Why don't you rent a place here to stay in?"

"We're considering it, but at the moment we haven't decided on how long we're going to stay in England. Finding accommodation in Oxford is not easy."

"I have a suggestion that might help. In three weeks' time I'm going on a six-week lecturing tour of the United States and Canada. Our house will be empty. Would you and your family like to stay in our home while we're away? You would be our guests and there would be no expense to you."

Without hesitation, Elaine agreed with the proposal. Our six weeks' living in Mr. Stallworthy's house, which was called "Shotover Edge", was the highlight of our return to England. Elaine, Kathryn and Patrick came down but Helen stayed with my parents; she had started school. The house came with a cook, maid, gardener, and chauffeur-driven Rolls had I wanted to use it! A large two-storey Edwardian house, built from grey stone and partly covered by ivy, it was situated on the top of a hill to the east of Oxford overlooking the city with its numerous church spires and surrounded by a large terraced garden which was big enough to accommodate a tennis court with ease. There were all manner of shrubs, flowers, trees and a fountain. We enjoyed the lavish lifestyle. Mr. Stallworthy was an exceptionally successful specialist. But I had observed how hard he worked; I didn't see myself ever aspiring to reach those heights.

On Mr. Stallworthy's recommendation, Elaine was able to spend five weeks observing in the Department of Anaesthesia. She enjoyed the work and entertained the idea of becoming an anaesthetist. Unfortunately the six weeks soon came to an end. Elaine and the children returned to Saltburn and I went back to the Nissen huts. The good news was Elaine had found a branch of medicine she was interested in and could look forward to pursuing in the near future.

In the meantime, I had written to the Canadian College of Physicians and Surgeons about taking the Canadian specialist examinations and had a reply stating that all my training was recognized but that I would have to do a further six months of general surgery before I could sit the exam. This was a bit of a blow because I had now spent five and a half years in recognized training, taken the British examination, and spent two years working in Uganda. I felt it was time I settled into a permanent job.

Since leaving Canada I had kept in touch with Marty Robinson and Dr. Walter McCord. Marty had moved back to London, Ontario, and was a busy obstetrician there. When I asked them, they both said my prospects in Canada were excellent, and Marty said he could arrange for me to do the six months of general surgery at the Westminster Hospital in London, Ontario. He said the job wasn't too stressful and that it would give me an opportunity to work towards the Canadian fellowship exams which, he warned me, were not to be taken lightly. I had also maintained my medical registration in Manitoba and knew that if worst came to the worst I could still practice there as a general practitioner.

In 1967 we decided to move back to Canada.

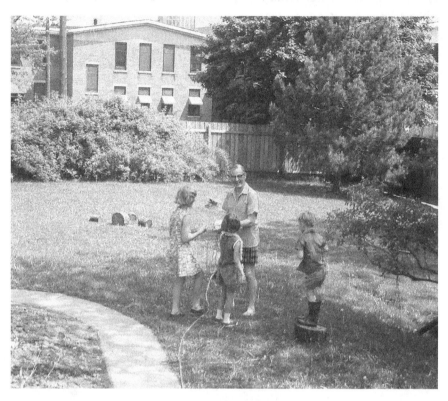

The family in the backyard in London, Ontario, in the late 1960s.

Chapter 11
Back to Canada: Private Practice

Returning to Canada occasioned some regrets. Once again we would be saying goodbyes, but this time we would be making a long-term move. Elaine would be leaving her parents in the Wirral and two sisters with families in Cheshire. My parents were now permanently based in Saltburn; my aunt, Alice, in Birmingham; my sister with her family in Dunfirmline, Scotland; and my cousin, Anne, in Guilford. The distance between Canada and the UK was great, and travelling back and forth, expensive. Seeing each other in the future would be dependent on our travelling back to the UK. Our relatives could not afford the trip to Canada. In addition, our parents were no longer young and my parents had no desire to travel outside the UK again.

We also wondered about the quality of education our children would receive in Canada. Another concern of mine was losing easy access to the history and culture of continental Europe. Amsterdam, Geneva, Paris, Berlin, Rome, Vienna, Madrid, Lisbon, Oslo, Stockholm, Copenhagen, Helsinki—all these names conjured up sights and smells to be savoured and lingered over. However, once we'd made our decision, the excitement of returning to Canada took over.

We were in our early thirties with a young family, looking to gain security for the future; Canada offered it.

During our early married years, Elaine and I had accumulated a surprising collection of belongings, including our car. After doing research into costs we found that the cheapest way for us to get to Canada was by ship. We booked passage on the *Empress of Canada*, a Canadian Pacific steamship that sailed between Liverpool and Montreal. Because of the high cost of tickets we could only afford to travel third-class. I would have to share a cabin with three other men, while Elaine and the children would have their own cabin. We would get together as a family on the decks, and during meals.

We sailed from Liverpool on the twentieth of June, 1967. Elaine's parents and sisters were on the dock to say goodbye. The voyage lasted for five days. The jade-green ocean was tranquil, the weather sunny and warm. The children enjoyed a fancy dress event and had lots of activities on deck to keep them busy. Adults were less fortunate; there was not much to do. On three afternoons I played bridge in the first-class dining room, with a man who was a bit of a "dandy" and who, I was later told, competed for high stakes in Toronto. I had never partnered with someone as good as he was. We did well and won a prize.

Sailing up the St. Lawrence River was a new adventure. On our first trip we'd not seen this older part of Canada. The bank of the river on the Canadian side was lined with picturesque French-style farms and small villages and houses. By contrast, development on the American side was largely industrial. The factories were impressive but dirty, similar to those found in Middlesbrough. A heavy layer of pollution blanketed the landscape around them. The ship stopped first in Quebec City, a four-hundred-year-old walled city built out of stone that looked like granite and through which ran narrow cobbled streets. Briefly I felt like I had been transported back to the Old World.

All passengers had to go through customs and immigration before being allowed to continue on to Montreal where they would disembark.

The immigration process turned into a nightmare. The ship's steward, an officious little man, told us that we had to go down to the dock and line up with several hundred other passengers of different nationalities. We found ourselves in a long line-up that moved at a crawl. Helen, Kathryn and Patrick got bored. It became impossible to keep them entertained much to the annoyance of the other people in the queue. We missed lunch. The hungry children grew even more irritable. Eventually we got to the desk and the immigration officer got increasingly agitated when he couldn't find our papers anywhere. After looking through his stack of paper a couple of times he went over to a colleague's desk. They went through his papers as well. By this time, I feared we would not be allowed into Canada.

"Show me your passports again," said the immigration officer in a strong French Canadian accent. "We can't find your papers so we can't stamp them to let you into Canada. You'll have to go back onto the ship and see the immigration officer there, get some new papers, and come back."

He said this while eyeing our nagging children with disdain. My composure, which was already strained, snapped.

"Oh, for God's sake, we've been waiting in line for over two hours and you're sending us back to fill out some forms I've already given you?"

"My apologies," he said. "There's nothing else I can do here. You'll have to go back on board. Here are your passports," and he slapped them in my hand. "Thank you. Next."

We returned to the ship, a dejected troupe, to find the ship's immigration officer. When I gave him our names and told him the sad story about our missing papers, he, to my astonishment, gave a big sigh and smiled with relief. "We've been looking for you. Your papers are here with the Canadian citizens. You're a mixed family because Kathryn, your daughter, was born in Winnipeg. I'm sorry you got into the wrong line up. Here are your entry permits. I can stamp your passports for you here." As I recall, I was the more relieved of the two of us. Gratitude replaced anger.

The next morning, when the ship arrived in Montreal, the sky was dull and the streets damp. We travelled past the Expo 67 site, which exuded a sense of pride. We lined up on the deck and watched the luggage being unloaded with cranes from the large holds. Eventually we saw our car being lifted out. Once our baggage was ashore we were allowed off the ship and onto the dock to retrieve our belongings. Our car had to be steam-cleaned to ensure that no unwanted insects immigrated with us into Canada. Our destination was London, Ontario, where I had accepted a position as an intern at Westminster Hospital. Elaine was going to enter the anaesthesia residency program at Victoria Hospital.

The last of the paperwork was relatively simple and we got away by ten o'clock. It was over six years since I had driven on the right side of the road; however, I was surprised by how quickly I adapted. The problem was, we didn't have a map of Montreal. All I knew was that we had to head west. I had asked for directions when we picked up the car and the man said to be sure to turn left when I got off the docks. His directions sounded simple enough. Nonetheless, I soon got lost. While stopped at a traffic light I asked a taxi driver in the next lane, how to get to London, Ontario. He seemed to think this was funny. He waved his hands in the air and answered in French. When he realized I didn't understand a word, he spoke in English.

"You must be just off the boat." He laughed and pointed. "Keep going on this road for five hundred miles. *Bon voyage.*"

We had arranged to stay in London with my colleague and friend, Marty, and his family for a week or so, while we waited for the hospital married accommodation to become available. The city, whose name would continually remind us of home, had been founded in 1826 and was, fittingly, located at the forks of the Thames River and the North Thames River. Like its namesake, the city was originally intended to be a capital, in this case, of Upper Canada. We soon discovered that London was very different from Winnipeg. The trees were bigger and the roads twisty and hilly. The power and telephone cables hung freely in loops above ground and formed helter-skelter patterns against the sky. When we arrived it was summer, extremely hot and humid, likely due to the close proximity of Lake Huron. Fortunately, Marty's large house was air conditioned, and we were housed in his cool basement.

As Marty and I drove around various neighbourhoods I noticed that most of the houses were wood-frame structures showing a strong European influence. Most of the roads in the suburbs were wide and lined with sidewalks and leafy, deciduous trees, largely elms, maples and oaks. He showed me around the city of just under 200,000 people, with its typical North American "downtown" business area. Some of the buildings had ten or more storeys, a scale unfamiliar to me. There were the Simpson's and Eaton's department stores as well as other major businesses, including London Life, 3M, Imperial Oil, Canada Trust, and London Life. He then took me to the impressive University of Western Ontario campus where the undergraduate portion of the medical course was offered.

The clinical portion of the course, the senior years, was offered at the older Victoria and Westminster hospitals. The Departments of Medicine, Surgery, Obstetrics and Gynaecology were housed at the Victoria Hospital. Marty explained that there were plans to build a new University Hospital on campus in the near future. Once again I was increasingly aware of the greater emphasis placed on an academic approach to medical education in Canada and the US when compared to the British system.

Our new home was on Commissioners Road, within easy walking distance of the hospital. This accommodation was a comfortable old furnished house with a fully operational kitchen. This was a godsend as we didn't have much money in the bank to buy household items. The girls started school and Elaine found a daycare nursery for Patrick so that she could start in the anaesthesia residency program at the Victoria Hospital under Dr. Spurrel.

My job was as an intern to Dr. Johnston, an accomplished surgeon. Once again I was cast in a junior position, but the workload was not demanding and I had plenty of time to prepare for the Canadian Fellowship exams. I was expected to attend two teaching sessions a week in the Obstetrics Department at the Victoria Hospital. This gave me the opportunity to meet many of the practicing OB-GYN consultants and I was able to get a feel for how things were done in central Canada. Unlike Winnipeg, where many consultants had spent time in the UK, here most of the local consultants had part of their training in the large teaching centres in the USA.

Since my last time in Canada, the remuneration of physicians and patient costs had changed radically. There was now a national health-care program in place and the costs were divided between the federal and provincial governments. Physicians were paid on a fee-for-service basis and most medical services and all hospital costs were covered by medicare. There were some inter-provincial differences in how the services were run and financed, but there was reciprocity. The physicians seemed to be comfortable with the changes although I heard much discussion and debate about the future. As far as I could determine the public thought that the national health care service was a good idea.

Having been brought up in the National Health Service (NHS) in England, where doctors were salaried, I had never been faced with the implications of working as a private physician and charging patients for my services. I, too, thought a national health system was a good idea, no matter how it was structured, and fair to both the patients and physicians. I had seen how universal health systems could be abused by both patients and physicians but felt that universality, in spite of these problems, was better for society. Under universal care, poor people who needed medical attention were spared the horrendous burden, embarrassment and ignominy of trying to pay an expense they couldn't afford. Illnesses often worsened because patients delayed seeking medical care. From what I understood, it was the inequalities of treatment of the rich and poor that had spurred Tommy Douglas and the CCF to first establish medicare in Canada.

Once I was settled in my new job and after discussion with Dr. Johnston and others, I came to the conclusion that it would be wise for me to take the Certificate and Fellowship exams in my specialty and the LMCC (licentiate of the medical college of Canada) in order to have mobility in Canada. The provincial medical boards were getting more and more restrictive about who could practice medicine in their provinces and without the LMCC I would not be able to practice in Ontario, Alberta or British Columbia. And to practice in Quebec I would have to take the exams in French!

I was not alone in having to write the LMCC. Another intern, David Downham, faced the same dilemma. His field was urology, which was even more specialised than obstetrics and gynaecology. We spent many hours reviewing our medical knowledge and signed up to take the LMCC together.

We drove to Montreal in the fall when all the trees were changing colour. Both of us marvelled at the explosive reds and yellows that dotted the hills and valleys. We arrived in the city in the early evening and thought that we should go and find where the exams were being held. After studying the map we decided that the simplest way was to use the freeway system. This was a mistake, especially for me as the driver. I took a wrong turn and got lost. It was rush hour and I was unaccustomed to Montreal drivers who honked their horns when they felt annoyed or aggrieved and manoeuvred aggressively. Madness, absolute madness, I said to David. Eventually we came to a stop at the American border and quickly got off the freeway. On consulting the map again we found a different route and meandered back into the city.

The LMCC exams turned out to be very similar to the graduating exams that we had taken in the UK years before. We both passed, which was a relief, but David was told by one of the examiners that his pass was dependent upon his promise that he would never deliver babies!

There were two streams of specialists in Canada. One group had the certificate and the others had the more academic fellowship. There were two separate examinations, but both were set by the Canadian College of Physicians and Surgeons. On completion of the training, which was the same, and, depending on one's confidence and future aspirations, one could take one or both sets of examinations. To get into university posts it was essential to have the fellowship. Although I was not thinking of an academic career I felt I should take both sets of exams while I had the chance. The certificate exam turned out to be very similar to the English ones I had taken while in Oxford with its practical bias. The fellowship exam was far more academic with its North American emphasis on theoretical questions.

Although I tried to adapt to the North American way of thinking about certain topics I was not successful when I wrote the fellowship paper. One of the areas where my answers did not meet the expectations of the examiners was my opinions on caesarean sections. The North American practice at the time was "once a c-section always a c-section." This was not my experience and, therefore, I didn't give it as my answer. Other areas of disagreement concerned the handling of breech presentations and the investigation and use of isotopes in the treatment of thyroid disorders. I did, however, pass the certificate exam and could now practice as a specialist in Canada.

It was during this time that I faced another personal health issue. One night, when I was called to see a patient in hospital, I could barely get out of bed. My joints had seized up. My knees, hips and wrists were incredibly sore. Once I had dressed and made my way into the hall, the pain lessened. I hobbled to the ward and saw the patient. I was still in a lot of discomfort but received enough relief from over-the-counter painkillers to continue working. After a couple of days, I talked to Dr. Johnson about my condition and he arranged for me to see the rheumatologist, Dr. Manfred Harth. After his examination and tests he concluded that I had a "non-arthritic rheumatism".

"What's that?" I asked.

"You have all the symptoms and physical signs of an acute rheumatic attack, but the X-rays are all clear. The blood tests are negative for a rheumatoid factor. You're mildly anaemic and you have a high sedimentation rate which could indicate an autoimmune disorder."

"What's the prognosis?"

"That's difficult to answer," he said. "Yours is a collagen disease, which is notoriously difficult to treat. As this is your first episode, which seems to be settling quite rapidly, I'm optimistic about the outcome. However, you could have another episode in the next few months and be semi-crippled in a year or so. I really can't say. In the meantime, I want you to take iron and aspirin daily. These might help. The other thing you might try is losing some weight and improving your fitness."

With this news, Dr. Harth altered my world view and perspective. For the first time I was the subject of observation and not the observer or analyst. Looking back I think this was one of the most worrying episodes in my life. Not only did I become acutely conscious of my own mortality, but I realized I could become disabled and unable to practice medicine. With severe rheumatism I would be unfit to operate. I'd be useless, my years of training a terrible waste. I remember now how forlorn I felt.

"I'd like to see you again in two weeks. You won't need a prescription today," he said. "Let's hope for the best and pray the condition settles down." This last comment did not sound optimistic or encouraging. At that moment, I felt totally disheartened, as if I had been disconnected from who I wanted to be. I even considered giving up obstetrics and gynaecology and going into pathology.

A few days later I was pain-free. At the time I was over 185 lbs. and had not done much in the way of exercise since leaving Uganda. I was sitting in the cafeteria nursing a cup of coffee, into which I'd poured two spoonfuls of sugar, in one hand and holding an "Oh Henry!" chocolate bar in the other. I was talking to the hospital parson, who was a fit and trim sixty-five-year-old. Canon Gardner.

"Do you play tennis?" he asked.

"I used to," I answered. "But I've not played in over a year, and not much since school. Why do you ask?"

"There's a tennis court in the hospital compound that belongs to the nurses, but the medical staff have permission to use it between 4 p.m. and 6 p.m. during the week. Hardly anyone plays and I enjoy the game. Perhaps you'd like to have a go?"

"I'd love to. When shall we start?"

"How about the day after tomorrow?"

"Sounds good," I said.

"Wonderful. I'll see you at four. The court is just down there," he said, pointing over my shoulder, "outside that window. I'd better be off now."

I was naïve and arrogant enough to think I could beat an old man like him without any trouble. I had played tennis for the school before I joined the swim team and was confident about my game.

My confidence was misplaced. The first day we played I won three games in the first set and none in the next. Plus, I was exhausted.

"I think you've had enough for today," he suggested. "I suspect you'll have a few sore muscles tomorrow. Perhaps we can have another game next week."

"I look forward to it," I said. "A little revenge, perhaps. How about Tuesday? I'm free then."

"That's a date. Thanks for the game. It was fun," he said and turned and walked away, smiling as if he knew a secret about why things happen the way they do. At that point I wondered if he knew Dr. Harth.

I was very sore over the next few days but by Tuesday I was feeling good and looking forward to giving him a better game. The outcome was similar except we played three full sets and I managed to win three games in each set.

"You played better today," he said. "I can see you've played before. Would you like another match next Friday?"

"Yes, please. I think it's doing some good. See you then."

We played once or twice a week for the rest of my stay in London. My fitness and game both improved but it took me several weeks and the loss of twenty pounds before I became competitive. Happily, all signs of my rheumatoid arthritis disappeared and did not reappear for some time. When I finally managed to hold my own I asked about his tennis background.

"You must have been a very good player when you were younger," I said.

"I used to think so," he said. "When I got to the finals of the Wimbledon Juniors I thought I might take the game up professionally, but at that time there wasn't a lot of money in the game. I thought becoming a 'Man of the Cloth' might be a better and more sensible career. I've never had any regrets."

After spending six months with Dr. Johnson in general surgery, I spent a year as a resident in pathology, a year that was less demanding because it was a nine-to-five job and did not require my performing surgery, responding to night calls and various other duties. Not only did I benefit from practicing another branch of medicine, but during this time of less stress I was able to recover my health. As the pain seeped from my body my mood changed and I was once again optimistic about my future career in gynaecology and obstetrics.

Elaine and I both kept busy, and our time in London passed quickly. When we had some spare time we explored some of the local sights, including a visit with the children to Niagara Falls. The volume of water cascading over the escarpments was breathtaking! Elaine and I drove to Stratford to see a Shakespeare play, the production a part of their yearly summer festival. We also purchased some camping gear and made family visits to several of the provincial parks in Western Ontario. We went to Orillia, which is famous for Stephen Leacock; and to Point Pelee, on Lake Erie, the southernmost point of Canada, where the Monarch butterflies congregated before heading south for Mexico. Detroit, just across the river from the relatively rural town of Windsor, was the first big American city we visited and I was impressed by it as the hub of the world's auto industry. Everywhere we travelled on the Canadian side we encountered tobacco, fruit and vegetable farms.

The summers in London, Ontario were intolerably hot and humid. The winters were cold and snowy, but we were told that London lay below the true "snow belt" where snowfall was literally measured in feet. The most striking weather phenomenon was the ice storms. I remember getting up one morning to walk over to the hospital. When I opened the door I discovered the porch, pavement, road, grass, trees, house tops, telegraph lines and power cables covered in one to two inches of ice. I slipped and fell several times getting to the hospital. When the sun rose the ice glistened and crackled. All the colours of the rainbow refracted through the ice and many tree branches snapped under its weight. The power lines stretched and hung dangerously low. Fortunately, the conditions necessary for ice storms were short-lived and only happened once or twice a winter.

In 1968 Elaine's father was seconded to a company in New York and visited us for a few days during our second summer. He was a chemist who was at the forefront of the development of plastics, working with the Americans to establish facilities for the mass production of plastics. His visit to London, Ontario was special. Elaine and I were both a bit homesick and it was fun for the children to see their grandfather again.

Once I had passed the certificate exams in the fall of 1968 I looked for a permanent job as a specialist. This turned out to be more difficult than I had anticipated. Unlike Winnipeg and Western Canada, most of the specialists in London worked on their own and none were interested in taking me on as a partner. There were over twenty consultant specialists listed and when I looked at their backgrounds and training, it became obvious to me that I was an outsider. They had all trained in London except for Professor Kinch, who was from Dublin, Ireland. I made some enquires about the other townships in Western Ontario, but there didn't seem to be any opportunities there either. I was faced with the prospect of setting up practice in competition with local consultants who were well known. This plan would have required borrowing money for an office, finding staff, getting support from the local general practitioners and receiving hospital privileges. The requirement to set up an independent practice was something I had no experience doing and I was not very confident. Looking at the bigger picture I didn't think I would be successful. I couldn't really see the need for yet another obstetrician gynaecologist in the area.

I wrote to Dr. McCord, my mentor in Winnipeg, to let him know I had passed my certificate exams and asked his opinion about where I might find work. He wrote back suggesting I could return to Winnipeg and join him as an assistant; they were looking for a third obstetrician in their group. After a trial year, if everyone felt I fitted in, I would be offered a full partnership. The salary was better than anything I had earned in the past and the position seemed to be an ideal way for me to get established in Canada. Elaine and I decided Winnipeg was our best option. It meant that she would have to give up the anaesthetist residency program in London, but Dr. Spurrel contacted Dr. Wade, a professor in Winnipeg, and they found space for her in their program at the University of Manitoba and its Health Science Center.

Our plan was to take three days to drive to Winnipeg. Early on Boxing Day, 1968, the Binns family left in a convoy which included two station wagons and most of our smaller, personal belongings. The movers had taken our heavier possessions three days earlier. Before they left I asked them which was the best route west. There were two possibilities, they suggested. One was a southern route through the States, and the other was a northern route through Canada. Either way the distance was just over fifteen hundred miles. The truck drivers said the weather was more stable on the northern route and there was less traffic. But since it was the middle of winter and we were going to have to stop twice because of the children, I decided we should take the more populated route through the United States. The illusion, I wonder now, of safety in numbers?

It was a dull, drizzly day when we started. Unfortunately, I had not checked the weather forecast and shortly after leaving London the drizzle turned into freezing rain. Yet we got through Sarnia and into the United States without much trouble. However, the driving conditions worsened and the cars were soon covered in two inches of ice. The road became treacherous and slippery. The traffic thinned. We managed to get to Flint, Michigan, which was approximately two hundred miles from London, and into the warmth of a motel. When we woke, we were shocked to see a further four to five inches of snow had fallen overnight on top of the ice on the cars. The truck drivers had been right.

The next morning, after breakfast and before we were able to continue on our way, we brushed away the snow and chipped away the ice that coated the windshields. The snowfall was light and the roads were in reasonably good condition. From Flint we headed north towards the Mackinac suspension bridge, two hundred and fifty miles away. As the hours passed the snowfall got heavier, and our progress slowed to a crawl. By three o'clock in the afternoon driving conditions had become impossible. Visibility was ghostly, at best. On the radio, all stations were broadcasting weather warnings. Travellers were advised to get off the roads. We pulled over at the next town to look for accommodation. When we had planned our journey, we had not appreciated the fact that we would be travelling through a ski area on a public holiday. All the popular hotels were full. Ironically, we finally found accommodation in a rundown ski chalet; a very cold ski chalet. Never had the entire family spent such a miserable night.

When we got up in the morning the weather had improved and

we were able to continue on our journey. Once we got over the spectacular Mackinac bridge, an engineering masterpiece spanning five miles from shore to shore, we were driving over roads with towering banks of snow on either side. Most of the time all we could see was snow. Luckily snow ploughs had been out during the night and the roads were clear. We managed to make good progress that day, covering several hundred miles before arriving in Ladysmith, Wisconsin.

As we drove west we noticed that the temperature was dropping but didn't think much of this fact. Both cars had block heaters. On the third day we made it as far as Fargo, North Dakota. We spent the night in a comfortable and deliciously warm motel, but when we got up in the morning the temperature was below −30 degrees F. Although I had plugged the car block heaters in, neither car would start. As it turned out, the Ontario garage mechanic had failed or forgotten, who knows, to connect the leads to the engine blocks. A stupid mistake.

Eventually I found a garage mechanic who was willing to give each car a boost. The Chevy Beaumont started up without difficulty, but the Volvo was frozen solid and had to be towed into the garage to be thawed out. After lunch we set off once again. Now on familiar roads we reached Winnipeg shortly after nightfall. We survived the trip in good spirits except for our pet mouse, Thomasina, who developed a cough during the trip and later succumbed to pneumonia, in spite of two attending physicians!

Dr. McCord had arranged accommodation for us in one of the hospital flats adjacent to the New Grace Hospital. The apartment was quite cramped, but adequate for our needs. We stayed there for two months while I settled into working at the Abbot Clinic and the hospital. During the Christmas holidays, Dr. McCord and his family, invited us over for a turkey dinner. Happy to be back in the company of old friends, we relaxed into the familiar surroundings of Winnipeg.

Situated on a small hill, just north of Portage Avenue on Sturgeon Creek, the New Grace Hospital had been built two years before we arrived. The Salvation Army still ran the new hospital of two hundred beds. There were the usual departments, including Obstetrics and Gynaecology. The Maternity Department had three delivery rooms and four first-stage rooms. One of the delivery rooms could also be used for caesarean sections. The ante-natal and post-natal patients were placed in a women's ward of forty beds which we shared with the general surgeons. The maximum number of patients in any room was four and there were several double and single rooms for special care. The maternity unit delivered fifteen hundred babies a year. Most babies were delivered by family physicians, the rest by consultants.

Although some of the nurses on the Labour and Delivery floor were trained midwives, midwifery was still not a part of Canadian practice. The babies were looked after on the same floor in two nurseries and there were several state-of-the-art incubators for premature babies. Six on-call paediatricians were expected to come in to attend caesarean sections. There was a modern Emergency Department and an Intensive Care area, twenty-four-hour anaesthesia coverage, laboratory support, and X-ray facilities. Dr. McCord showed me round the hospital, happily explaining many of the new features incorporated into the design. His enthusiasm for the facility was obvious. I realized then how outdated and primitive some of my past placements had been and how fortunate I was to be able to practise here.

Within the Department of Obstetrics and Gynaecology, twelve consultants were listed. However, only five of them used the Grace Hospital as their main practising hospital. Most of the consultants working in Winnipeg had operating privileges in more than one location—in the peripheral hospitals and usually in one of the teaching/tertiary care hospitals (either the Health Sciences Centre or the St. Boniface Hospital).

The arrangement of hospital privileges that included both peripheral hospitals and teaching hospitals was a new system to me, but I soon got used to the idea and could see its advantages, the foremost being the creation of a closer relationship between family physicians, consultants and patients. The general practitioners regularly came into hospital to see their patients and were responsible for much of their post-operative care. I liked this intimacy.

And so, in 1968, at the age of thirty-five and ten years after qualifying in medicine, I was now a consultant Obstetrician and Gynaecologist in Winnipeg, Canada. Over the past ten long years I had gained considerable experience and had seen different parts of the world. I had personally observed the practice of medicine in the United Kingdom, Uganda, and Canada and I felt I had a lot to offer my colleagues. Our travels had enriched us all; had made our lives larger.

In 1969, Winnipeg had a population of about half a million, with an additional half-million scattered across the province. Apart from two obstetricians working in Brandon (population 50,000) all the obstetricians and gynaecologists were based in Winnipeg. There were several large clinics with multiple specialists. The two largest were the Winnipeg Clinic and the Manitoba Clinic with consultant staffs of fifty to sixty. There were three smaller consultant clinics, the Mall Clinic, the Abbot Clinic, and The Group. The total number of obstetricians and gynaecologists for the province was twenty-seven which included six full-time university staff, who worked and practised at the two tertiary centres when not teaching. This ratio of consultants to patients contrasted starkly with the situation in Uganda.

The Abbot Clinic, where I worked, consisted of twelve consultants with specialties in general surgery, internal medicine, urology and obstetrics and gynaecology. We had basic laboratory and X-ray facilities on site with part-time consultant radiologists who reported on the X-rays. To start with, I was expected to spend three half-days a week seeing patients in the clinic. Some of these were "clinic patients" who didn't have a private doctor and others were referrals from general practitioners. I was also expected to spend one morning a week in the staff clinic at St. Boniface Hospital and another half-day a week looking after the staff outpatients at the Grace Hospital for Unmarried Mothers. Once a month I offered a family planning clinic for the provincial health services. I had operating privileges at the Grace and St. Boniface hospitals and the Health Sciences Centre, but did most of my surgery at the Grace.

When I had a patient who required surgery I would phone the hospital operating room clerk to book the patient in for surgery. Usually the patient's own doctor would come to assist at the surgery if it was a major procedure. "Staff" patients were people who did not have general practitioners they visited regularly. This was an especially serious problem for people who lived in remote communities or off in the wilderness on their own. Many came from Indian reserves and the North West Territories. This practice was completely different from what I was used to, but very easy to adapt to.

My practice grew rapidly and after six months I was invited to join the Abbot Clinic as a full partner. Although the type of practice differed from what I'd experienced in the UK, the volume of work I was doing by the end of the year was comparable to that of the consultants I had worked with in England. A major difference was that we performed many more normal deliveries, essentially functioning as midwives.

My gynaecological expertise in the areas of pelvic inflammatory disease, infertility, myomectomies for fibroids in young patients, and some other unusual gynaecological problems, such as transsexuals and gender anomalies, gradually became known and became a significant part of my practice.

My Ugandan experience instructing midwives had kindled my interest in teaching, so whenever the opportunity to teach arose I volunteered. This passion meant I spent as much time as I could working at the St. Boniface and Health Sciences Hospitals.

The University Department of Obstetrics was always looking for consultants and general practitioners who were willing to teach medical students practical skills in their offices. Showing students the real world of medicine off-campus was something I liked to do, but there were some drawbacks. I saw fewer patients because I had to spend time discussing details of patients' problems with the students. Even though my teaching affected the number of patients I was able to see, I was fortunate that my partners were understanding and valued my teaching contribution.

In addition to the time I spent with patients, I attended monthly administrative meetings at the Grace and Boniface Hospitals, and at the Health Sciences Centre. I continued to attend weekly grand rounds at all three hospitals. My day usually started at seven-thirty in the morning and I rarely got home before six in the evening. Somewhere in the middle of all this I used to average three or four weekly games of squash in the winter and a round or two per week of golf in the summer months.

After two months in the cramped apartment near the hospital, Elaine and I decided to buy a house. We needed four bedrooms, one for a live-in-nanny to look after the children while Elaine was working in the anaesthetic residency program at the Health Sciences Center. In the dead of winter we set off on our search.

There were two large building corporations building new homes in Winnipeg. After looking at several of these houses, Elaine decided that she didn't like them. She thought they were poorly built and drafty, something to be avoided in a Winnipeg winter. After a lot of searching, we eventually found a four-bedroom house that had just been built by a reputable Mennonite builder. The house was a bit more expensive than the others in the area but it was within walking distance of the Grace Hospital. In March 1968, we took possession of our first house on Frost Avenue, a fitting but ironic name, and for the first time in my life I was no longer an itinerant wanderer.

Part of Elaine's requirements in the anaesthesia program meant she had to stay at the Health Sciences Centre overnight several times a week. To ensure that someone was home when the children returned from school or when I was called out in the middle of the night to deliver babies, we thought supporting a student looking for a place to live might solve both problems. We posted an advertisement at a technical college near us, offering room and board in exchange for child-minding in the afternoons, evenings and overnight when required. Our first applicant was Peggy, a farm lass from Saskatchewan, who had never been in a big city. We liked her immediately and hired her. Initially she missed her close-knit rural community and had trouble making friends with her classmates. Yet she was great with the children and it was fun watching her adapt to the world of Winnipeg. By the time the end of the school year came, she had settled into college life and had a healthy social calendar. Not surprisingly she left us for a more permanent and independent accommodation.

Our second student boarder was Mahindra, a young woman from the Caribbean. She was a lively person, who loved to dance and sing, and party in the evenings. While we loved her energy and spunk, her lifestyle defeated the purpose of having her stay at our house. By the end of Mahindra's time with us, Helen was old enough, thank goodness, to take responsibility for Kathryn and Patrick after school, and our days of student boarders ended.

Partnership in the Abbott Clinic came with some perks. One of these was a membership at the Winnipeg Winter Club, where a lot of our friends were members. This was a family club with facilities for badminton, squash, curling, five-pin bowling, skating, and gymnastics. The site included a twenty-metre swimming pool and tennis courts in a bubble. The club had a cafeteria for casual food and a dining room for more formal meals. Other amenities included an area for duplicate bridge and a reading room. Over the next twelve years our family took full advantage of these facilities.

Helen and Kathryn excelled at badminton. They trained with the professional badminton coach, Pal Chawla, and played in tournaments in Manitoba and across Canada. They were both provincial champions and competed at the national level. Helen won a silver medal in the junior U19 nationals in singles, became the Quebec provincial champion, won the New England Open in Boston and the Bermuda Open, and played for Canada in Sweden. Kathryn reached the top four in doubles. Patrick learned how to play squash, taking lessons from the professional on staff. I began to play squash again and discovered that the game in North America was slightly different from the game I'd known in the UK. The court was smaller and the ball had a different texture and bounce.

Once my squash game was back up to scratch, Charlie Ives, who worked at both clubs, suggested I should join the Winnipeg Squash

Club where all the serious players played. After a few visits there and talking to the members, I decided to play competitive squash again and I joined. This club had plans to build new courts to host international squash tournaments, which for all of us was an exciting prospect.

The Winnipeg Squash Club was an all-male club whose membership included people from a range of professions. Despite being an all-male establishment, not a policy with which I agreed but one to which most members clung—it was actively criticized by several equal rights organizations in Winnipeg—the club survived and was never sued. The club held many tournaments including the annual Manitoba Open. These Open tournaments attracted top ranking international professionals who stopped off in Canada when travelling to and from tournaments in Australia, New Zealand and Europe. Over the years I had the pleasure of seeing many of the top ten world-ranked players including Hashim, Jahanjar, Sharif, and Rosham Khan, Jonah Barrington, Geoff Hunt, Jonathan Power, and Murray Lilley compete, as well as a few top females such as Susan Devoy and Heather McKay. Few members saw the irony!

Once again we enjoyed Winnipeg as a centre for the performing arts. The Royal Winnipeg Ballet was internationally renowned for its world-class productions, both classical and modern. We supported the ballet as well as the Winnipeg Symphony Orchestra and the Manitoba Opera by purchasing season tickets for our family. There was a continuous stream of visiting musical groups and solo singers who performed at various venues around town. Two live theatre groups put on plays in the winter that included everything from Shakespeare to contemporary Canadian plays. Last but not least, there was the Winnipeg Art Gallery, affectionately known as the "WAG", where an active and dedicated art group ran classes in all the visual arts. After a visit from Donald and Lillian Fisher, friends from our London student days, Elaine became interested in these classes and took up painting seriously. Don now worked for Elstree Studios, a TV and film company in London, as a set designer/director.

When summer arrived I discovered that some of my medical colleagues played golf. They took me to several golf clubs in Winnipeg and I started to play regularly on Thursday afternoons. By the end of my first summer I was hooked on the game and applied for a family membership at the St. Charles Golf and Country Club. This became an activity the entire family enjoyed for decades. Elaine and I played on a regular basis during the summer months. One nine was designed by Alistair MacKenzie and the other by Donald Ross. The third, the "West" nine, was meant for beginners and it was here where our children learned how to play.

Two years after we joined, the club rezoned land that had been originally set aside for a second nine-hole course and created a new subdivision for housing. When the building lots were surveyed, club members had first option on the lots that surrounded the golf course. This was an opportunity for us to build a larger house directly fronting the golf course. We chose a lot facing onto the fifth green on the "West" nine. The house we designed and built there became our home for the next twenty years.

While many of our friends had lake cottages to which they migrated during the summer months, to boat, fish, swim, socialize and relax, we never opted for this lifestyle because of our time commitments at work. Since Elaine and I were on call every third or fourth night and often on weekends, we were rarely off together. Besides, some cottages were over a hundred miles away from Winnipeg and the prospect of commuting back and forth all summer long didn't appeal.

Planning holidays each year for the whole family was often a cause of strife. Inevitably Elaine or I had other commitments. On family outings, we tried our hand at fishing, at first casting from shore, but we were usually skunked. So I bought a twelve-foot aluminium boat, which we loaded on the roof of the car, and a seven-horsepower motor to see if fishing from a boat would improve our luck. It didn't. Manitoba lakes and rivers are replete with pickerel, lake trout and jackfish (pike). Unhappily we mostly hooked jackfish. Although tasty, their flesh was chockful of Y-shaped bones.

Every fall several friends and I went hunting for upland game and water fowl. For five to six weekends we headed out into the wilds, dressed in colourful gear, mainly plaids, with bird whistles dangling around our necks. Once in our blinds we would place the whistle between our frozen lips and mimic the sounds of birds. These excursions required getting up before the crack of dawn and driving vast distances north only to wait patiently in cold, wet, windy conditions for the birds to fly by—migrating south. To this day I don't understand why we did it, but everyone was convinced we were having fun. Perhaps we felt we were asserting some primitive instinct, as hunter-gatherers from a past that was lodged in some remote part of the brain.

I remember when my son, Patrick, at the age of seventeen, tried to work out what the value of the total hunt was in dollars per pound of bird. His final figure came to several hundred dollars when he included the price of gas, appropriate clothing and boots, guns, ammunition, depreciation, licences and, last but not least, paying farmers to pull our vehicles out of bogs and wetlands. After a few of these mishaps, Elaine predicted that I would definitely run out of gas at least once and no matter how good the latest 4 x 4 was supposed to be, I would manage to get the vehicle mired in mud. Our expeditions proved her right.

We also invested in a black Labrador Retriever we named Belka. He eventually became a house pet, but initially he was supposed to be a working dog. A part of the hunting team. Belka's and my early training routine was a constant source of amusement for my hunting friends. I spent many hours attempting to train him to retrieve. While he had all the characteristics for which his breed is renowned, fetching didn't appear to be one of them. Then, suddenly, instinct kicked in, and he retrieved anything and everything. Once he had been taught to swim properly—I was surprised to learn you needed to teach a dog to swim—he loved water, especially if it was cold. He didn't hesitate to break ice at the edge of frozen sloughs in order to retrieve birds and there were occasions when I thought he would drown from enthusiastic determination. He was a great companion.

When he went deaf at seven years, he used to go off after fallen birds, didn't respond to the whistle, and wouldn't look back. I had failed to teach him to turn around. We tried all manner of tricks to get his attention. We shouted, waved, jumped up and down, even hurled stones and sticks in his direction. This, of course, was when the next flock of ducks or geese flew over, the one for which we had been waiting for several hours, and they immediately changed course and flew away from the ruckus below.

After a few Winnipeg winters I noticed a pattern developing in myself and my golfing friends. By February we all suffered from golf deprivation. Snow covered our golf courses from October to April. To escape the snow and to get ourselves ready for the new season, Jerry Morrissey, a golf professional, came up with the idea of spending a week golfing on Vancouver Island where the weather was mild enough to play golf all year round. These trips afforded a welcome relief from the stress of work and introduced me to the place where Elaine and I would eventually build our retirement home.

It was not until 1971 that we, as a family, travelled to the United Kingdom to visit our relatives and some of our old friends. We spent three hectic weeks scurrying about the country to see Elaine's parents, my parents, my sister in Dunfirmline, Scotland, Mike and Jean in Welshpool, and some friends in London. Helen, Katherine and Patrick were spoiled by doting relatives who stuffed them with tea, cakes and sweets while Elaine and I soaked up the familiar delights of a long overdue homecoming.

On this visit it was obvious that my mother's health was not good and as we were leaving Saltburn I had a premonition that I would not see her alive again. Sadly I was right. She died the following January, a few days before her seventieth birthday. Father telegraphed me the news a day or so after. When I phoned him he insisted that I not try to get back for the funeral. This was a little difficult for me to understand, but it turned out that I could not have arranged the trip anyway because of airline schedules. Much to my dismay I was unable to attend my mother's funeral, a celebration and leave-taking I never thought I would miss. As a consequence of this loss, over the next twenty years I made a point of visiting my father, my sister and other friends and relatives in the UK at least once every eighteen months.

I combined many of these visits with attendance at professional meetings such as the Royal College of Obstetricians and Gynaecologists, the International Congress of Obstetrics and Gynaecology, and other scientific meetings and college reunions in Europe. When possible Elaine would accompany me and she would go to anaesthesia meetings. Over the years we also managed to arrange trips so our children could visit England, Scotland and Wales to see relatives and to connect with their cultural heritage.

At the Grace Hospital I soon became involved in most of the administrative committees that were responsible for the day-to-day running of the medical side of the hospital. Initially this meant being a regular attendee at the departmental meetings and later, when I became head of the Department and then Chief of Staff, I was required, when invited, to sit in on Hospital Board meetings. Surprisingly there were many similarities between the Grace Hospital administrative problems and those I had witnessed at the Churchill Hospital in Oxford.

Between 1970 and 1980 significant changes occurred to the way obstetricians were able to practice. These included economic, political, and academic pressures. Three of the peripheral hospital maternity units were closed which directly affected patients living in the suburbs. The Grace Hospital maternity unit survived the longest because of its geographic location, the strong support of the local physicians, and the Salvation Army. The trend to consolidate specialized services was obvious and eventually all maternity care was concentrated in the two major hospitals, St. Boniface and the Health Sciences Centre. This meant that the doctors who had practices in peripheral hospitals, with individualized care, lost the ability to follow their patients after diagnosis, because all patients had to be sent to the tertiary care hospital.

During this time, when the government's focus was on fiscal responsibility, there were many meetings to discuss the best way to achieve an economic and efficient service. Some of these meetings were quite contentious. Patients needed to transfer from small towns to Winnipeg and away from their supportive families, which was a particularly serious issue in the Aboriginal populations. The general feeling was that removing primary care doctors from the team of caregivers might result in negative outcomes because a specialist might not know the full case history when making a decision.

Theoretically the risk to mothers and babies was foremost in the minds of government officials, but their decision to centralize services ignored individual and special concerns. Unfortunately, the "bean counters" could not really understand the unpredictability of running a maternity ward and their decisions to decrease beds based on occupancy rates was an example of this oversimplification—their "one size fits all" model simply didn't work.

The closing of peripheral hospital maternity units was accompanied by an expansion of the full-time University Obstetric and Gynaecological Department which specialized in the areas of ultrasound, cervical screening, gynaecologic oncology, infertility, and perinatology. The impact of these changes on non-university specialists, who did not have privileges at St. Boniface or Health Sciences, changed the way they practiced. They were no longer included in the loop; they were often no longer participants in the care of their own patients.

The effect of these changes was gradual and frustrating at times. For example, I had been trained to diagnose and treat gynaecology patients with all kinds of cancer and had been doing this since I started my specialist practice. I performed surgery and followed up with these women throughout their chemotherapy and/or radiation treatments. Over time, with the advent of new radiology technology and chemotherapy regimes, as well as specific glandular surgeries, a new speciality developed within the field of gynaecology—the gynaecological oncologist. Whereas before I was making decisions to help the patient, now the gynaecological oncologist took over total care of these patients and frequently I never saw them again. The other change I noticed was a reduction in the number of medical students visiting our offices and the hospital maternity unit at the Grace Hospital.

As these changes were implemented I became frustrated and bored with my routine clinical practice. I was no longer involved in

complicated cases. I liked seeing patients but I tired of the practicalities, restrictions and routine. The job had lost much of its appeal. I
felt more like a robot than a physician. The challenge was missing.
The prospect of continuing to work in an environment that was not
going to improve and over which I had no control eventually persuaded me to look at new options.

One of these options was to move to Australia where Elaine's sister
and family were already established. They had started in Melbourne
in 1970 and moved to Sydney two years later. The family loved their
new lives in Australia. Now the country was recruiting consultants to
service the growing population. As attractive as such a change might
be, I was reluctant to move because of the disruptions *I* had experienced as a schoolboy. I did not feel it was fair to subject our children
to the stresses of having to make new friends and establish themselves
in a new school system. I remembered how emotionally distraught,
fractured and out-of-place I'd felt when my parents decided to return
home.

Elaine's speciality was not affected in the same way as mine was.
She was quite happy to continue working at the Grace Hospital and
eventually became head of her department. On the other hand, I felt
disconnected, as if the glue that had kept my world together had lost
its hold, its bond.

The next event to impact my life long-term was a change in the
professorial head of the Obstetrics and Gynaecology Department at
the university.

After lengthy discussions with Elaine and some of my colleagues
I decided to approach the University of Manitoba with a view to joining the Department of Obstetrics and Gynaecology as a full-time
member. I felt a switch to an academic life might just provide the
intellectual stimulus I craved. I made an appointment to see Dr. J. —
known as "the Jet"—the new head of department.

"Dr. Binns, what can I do for you today?" he asked once I was
seated opposite him in his office, his long legs stretched out beneath
his desk. I had met him briefly before at a social gathering and had
been struck by his enthusiasm, energy and interest in improving and

expanding the Obstetrics and Gynaecology Department at the university.

"I'm interested in making a career change and teaching and research are at the top of my list. One area that's fascinated me for years," I answered, "is infectious diseases as they affect both gynaecology and obstetrical patients. I had considerable experience dealing with these problems in Uganda, where I practiced for two years, and in Oxford where Mr. Stallworthy, the senior consultant, had a particular interest in infectious disease as a cause of infertility. At the present time I'm not aware of anyone pursuing this health issue in Manitoba, or Canada for that matter."

"True." He paused, his blue eyes studying me, and then continued, "I hadn't thought of that before. There's a Department of Infectious Disease within the Medical School but our Obstetrics and Gynaecology Department really doesn't have much contact with them. If you're really serious about this I suggest you go and talk to Dr. Alan Ronald, who is an associate professor and Head of the Infectious Diseases Department."

For the first time I was encouraged to believe that a dream I had long harboured might be feasible.

"I'll do that. Perhaps you could also ask Dr. Ronald if lectures on obstetric and gynaecological infectious diseases would be valuable to the students and residents within the Medical School."

Within ten days I had a call from Dr. Ronald's office asking me to come for an interview. Although he and I had both worked in the same hospitals for several years we had never met.

"Bernie, I gather from Dr. Tyson that you want to become an academic and that you have a particular interest in infectious diseases as they affect women. As a trained Obstetrician and Gynaecologist you would certainly have an understanding of the field. Someone with your knowledge could be of great value to both our Departments. However, I'm not sure you have the formal skills and training that somebody in such a position requires. Before recommending you for a teaching job at the university I feel you would require further training in infectious diseases. I'm wondering whether you've really considered the financial implications of what you're considering. It strikes me as being a little mad."

"I was hoping someone would ask me that. I've given a lot of thought to my request. I've discussed it with my wife and several friends. The conclusion I've come to is that I really need to change my present situation. With the closure of community maternity units and the recent changes to gynaecological practice, much of the joy has gone out of the job. I've always been interested in teaching and the academic side of medicine. I was fortunate to spend time with an enthusiastic teacher in Oxford and would have pursued an academic career if it hadn't been for the pressures of earning a living. My wife, Elaine, is now working as a full-time anaesthetist and is comfortable with the idea of supporting me."

I watched as he raised his eyebrows.

"You're a lucky man. However, to give you some idea of how difficult this might be, here is what I would suggest. To start with you would have to take a year off and work as a fellowship student in my department. This will involve working in the bacteriology laboratory with the technicians. You will have to relearn your basic bacteriology as well as learn about the newer research on infectious diseases. At the end of the three months I would like you to spend three months with William Schachter in San Francisco, specifically to learn everything there is to know about the chlamydia bacterium. When you come back I will expect you to continue to work as a fellowship student for six more months. This will involve consultation work in Infectious Diseases as well as working within our department. At the end of this time you should find yourself in a position where you will be of value to both the departments of Obstetrics and Gynaecology and Infectious Diseases. I would hope you could become a bridge between the two departments.

"I can only afford to pay you $27,000 a year as a fellowship student. I suggest you consider this information and think hard about whether you can cope with going back to basics. I warn you right now that what you are contemplating is not going to be easy."

I knew he was right but I would not be deterred.

My colleagues at the Abbot Clinic were disappointed to see that I might be leaving them but they also felt that if this was what I wanted to do I should do it. I contacted Dr. Ronald again and had a further interview with him. I told him I was prepared to learn a new specialty—I was ready to give it a go.

At this interview he informed me that he felt I should really spend two years as a fellowship student in infectious diseases before starting to teach the topic to students. On the other hand, Dr. Tyson wasn't willing for me to be away that long. He wanted me back in the Department of Obstetrics and Gynaecology within one year. Dr. Ronald finally agreed to this timeline and I started a fellowship in the Department of Infectious Diseases in the fall of 1980.

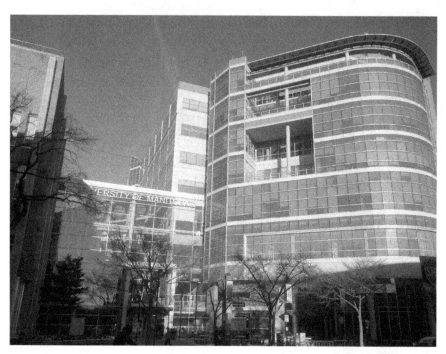

Top: The medical school at the Health Sciences Centre, University of Manitoba, in November 2019 (Credit: Jimj wpg/Wikimedia Commons).
Bottom: Bernie (top row, far left) and his colleagues in San Francisco.

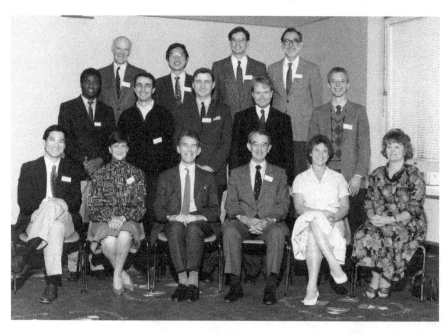

Chapter 12
Switching Focus: Teaching

On the morning of January 2, 1980, Dr. Ronald took me to the Bacteriology Laboratory at the Health Sciences Centre and introduced me to Katherine, the head technician, a tall lady wearing a clean white lab coat.

"This is our new Fellow," he chortled, "the *ancient* post-graduate student I mentioned the other day. Bernie needs to learn as much bacteriology as he can in the next three months. His basic knowledge of the subject is a bit rusty and old-fashioned. He last worked in a lab years ago in the UK. He is, however, an experienced obstetrician-gynaecologist who has, for God knows what reason, decided to pursue an academic career."

I could tell that he took some pleasure each time he mocked me.

"I'm pleased to meet you, Bernie," she replied. "I've heard about you from mutual friends. If I remember correctly, you worked at the Abbott Clinic and the Grace Hospital," she said as we shook hands. "I hope you enjoy yourself here. We'll try to get your bacteriology up to scratch. I've already planned your curriculum, but three months is not much time to cover what Dr. Ronald has in mind. If there are any areas that you're particularly interested in that I've not included, please let me know. Then we'll see what we can do to fit it into your schedule."

I looked around the lab, impressed by its spaciousness, particularly when I compared it to the cramped quarters at Oxford.

"I'm looking forward to this new challenge. My specific interest is, of course, obstetrics and gynaecology. So all the bacteria that cause sexually transmitted diseases [STDs] are up there on my list."

"I'm sure we can help you with those," she replied.

"You're in good hands," injected Dr. Ronald. "Katherine will keep you on your toes," he said as he turned to leave.

"Thanks. Will I see you at rounds on Friday?"

"I'm sure Katherine can free you up. I look forward to seeing you there," he said as he closed the door behind him.

"Let me show you around the lab. It's quite large and has several sections," Katherine said with obvious pride. "We do all the bacteriology and fungal work for the Health Sciences Centre, but we also do outside work for some of the larger clinics and private doctors' offices. However, we are not the only bacteriology lab in Winnipeg. The majority of virus detection and identification is done at the Provincial Lab, which is close by. Because you need to learn some virology, I've arranged for you to spend a couple of weeks there."

As we toured the lab, Katherine explained the layout. "The lab has eight benches. Most of them are polished wood and have drawers down each side. Between the benches there are shelves on which you will see various chemical agents. Because they're quite toxic, they're always kept in glass-stoppered bottles which are well labelled.

"Each bench has its own sink with hot and cold water and a Bunsen burner. The drawers contain various other pieces of equipment required to handle bacteria safely. The first two benches near the door are where the specimen samples are brought in, labelled and then separated into batches depending on what tests the physicians have requested. Some samples will go to the aerobic benches, others to the anaerobic benches, and some will be sent to the specialist benches.

"We receive a variety of specimens, which include spinal fluid, urine, faeces, blood, and swabs from various areas of the body. You'll spend your first week on these benches. I'm sure you appreciate this is an exceedingly important part of the lab. Marie," she said, introducing me to a petite young lady with bright red hair and green, mischievous eyes, "is in charge of this area. She'll teach you our procedures and techniques for labelling specimens, categorising them and sending them off to the appropriate benches. We don't want results going to the wrong doctors."

"That's certainly true," I agreed. "When this happens it causes all sorts of problems, particularly if the mistake's not caught immediately."

"I look forward to starting work with you tomorrow," Marie said. "I hope your handwriting's legible," she added with a wink as Katherine and I moved on.

Katherine then showed me around the rest of the laboratory, stressing the specialised areas which handled potentially highly infectious and dangerous organisms. These areas had a one-way air-positive pressure-flow system and the specimens were handled very carefully behind glass barriers.

"We do have a separate bench for sexually transmitted diseases. In view of your interest you will spend longer there. The organisms studied are chlamydia, gonorrhoea, *trichomoniasis*, monilia and syphilis, which we see occasionally. Other unusual organisms that we look for include tuberculosis and unusual fungi. These may take several weeks to culture and identify."

Finally she stopped, clearly signalling that our tour had come to an end. As we stood there, I sensed she had a passion for her job, an enthusiasm that would be impossible to replace. Something, in its way, approaching elegance and precision.

"I don't think there's anything else I can show you in the lab today. However, I do have some useful information and procedures on general bacteriology which you might like to read before coming back tomorrow," she said as we walked out of the laboratory.

In her office she handed me a large manila folder an inch thick that contained sheets of paper with various protocols, bacterial classifications and procedures for identifying different kinds of bacteria.

"There's a fair amount of reading here and I don't expect you to do it all in one day," she said.

Chlamydia, the organism that I was primarily interested in, was a bacterium that was especially difficult to identify in those days. It had to be cultured in cells lines as we did with viruses. It was a very small bacterium which lived inside the cells of the tissue that it was infecting. It was not a virus but had some properties that resembled them. Chlamydia was recognised as an infectious agent before the Second World War when scientists were able to stain and identify specific inclusion bodies (proteins) in samples taken from patients with trachoma, a common cause of blindness in Third World communities. With the identification of a bacterial agent as the cause of trachoma, doctors were able to treat the infection with antibiotics and decrease the rate of blindness.

The sexually transmitted strains of this bacteria family were recognised a little later and were first found to be the underlying cause of inflammation in the cervix. The bacterium was then identified by some researchers as the cause of non-gonococcal urethritis in men, neonatal conjunctivitis, and was thought to cause some forms of arthritis. It was also a major cause of epididymitis in men and salpingitis in women, both of which could lead to infertility.

I was fascinated by the bench work I was involved in during the next three months and I certainly learned a lot. Apart from culture, the other method of identifying chlamydia was to search for its inclusion bodies with special stains in biopsy specimens or scrapings from the cervix. Bacteriology was very much a search-and-identify field and it could be exceedingly difficult to identify a specific organism. There were thousands of them. Many bacteria had similar properties and it usually took twenty-four to forty-eight hours to identify an organism and its antibiotic sensitivity. Other pathogens grew very slowly, for example, tuberculosis and fungi. Many were difficult to grow and required specialized media with additives such as blood, chocolate, and other nutrients or elements. Some required special broths to grow in and others needed special atmospheres and temperatures.

The problem of time was paramount. The patients were sick and their physicians were waiting for the results before they could order the most effective antibiotics. It often amazed me how quickly the technicians correctly identified the pathogens and their response to various antibiotics. The work required many skills, including manual dexterity, visual perception, a good sense of smell, use of microscopes and a knowledge of bacterial behaviour. It was not until I had spent time on the benches that I really appreciated how difficult lab work could be.

During my introductory three months I attended all the infectious diseases teaching rounds and Friday afternoon Grand Rounds.

Although I was only spending a year in the Department of Infectious Diseases I was officially one of the fellows in the Department. The program was designed for post-graduate doctors who had completed their four-year internal medicine training and who wanted to become specialists. After a further two-year fellowship they could take an exam and become infectious disease consultants.

The infectious disease fellowship program was run by Doctors Ronald, G. Harding, F. Aoki and T. Williams. The number of fellows varied, but there were usually five or six of us. We were all expected to spend time in the laboratories while the rest of our training involved various areas of clinical medicine with particular emphasis on infectious diseases.

Although the other fellows were considerably younger than I was, they were very supportive. Given our different focuses, our paths did not cross that often. Once again I had to think like an internist and not like a surgeon; I was no longer required to make a diagnosis that could be surgically corrected.

After I'd spent three months in the laboratory, I was sent to San Francisco to work with Dr. Richard Sweet and Dr. William Schachter at the University of California. Dr. Sweet was a gynaecologist at the University Hospital. He specialized in infections of the female genital tract, in particular the effects of chlamydia on fertility rates, and went on to study AIDS infections in women during pregnancy and childbirth. Dr. Schachter was a research scientist who concentrated on both genital and non-genital chlamydia infections.

When I set out, my plan was to drive south as far as Fargo and head west through Montana, Idaho, Nevada and then onto California. I left Winnipeg on a clear, crisp morning at the end of March. Driving conditions were good. Fortunately I had the radio on when I arrived in Fargo and heard there was a blizzard raging in the west, near Butte, Montana. I made a quick decision to carry on south as far as Omaha, Nebraska, where I turned right and carried on through Colorado, Utah and Nevada. The lack of traffic on the roads and the vastness of the unpopulated countryside surprised me. Until I reached California.

I arrived at the top of the escarpment between Sacramento and San Francisco on a Sunday afternoon. The drive from there into San Francisco was one of the most hair-raising experiences I had had in many years. Keeping up with American drivers heading home after a weekend of skiing and gambling was harrowing. The tortuous road had concrete barricades on either side. The number of skid marks on these alarmed me. Were they evidence of accidents by drivers going too fast?

Eventually I found sanctuary in the accommodation Dr. Sweet had arranged for me in a private house within walking distance of the Moffitt Hospital, a part of the larger University of California complex. In the house, I had a single studio room on the second floor which reminded me of my digs as a medical student in London.

I spent two mornings a week in Dr. Schachter's research laboratory, which was on the seventh floor of the Moffitt Hospital and had a magnificent view of the surrounding city. I worked with him and his technicians on both genital and non-genital chlamydia. Dr. Schachter had specimens coming in from all over the world and I learned about some of the problems related to transporting these particular bacteria.

New techniques for recognising certain bacteria, including chlamydia, had been recently developed. They made the whole identification procedure much simpler and quicker, using antigen or nucleic-acid detection of the organism in swabs. Serology, the scientific study of serum and other body fluids, was also beginning to be used to recognise the serotypes of disease causing strains of bacteria and viruses. The use of these new technologies for identification was extremely helpful because it meant that results could be sent out to doctors' offices within hours instead of days. However, cultures were still used by many laboratories as the gold standard of diagnosis.

I had been in San Francisco about two weeks when Dr. Sweet asked if I might be interested in moving into a small house that one of the anaesthesia nurses wanted to rent out for three months while she went on a trip to Europe. By this time I was bored with living in a cramped room and having to eat out every evening. In spite of the seven ethnic restaurants within easy walking distance of my room, I longed for some home-cooked meals. The nurse's house had a bedroom, a living room, a small kitchen and a bathroom and was situated between the two hospitals in which I was working. It was just off Castro Street, in the heart of the gay community. While I had a glimpse of the unique character of this community, my contact with neighbours was limited; I was far too busy working during the day and staying home with my nose buried in books in the evenings.

When I thought about it I realized I had never lived alone, even during my student days. I had to learn how to cook and do basic housekeeping chores. Luckily the many house plants had instructions on them telling me how and when to water them. A Stagg horn cactus sat on a board and the instruction card said, "I like a cold shower once a week, in the bath!" Notes on the other plants told me either to spray them or give them a specified amount of water from a watering can. All was going well until I discovered one plant I had been merrily watering was artificial!

The time I spent at the San Francisco General Hospital was far more rewarding than the time I spent in the laboratory—because I was seeing patients again. I was surprised by how much I missed this contact. And my old practice.

The hospital was a newly rebuilt concrete structure. It was part of the University of San Francisco and had a large contingent of physicians in training (residents and interns) with whom I had the pleasure of working. A big hospital with over five hundred beds, it serviced all branches of medicine, including active psychiatric and emergency departments. In fact, it had one of the few emergency departments in San Francisco that remained open twenty-four hours a day.

The hospital was an exceedingly busy place. I dashed between the maternity department, the operating rooms, and gynaecological outpatients, while making the occasional detour to the emergency department. Dr. Sweet, the senior gynaecologist, spent much of his time at the Hospital where he taught me the principles of identifying infections in the female genital tract. During my time there I was able to observe and help care for many patients with acute pelvic inflammatory disease. Dr. Sweet was particularly interested in trying to find out what the incidence and significance of chlamydia infections were in these patients. Specimens from the outpatient department, the labour floor, as well as the operating rooms, were collected and transported, often by me, to Dr. Schachter's laboratory.

In 1980 the AIDS virus surfaced. Initially the main concern was with the male gay community in San Francisco, but the implications of this virus for women and newborns soon became apparent. I was at San Francisco General Hospital when one of the first cases of the transmission of the virus from a mother to the in-utero fetus was recognised. Dr. Sweet was one of the physicians involved and he published a paper outlining the dangers. I witnessed firsthand the development of the strict isolation techniques that became imperative for the care of these patients. All the protocols I learned in San Francisco proved indispensable when I returned home and faced the problems of caring for AIDS patients in Winnipeg.

As part of my training in infectious disease, both Dr. Sweet and Dr. Schachter taught me the principles of how to set up research projects. Good research is complicated. The specific area of research needs to be chosen and defined, project plans outlined, and budgets prepared. Then comes the search for funds.

Budgets contained a surprising amount of detail, from the expected number of swabs, culture plates, test tubes, agents, broths, other special materials, and so on, to technicians' salaries. Some research projects were planned over several years and required considerable amounts of money. Governments, drug companies, foundations, and, sometimes, private donations were all sources of funding. Each had their own agendas, requirements, and expectations as to how the results of the research would be used. As I entered further and further into the funding maze I realized how political and biased applications could be.

Relatively small projects were often combined with others so that the same technicians could be used for several projects at the same time. At the end of a project a detailed description of the findings, with validated conclusions, had to be written up and published. This was all new to me. Previously I had dealt only with the clinical application of research. Until now I had focused on post-procedure outcomes; how patients responded to research results. Because I was going to have to become involved in researching chlamydia and other gynaecological pathogens when I got back to Winnipeg, I paid particular attention to the projects being developed by Dr. Sweet and Dr. Schachter.

Working with young interns and residents stirred up a lot of memories. While our early careers shared much in common, I sensed that the financial stresses these young physicians faced were greater than in my day. They all seemed to have their careers well plotted. Many planned to specialise and were looking forward to several more years of training before going out to practice. A high percentage of the interns and residents were married with children. Many were supported by their partners and families but all appeared to have already amassed large debts.

Shortly after my arrival I came face-to-face with some of the less pleasant aspects of living in a large American city. I had only been in the Hospital a few days when I came out of the stairwell opposite Dr. Sweet's office. He was standing at the door and looked at me with concern.

"I wouldn't recommend using the stairs, Bernie. The stairwells aren't safe. Haven't you noticed, even the security guards go around in pairs?"

"Really? No, I hadn't even noticed the guards. And certainly not that they worked in pairs. I'm used to climbing stairs to keep myself fit. But now that you've alerted me to the danger, I'll use the elevators."

"Good. I'd hate to have to report to Dr. Ronald that we'd lost his fellow in a fight or a hold-up," he said with a chuckle.

One day I was sitting in the Common Room where residents gathered for coffee to escape the hectic wards. I was telling them about my medical training in the UK. A senior resident, who was already looking forward to working in Hawaii, mentioned that he came from New

York. "Are all the stories we hear about the dangers of living in New York true?" I asked. "The murders, the muggings, the robberies?"

"Yes, they're mostly true, but New York is a big city. People do exaggerate. Some even call it an urban jungle."

"Why would anyone live there then?" I asked.

"Well," he said, and then paused, "it's home. What else can I say? We were brought up in it. We knew how to avoid trouble. It's often outsiders and tourists who get into difficulty with petty and violent crime. I'm sure the same applies to London, where you trained, and other big cities in Europe."

"Perhaps you're right. There are areas of London I'd avoid after dark. The hospital where I trained was in the heart of the East London dock area. It had a bad reputation."

One evening Dr. Sweet invited me to his home for dinner. When we finished working in the outpatients department he said, "I'll meet you down at the car. It's in the doctors' parking area at the back of the Hospital, in stall H35. It's a red Porsche but don't touch it when you get there."

"Why not?" I asked, curious about what would happen if I did.

"If you touch it, it'll set off the alarm and either the police or hospital security or both will surround you wanting to know what you're doing. They can be uncompromising and short-sighted. Not that anything is likely to happen." He went silent and thought for a moment. "I'll see you there in fifteen minutes," he said heading off to finish his paperwork. Car alarms were new in the 1980s and I didn't know of anyone in Winnipeg with this feature.

Dr. Sweet lived in a beautiful house in Marin County. To get there we had to drive through a park called the Presidio of San Francisco, then across the Golden Gate Bridge. The Golden Gate National Recreation Area on the other side of the bridge was pristine, the road winding through it spectacular.

When we arrived at his house, I was struck by the number of security systems I could see. The place was like Fort Knox. A massive wrought iron security gate barred the entrance to his driveway. The house was outfitted with the latest alarm systems. In fact, as far as I could see, the whole neighbourhood was similarly secured. It was difficult to tell if they were locked in or locked out.

Towards the end of my stay, Elaine and Patrick came to visit me for a few days on their way back from a holiday in Australia. They had been to see Elaine's sister. I was delighted to see them and together we took in the main tourist attractions of Otis Redding's city by the bay—Fisherman's Wharf, the multiple markets, the observatory and the cable and street car lines that started near the wharfs and climbed into the hills. In the distance we could see Alcatraz through the masts of the fishing and sailing boats at anchor in the harbour. One day we drove to Lake Tahoe, a resort lake two hours' drive away and high in the Sierra Nevada Mountains, renowned for its deep, clear water and year-round recreation. I realized then how much I had missed the companionship of my family. Family was at the centre of all the important things I knew. It always had been. My trip to San Francisco had taught me a lot, not least of which was something about my own curiosity and determination.

When I returned to Winnipeg I was still expected to work as a fellow within the Department of Infectious Diseases. I was placed on the duty roster and put on call. I was often the first physician to see new patients. Usually, these patients had already been assessed and treated unsuccessfully for their infections and had been referred. Some were general medical patients, others were postsurgical, some were from the Children's Hospital and some were gynaecological patients. Prompted by their symptoms, others arrived in emergency, on their own.

As a fellow I had to assist in the setting up of new research projects. One important long-term project I worked on was to assess the value of prophylactic (preventative) antibiotics in patients who required emergency caesarean sections. In other research projects, I helped examine the role of chlamydia in infertility, acute pelvic inflammatory disease, cervicitis, and neonatal conjunctivitis. As the gynaecology specialist in the department I was responsible for identifying the patients and collecting the necessary specimens.

As part of my fellowship responsibilities, I was also expected to present the results of our research at international conferences. Condensing the results of a research study into a ten- to fifteen-minute talk required a lot of work. Fortunately I had excellent guidance. I was soon presenting papers to large audiences in North America, Europe and Australia.

In time I became aware of some of the pressures that were brought to bear on academic researchers by their department heads. The University expected its departments to produce research material for publication and presentation at international meetings. Good research and publications in peer journals enhanced the University's status and credibility. A first-rate reputation for research increased undergraduate enrolment, attracted more top researchers and increased long term revenue streams. Presentation of these papers was my first exposure to the politics of academia.

The relationship between research centres and major drug companies was complicated by the need to produce positive findings. Dr. Ronald advised us to be extremely cautious about accepting funding from any source with the potential for a conflict of interest. He was particularly concerned about any sort of restrictions that could be attached to the grants. The catch was that the companies which funded drug research often insisted that they review any papers before they were published. Occasionally this led to restrictions on the data presented and consequently on the conclusions reached. This potential manipulation of data raised ethical questions related to the ownership and subsequent disclosure of information within the healthcare field.

By the end of 1980 I completed the requirements of my fellowship. The plan of working across two departments appeared to be viable and in January 1981, I returned to the Obstetrics and Gynaecology Department.

* * *

When I joined the University of Manitoba's Medical School it had two large teaching hospitals under one faculty—St. Boniface Hospital and the Health Sciences Centre. Inevitably there was a duplication of services between the two. This resulted in competition for beds and funding. Some specialities were unique to each hospital because of the doctors and researchers who worked there. Obstetrics and Gynaecology services were split equally between the two facilities. Students spent time at both places and were assigned to professors and part-time faculty, depending on their availability.

I was officially a member of the Obstetrics and Gynaecology Department within the University as they had more funds than Infectious Diseases for full-time staff. I did not receive a salary or stipend from the Department of Infectious Diseases. Initially this was not a problem. My duties within the Infectious Disease Department were outlined in my contract. I would be responsible for teaching undergraduate and postgraduate students at all levels; I would give lectures, seminars and courses on clinical procedures in my area of expertise. I would also update nurses, doctors and other health care providers on infectious diseases within Obstetrics and Gynaecology.

My hospital position had the grand title of "Head of Section and Chief of Gynaecology Services, Director of Obstetrics and Gynaecology Infection Control Program and Ambulatory Services." A real mouthful, to be sure. I was based at St. Boniface Hospital, but I was also expected to manage and take care of consultations on patients with infectious complications at the Health Sciences Centre. In addition, I had two outpatient clinics a week at St. Boniface and one at the Health Sciences.

Dr. Tyson had been generous in his allocation of a continuing salary for my assistant professor position. I was completely comfortable with what he proposed and was keen on developing a research and educational program which would increase the awareness of the long-term impact of gynaecological infectious diseases on women.

I was also expected to present research findings and studies in two specialities. I attended gynaecology conferences as well as infectious diseases conferences. There were usually four major meetings in the areas of infectious diseases and sexually transmitted diseases a year and a similar number in obstetrics and gynaecology—in sum, a major commitment. Even so, I was keen to make my dual role a success. At this time I also became captivated by workshops on undergraduate education.

How medicine was taught was beginning to intrigue me.

My field of interest was a relatively small area of practice in obstetrics and gynaecology. At this time I was one of only four or five gynaecologists in North America who had completed the basic infectious diseases and pathology training. Because the common pathogens (STDs and AIDS) triggered social taboos, my area lacked the broad appeal of some other developments, such as in vitro fertilization, gynaecologic oncology, ultra-sonography and improved neonatal care (although I was frequently asked to see patients in these areas when they became infected).

Regardless of its low public profile, I knew my research on the causes of pelvic inflammatory disease, infertility, and the prevention of infections following emergency caesarean sections was important. While attending the Inter-science Conference on Antimicrobial Agents and Chemotherapy in Chicago in 1981, I met Lars Westrome from Lund, Sweden, who was well known for his work on chlamydia in Europe. During our lengthy conversation, I learned that he was doing diagnostic laparoscopies (keyhole surgery) on all his patients with suspected pelvic inflammatory disease. Gynaecological laparoscopy had only recently become a recognized procedure in our specialty. I wanted to learn more about it so I arranged to visit Westrome's unit in Sweden later that year. The trip was productive from both a practical and philosophical view. Armed with my new experience, I was able to persuade my colleagues that laparoscopy was a valuable and safe tool in the treatment and management of patients with pelvic inflammatory disease. The department invested in the necessary equipment and subsequently trained gynaecologists in their use. To this day, women continue to benefit from the innovative use of this technology.

While the use of the laparoscope for diagnosis was a major improvement in obstetrics and gynaecology, the greatest change in practice I witnessed was the development and use of improved ultrasound scans. This change included pre-natal ultrasound screenings for obstetrical problems, and gynaecology scans for pelvic tumours, abscesses and cysts. Other applications soon followed. Much of the early work and publications came out of Winnipeg thanks to the research and innovations of Dr. Frank Manning.

These new technologies led to the establishment of a special section of gynaecological oncology, set up under the direction of Dr. G. Krepart and Dr. Lotoki at the two teaching hospitals. A section for the investigation of endocrine infertility and IVF (in vitro fertilisation) was formed at the Health Sciences Centre under Dr. Kredenser. Dr. Fernando Guijon started a major research project into herpes and HPV (human papiloma virus) and their effect on the cervix, with particular interest in their relationship to precancerous and cancerous changes of the cervix. Due to this innovative work, and that of Dr. J. Bowman and R. Feisen on Rh Disease in the newborn, the University of Manitoba Medical School gained a pre-eminent reputation and students enrolled in the program from all over North America.

These were exciting times for our department. Within five years the department expanded from five or six full-time faculty to a dozen.

Nine months after I started my position at the St. Boniface Hospital my job description and responsibilities abruptly changed. My office moved to the Health Sciences Centre but my title, teaching, and research responsibilities remained the same. Happily, I was now more involved in the running of the undergraduate program while my work in the Department of Infectious Diseases at St. Boniface continued. I saw consultations and continued to run an outpatients' clinic; and, crucial to me, I got to attend rounds.

One of the most transformative responsibilities I had during my time as an assistant professor was caring for patients in the Keewatin area of the North West Territories, along the west coast of Hudson Bay. These duties were organized by the University of Manitoba Northern Medical Unit. Faculty took turns going up to these northern communities to see patients, perform minor surgery, and teach the nursing staff and other health-care personnel.

My turn to go to Rankin Inlet came in 1981. I jumped at the chance to see something new. I had to fly to Churchill and spend the night there before flying on to Rankin Inlet. Since it was minus twenty in Winnipeg and Churchill was six hundred and seventy miles further north, I assumed it would be colder. The clerk in the Northern Medical Unit booked my flights and told me I would have to stay at Hilde's House. With these instructions I received a package that contained a dictating machine, plane tickets and a report form to complete on my activities during the trip. I packed some warm clothes in a light bag and carried my parka with me onto the plane. I would have to change planes in Thompson.

We flew from Winnipeg in a warm, comfortable Boeing 737 at 4:15 p.m. in January. By the time the plane arrived in Thompson the sky was pitch black. As we were coming in to land the pilot announced that it was minus thirty-two Fahrenheit and that there was a strong wind blowing.

The Thompson airport was small. It consisted of a one-storey wood frame structure and a single gravel runway. We deplaned from the rear, using the plane's own steps. Before I had reached the bottom I could feel the cold cutting though my pants. We walked about two hundred yards to the terminal building, the wind and snow, which felt more like fine hail, biting into the exposed skin of my face. Quickly I pulled up the hood of my parka. The skin on my legs began to grow numb. By the time I reached the terminal building the cold penetrated my entire body and I realized how quickly a person could freeze to death. With relief I stepped through the door into the hot smoky waiting room.

The next leg of my trip was with Calm Air, a smaller airline that served the North and had its base in Thompson. According to my itinerary I had an hour layover, but I soon realized that time didn't seem important in this part of the world. The plane was an additional hour late. By the time it was ready to depart I had taken the precaution of putting on some fur-lined ankle boots. The wind was still blowing and walking out to the plane I felt as cold as I had getting off the jet.

The twenty-five-year-old Hawker Siddeley, which carried up to forty passengers, had been standing on the runway for some time and was agonisingly cold. The seats, which folded back, gave little protection from the elements and felt as hard as a stone slab. The other fifteen to twenty passengers all looked more experienced than I was and appeared to be happy with the seats. Fifteen minutes after takeoff my arse was still frozen even though the "heat" had been turned up. When the stewardess served us peanuts and soft drinks still wearing her full-length parka, I lost hope. In fact, she didn't take her parka off during the entire flight to Churchill. On the walk to the terminal I felt like Otzi the "Iceman".

Churchill Airport was one of the biggest in northern Manitoba. It was built as a base for the shipment of personnel and equipment to areas further north to service the Distant Early Warning Line (or DEW Line) in the 1950s. The DEW line was operational until the late 1980s when it was replaced by the North Warning System (NWS), which remains in operation today despite the fact that the Cold War has long since ended. As the runway was built for large Air Force transport planes, Boeing 737 jets landed there on a regular basis. Unfortunately I discovered I had been scheduled to fly on a day when there was no direct jet service from Winnipeg. Churchill was a fairly busy town of 1,200 people, a sea port that was operational in the summer with a railway that linked the community with the rest of Canada.

It was midnight when the plane landed and I was unable to see much outside. The inside of the airport was a concrete American Forces building, functional but cold. I was not sure how I was supposed to get to the Hospital or to Hilde's House so I asked the clerk at the desk.

"Oh, someone, probably Joe, will come for you," he said.

I had no idea who Joe was or how I was supposed to recognize him but I needn't have worried. He spotted me quickly enough. He was a short man, well bundled against the cold. He hadn't shaved for a few days and had a cigarette in his mouth.

"Are you the doctor?"

"Yes," I said. "I'm supposed to be spending the night at Hilde's House."

"Good trip?" he asked.

"Bit cold," I replied.

"It's down to below forty outside and the wind's been blowing all day. They say it might get worse tomorrow. Is there anyone else with you?"

"No."

"Do you have any bags to get off the plane?"

"No."

"Do you mind if a couple of other people come with us?"

"No."

"It'll only take them a few minutes to get their bags," he said, as he wandered off to find his other passengers.

This gave me time to look round the airport and eyeball some of the people who had come to meet the plane. The area was crowded and hot. Everyone seemed to be smoking. The scent of tobacco smoke mixed with the smell of sweat and animal skins. Most people still wore their outdoor clothes—parkas, animal skin coats, and well-used fur or felt-lined boots which gave off their own pungent odour.

The airport facilities were adequate but simple. They consisted of a single rectangular room that was approximately thirty by one hundred feet. It housed two airport desks, one for Calm Air and the other for CP Air. Two plastic benches sat three people each. There was standing room for fifty to seventy-five people. Next to the exit was the baggage collection area, which was covered in frost, inside and out. Every time the doors opened a blast of cold air blew in reminding me of the deep freeze outside.

The driver soon found his other passengers, two men and a young woman, who seemed to know each other and took no notice of me. We went out and found the "bus", an old-fashioned machine that seated ten and was a bit the worse for wear. Although it had been left running with the heater on full, the inside was covered with frost. The only view out was through the driver's side of the windshield. This didn't matter much; it was dark and visibility was down to less than one hundred feet because of the blowing snow. We started to move with a firm, bouncy motion. The wheels and shock absorbers were frozen solid—a sign, Joe said, that the temperature outside was minus forty.

I looked through the cleared area of the windshield. All I could see was a snow-packed road. I hoped the old bus wouldn't break down. After driving for about fifteen minutes I could see the lights of Churchill over the driver's shoulder. When we got into town I saw the effects of heavy blowing snow for the first time. It was piled up against solid objects like sand blown against stones on the seashore. Here I was looking at snow blown over cars, trucks, and single-storey homes. The snow swirled around solid objects, making abstract patterns in the bus's lights, reminding me of Henry Moore's dynamic flowing figures. Soon the other three passengers got out. The driver made a few more turns and came to a stop.

"Here you are. Hilde's House, 110 Simpson Street. I'll pick you up for the airport at seven-thirty tomorrow morning," Joe said.

I assumed this meant I had to get out of the bus, not a prospect I relished. I grabbed my carry-all bag. To get to the front stairs of the house I had to climb over a snowdrift, feeling colder by the second. Obviously no one had been up the steps that day and I fought my way through drifts to the front door. I had to take one mitt off to open the latch on the storm door. Once again I experienced the curious sensation of bare skin sticking to metal. I tried to open the main door and discovered it was locked. Suddenly it occurred to me that I could be in a dangerous position. I had no idea where the key was, where the hospital was, and I knew nothing about Churchill. In addition to this, I was not clothed well enough to go walking around a strange town looking for help at one o'clock in the morning. There was a sudden gust of wind as I looked up to see if there were any lights on in the houses down the street, but it was impossible to see anything at all through the wall of blowing snow.

In the midst of my desperation, the wind died down and the lights of the bus reappeared. Thankfully Joe had waited to make sure that the southern city-dweller got into the house. Greatly relieved, I retraced my knee-deep tracks back to the bus and he opened the door.

"Didn't they give you a key in Winnipeg?"

"No," I said.

"Well, let's go and get one from the hospital."

"Is it okay to leave my bag on the porch?"

"Sure, we'll only be a few minutes."

A blast of warm air hit my face and body, like a chinook, as I climbed back into the sanctuary of the bus. I wondered what Joe was thinking about my futile excursion to the front door. True to his word, the trip to the hospital took only two to three minutes. The hospital was quiet, the lights dimmed, with only two nurses on duty. After explaining who I was, one of the nurses found a key for me and told me to give it to Joe in the morning.

The house turned out to be a typical wood-frame, semi-detached structure with a single living/dining room and a small kitchen area. There was a comfortable settee, a small coffee table, three stand-alone lights, a small dining table, four chairs, a telephone and an ancient television. Scattered around the room were old magazines. On the walls there were three beautiful enlarged photographs, two of polar bears, and the other of an arctic fox. Hanging over the television was an old green teapot with a dead plant in it. The room was warm. I could hear the gas furnace running in the background.

The next morning I got up at six-thirty. After shaving and washing I went downstairs to see if there was any food. The fridge was well-stocked with plenty of canned and packaged items to eat. The fresh milk was in the freezer so I had to do without. I made toast and tea. Outside it was still dark but the wind had died down. Through the kitchen window a single streetlight lit up a rounded outcrop of rock piled high with snow. There were no houses or other signs of habitation in that direction. Through the front window, I could see yellow light from several streetlights. In spite of the early hour a few lights shone from some windows of a row of wood-frame houses. A dusting of snow fell but visibility was much better. Just as I finished tidying up, Joe and the bus arrived. I was the lone passenger.

When I gave him the key he asked, "Did you have a good night?"

"Not bad."

"It looks like a nice day coming up. Where are you headed to-day?"

"Rankin Inlet."

"It'll be colder there and the winds are usually worse."

"At least I've got my long johns on today," I said.

"Do you have any wind pants?"

"No, what are they?"

"We use them a lot up here. There are different kinds but the best and easiest are the ones with long zips down the outside of the legs. They're lined and sure keep the cold out. You put them on over your other clothes."

"Where do you buy them?" I asked.

"The Bay carries them. There's a store in Rankin but they cost more up there."

There were about twenty people in the waiting room at the air-port, most of whom were Inuit. I had treated the occasional Inuit pa-tient in Winnipeg, but this was the first time I found myself in the midst of a large group. There were at least two families, ranging in age from a few months to three seniors, one of whom, a woman, sat in a wheelchair and was attached to a portable oxygen cylinder and breathing mask. Two babies were on their mother's backs, tucked in-side enlarged coat hoods. Everyone chattered away in Inuit, a lan-guage new to me and different from anything I'd previously heard. I was struck by their easy camaraderie, their quick smiles, and their sense of rootedness. This initial impression has stayed with me over the years. Most were smoking and all the young adults were missing a lot of teeth. Two of the children had dark marks on their faces over their cheekbones. I found out later that these were due to frostbite. Skin can freeze in less than a minute when a stiff wind combines with minus forty degree temperatures.

While I observed the group, a young man approached me and introduced himself as one of the physicians working in Churchill. He asked if I was taking the flight to Eskimo Point (now known as Ar-viat) and if I would be willing to supervise the elderly lady on oxygen.

He assured me there would be someone to look after her when we got to our destination. He explained what had to be done and confirmed she had enough oxygen to last the trip. Then with the help of an interpreter, he told the old woman that I was another doctor and that I had agreed to look after her.

Shortly after he departed we learned that there were some mechanical problems with the plane and we would be delayed thirty minutes. This news did not seem to surprise or upset any of my fellow passengers, so it must have been a common occurrence. An hour later we were let on to the plane, another Hawker Siddeley. All but the back twelve seats were folded away to make room for cargo.

The passenger compartment was icy, probably because the crew had been working on the plane with the doors open. I found a seat for my patient and took a seat across the aisle from her so that I could keep an eye on things. Once we were settled I heard some banging and clattering from the back of the plane. The stewardess was having trouble getting the door closed. She fetched the pilot but even with his help the door wouldn't budge. They struggled on for about ten minutes before giving up and asking us all to go back to the waiting room. They were going to have to get what I heard someone call the "steam enema". This equipment was needed to get rid of the ice that had frozen around the door.

Back in the waiting room I asked the clerk at the check-in desk if there was anywhere to get coffee.

"Not at this time of day," she said. "I've not seen you before. Is this your first time in the North?"

"Yes."

"Well, don't worry about these 'mechanical delays'. Most of them turn out to be small problems. This morning's typical. The reason for the first delay was that they couldn't get the valves on the fuel tanks open. The plane had been out all night and had frozen tight. They tried steam but it was too cold, so they had to go into Churchill to get different equipment."

I realized then that we had been delayed for at least two hours and that the old lady's oxygen cylinder could be close to empty. When I checked the gauge, I found it was down to a quarter-full. I decided to get a replacement from the Churchill Hospital and this took another half hour. We finally got back onto the plane two and a half hours after our scheduled departure time.

The flight to Eskimo Point took fifty minutes and the pilot announced that the temperature had dropped to minus forty-three with a moderate wind. He said the stop would be short and that only those passengers who were disembarking at Eskimo Point should get off. When I saw the old lady was deplaning I decided to use her departure as an excuse to stretch my legs. The airport consisted of a converted mobile home, the type often used on large construction sites. There wasn't much else. I lowered my head and shoulders against the wind and walked quickly to the trailer. The small room had a counter and a place for checking baggage at one end. People crowded onto a wooden bench which ran along one wall. The room was hazy with cigarette smoke.

The only non-Inuit female in the room approached me.

"Hi, I'm Judy," she said, glancing up at me. "From the nursing station. I gather you have Mrs. Akutuk with you. How did she make out on the flight?"

"Fine, it didn't seem to worry her at all," I said. "There's plenty of oxygen left in her cylinder. We got a new one just before we left Churchill."

"Her lungs are pretty bad. She got pneumonia last week. We didn't think she'd make it to Churchill this time. This is the third time in the past six months we've had to send her out."

"She seems remarkably cheerful about it all."

"She's just pleased to be home with her family. I think she knows that she's not going to last much longer. I don't think she wanted to leave last week. She probably won't tell us next time, until it's too late." She turned to look at Mrs. Akutuk who was surrounded by family. "Is this your first time up here?"

"Yes," I said, almost apologetically. The confidence I felt in my medical training seemed superfluous. Everything here was much more straightforward.

"How far are you going today?"

"Rankin Inlet. I gather it's the next stop."

"Yes, but from the look of the weather out there, you might not get out of here today. A sea fog has just started to roll in and planes won't take off if the ceiling is too low."

I looked out of the window. The other four passengers had just got off the plane and were headed for the "terminal".

"It looks as though you may be right. Is there anywhere to stay in Eskimo Point?" I asked.

"We'll find somewhere for you to stay if the hotel is full," she re-assured me. "I better get Mrs. Akutuk back to the station and perhaps home. Phone the nursing station if you're stuck. We can probably find something for you to do while you're here. It's nice meeting you. We'll probably meet again if you start coming up on a regular basis."

She collected her gear, got her charge in tow and went out into the cold. The old lady gave me a broad, toothless smile as she wheeled past in her wheelchair.

Five minutes later we were told by the desk clerk that we could get back on the plane. A few minutes after getting airborne the low cloud cleared and I was able to see what the Keewatin portion of the North West Territories looked like from 10,000 feet. The prospect was very bleak. All I could see was large drifts of snow and ice, the occasional snow-covered lake and some outcrops of rock, which broke up the blinding white of the landscape. There was no evidence of man. And no trees. I learned later that some animals—foxes, wolves, caribou, musk ox, rodents, ptarmigan, owls, and some other hardy birds—can survive in this bleak world, but I didn't see any sign of them.

In less than an hour the plane banked to the right and started to descend. The pilot made a circuit of Rankin Inlet before coming in to land. I saw an oasis of various-coloured houses, some well-looked after and others not, in the sea of white snow which washed up to the town's outskirts. I could identify the inlet, which adjoins Hudson Bay, and I was surprised to see a rusty old steamboat lodged in the ice. I found out later that it was derelict. There was one large new build-ing on a small hill and in front of it I could see children playing. A few people walked around the half-dozen streets, while a few snow-mobiles, throwing up short rooster-tails of snow, scurried about. A single bright-red half-ton truck came to a stop at the main crossroads of the settlement.

The airport was crowded with Inuit. They were all in good spirits; they had come to meet their friends and relatives or to collect goods off the plane. Unable to understand a single word, I felt as if I were visiting a foreign country. Once the luggage had been delivered, and people were drifting out of the waiting room, I began to worry how I was going to get to the nursing station or the hotel. At that point an Inuit man, over six feet tall, dressed in dark blue overalls and an open parka with the hood up, came through the door and looked round the room. Spotting me, he waved, as if greeting an old friend, then came towards me, his wide grin revealing toothless gums.

"You want taxi!" This was more a statement than a question. I was not sure if any arrangements had been made for my transport, so I replied, "I'm the doctor. Do you know if anyone is coming to meet me?"

"They didn't tell me to get you, but the nurses' station vehicle isn't here."

"Perhaps I should come with you, then."

"Okay, I go and find more passengers, then come back and get you." He smiled, as if tallying up figures in a ledger, and went off, leaving me wondering if I had been conned into something.

Minutes later, after the luggage had been gathered, six passengers surrounded the "taxi," a battered van that could seat six in a pinch. The trip into Rankin Inlet only took five minutes and I was charged seven dollars. This was a lot in 1981 and illustrated the high cost of living in the north.

The hotel was situated at the bottom of a small incline just below the main road. Because of its situation and the prevailing winds, a lot of snow was piled up around the building, preventing the van from accessing its driveway. The front door opened into a bare wooden room with a few coat hooks on the wall. A second door led into the reception area where a portly, middle-aged man sat behind a desk. He looked up as I came through the door.

"Hello, sir, how can I help you?"

"I think you have a room for me. I'm the doctor and I'll be working at the nursing station for the next three days."

"I don't think we're expecting you," he said checking the register, "and we're full today because of the council meeting."

"Are you sure?"

"Let me double check," he said, and wandered off into a back room.

The reception area was part of a corridor. To my right I could see a stairway leading up to a dingy looking hallway. Beyond the stairs I could make out the entrance to the dining area. I could smell cooked food and hear the clatter of knives and forks. It was just past one o'clock in the afternoon. To my left there was a large room with some battered old sofas and stuffed chairs, plus half a dozen tables with wooden chairs. There was a bar at the far end of the room. This surprised me as I had seen a notice at the Eskimo Point Airport warning passengers not to bring alcohol into the Keewatin. There was a $500 fine for doing so. Rankin Inlet, on the other hand, was not dry to travellers. While I was thinking about the implications of a dry community, the receptionist returned.

"I think I've sorted this one out. I called the nurses' station and they tell me that they're expecting you over there at two. You'll be staying here for three nights. I'll have to fit you in with someone for the first two nights. Hope you don't mind?"

I was stunned to learn that the room rate was $160 a night, including meals.

After dropping my things onto the unoccupied bed in Room 12, I put on my parka and fur boots to walk to the Nursing Station, a blue building, number twenty, the receptionist told me, up a small hill, opposite the hotel. I slid onto the road and was nearly run over by a speeding snowmobile. One of the problems with parka hoods was the restricted view. It was like looking down a tunnel. Hearing was also a problem, so I made a point of looking both ways twice before continuing.

While climbing the fifteen slippery snow-covered steps I wondered how really sick patients got into the station. Entering through a double set of doors into a small waiting room, I was met by a petite, dark-haired young woman in a white lab coat. She introduced herself as Joan, the nurse in charge. I introduced myself, explained that this was my first time in the North, and asked what they had in store for me.

"We have plenty of patients for you and they should be arriving in about ten minutes. Would you like a guided tour of the station first?" she asked.

"Thanks."

"Basically we're a self-contained unit. Everything is under one roof. We have four examining rooms and a larger room at one end of the station. It has two beds for overnight patients. It also serves as an emergency room, and we use it for minor surgical procedures, delivering babies, and keeping patients under observation while they're waiting for transport."

"How do you get the really sick patients up and down the steps?" I asked.

"Oh! You noticed that. Well, we have a couple of strong Inuit men who bring them up on stretchers."

We moved down the corridor a few steps and arrived at the hub of the station, where the charts were kept and paper work done. I could see that there was just as much paperwork dealing with patient care in Keewatin as anywhere else. Perhaps more! As we continued our tour I saw a small room to the left in which there was an X-ray table. Past this we came to a fairly wide corridor that shot off at a right angle. Down this corridor there were three examining rooms. Then came the larger room. In it were the two beds she had mentioned, but I was surprised to see an incubator for newborns with oxygen and resuscitation equipment. There was a good supply of IV fluids and other equipment for emergencies. Shelves were stocked with various pre-packed and sterilized bundles. Some supplies were for delivering babies, some were for suturing and others were for medical emergencies.

"Who uses all this stuff?" I asked.

"We have to when there's no doctor around."

"And how often is that?"

"We're lucky in Rankin Inlet. We have a resident doctor who's here sixty percent of the time, but the other stations only see a doctor for a few days each month. Things can become pretty daunting and frantic when blizzards isolate us for days. Then our only contact for medical advice is by radio telephone."

"Who delivers the babies?" I asked.

"We do, if the doctor's out. At the moment we have a midwife working with us, but not all stations are so lucky. Our telephone lines are busy!"

"I thought midwifery was illegal in Canada?"

"That's true, but a few of the girls who work up here come from Britain and they have their midwifery training. Over the years, the Territories have tried to hire British nurses, so there are always a few midwives around to help out. But the situation is changing. The number of British-trained nurses in the North is dropping. I'm going to England this fall to do a midwifery course in Leicester. At the moment I feel really inadequate looking after pregnant women."

"You must like it here."

"Yes, but I'd like to see other parts of the Territories. I understand that the Western Region is completely different, both topographically and ethnically. We hear a lot of stories about the different parts of Canada from the RCMP. They're always being moved about."

Joan hesitated and glanced at her watch. "Let's have a quick look at the dental room and X-ray area. Then we should get to work."

On the way back towards the hub I noticed a door with pictures of children and a few adults demonstrating the problems of poor oral hygiene. The pictures reminded me of Uganda where similar pictures had been displayed. Joan opened the door to the dental room, a simple room, with a dental chair and all the modern gadgets. And yet, as if to twist my mind, I noticed an old foot-operated dental drill, standing in one corner.

"How often does the dentist come up?" I asked, staring at this relic from the past.

"He visits most of the stations once or twice a year, but he comes here monthly. There's a lot of work for him, particularly with the children and teenagers who seem to live on junk food."

"What's the old portable drill used for?"

"Oh, he takes that with him to some of the smaller settlements where they don't have any electricity or equipment. Apparently it works quite well."

Then she showed me the X-ray room, which housed a small but effective machine for taking routine X-rays of the chest, abdomen and limbs.

"Who takes the films?" I asked.

"One of the locals has been taught to take them but if necessary we can. After we or the resident doctor have looked at them, they're sent down to Winnipeg for additional assessment. We use X-rays a lot and find them very helpful. Next to this room we have the lab. It's basic but we can do blood work—haemoglobins, white cell counts, urines (including pregnancy tests), vaginal wet preparations and other common tests. The rest have to be sent to Winnipeg or Yellowknife."

"Do you have Uri cults for urinary tract infections?"

"Yes."

We returned to the main corridor. There was a locked door with the word *Pharmacy* posted on it.

"What do you keep in there?"

"All our drugs. And other valuable supplies. We're fairly well stocked with general medications, especially those we need on a day to day basis. Anything special has to come from Winnipeg or Yellowknife. Most things reach us in a few days. Larger items come by barge once or twice a year."

Opposite the Pharmacy there was a coffee room with a sink, stove, and fridge. In the middle there was a small table with four plastic covered chairs around it. "Up that way," Joan said, pointing up another corridor, "are our bedrooms and the doctor's office. And down this way we have a large common room, with some comfy chairs and a TV. It gets one and a half stations, in black and white. Usually with lots of snow," she laughed.

"How many nurses live here?"

"There are three bedrooms, but two of the nurses live out. They're married. But we're trying to get accommodation for all the nurses to live out. Getting away from this place when not on call is important. We also feel that it would improve recruitment. Then the bedrooms could be used to expand the station's facilities. Rankin's growing and will continue to do so. More and more Territorial administration is moving here.

"That's about it. Now we'd better put you to work." She led me back to the waiting room which was now full of patients. Most of them were women and all but two were Inuit.

"What have you got lined up for me?"

"Fifteen patients. They're a mixed bag of pre-natal patients and some gynaecological problems. Tomorrow will be really busy. We have you booked all morning and afternoon. Then at four o'clock we hope you'll give us an in-service on gynaecological emergencies."

"How many of you will there be?"

"Four nurses, a medical student, and the resident doctor if they're all in town," she replied.

She turned and started walking toward the door. Then stopped, as if suddenly remembering why we were here.

"Oh, I meant to say, this will be your examination room. Most of the things you'll need are on the tray. The speculums are in the drawers at the end of the examination table. If there's anything else you want come and ask me. I'm just down the corridor. Most of the patients you'll be seeing can't speak English, so they'll come in with the interpreter. When you're ready for a new patient just come out to the desk and the clerk will find the next one."

With these instructions I went up to the desk, requested the first patient's chart and asked the desk clerk to bring the patient to the examination room. The chart was completely different from anything I'd encountered before and the hand-written notes which went back for years were almost impossible to read.

The cliché about doctors' writing being illegible is often true, and at times makes life difficult for everyone concerned with patient care.

I would have to make do. Fortunately, I had had a lot of experience practicing medicine through interpreters in Uganda. This added hurdle was not new to me.

The obstetric and gynaecologic problems I saw that afternoon were similar to those found in any busy practice.

Several patients were concerned about sexually transmitted diseases and infertility. Infertility proved especially difficult to diagnose in these new patients because, as I was soon to discover, history-taking and social customs were different.

Fifty percent of the time infertility was the fault of the male. And yet examination of the partner (not necessarily the husband) was often not acceptable or possible. Sometimes transporting specimens could also be a problem. Thus infertility testing was particularly unfair to the women, who were subjected to investigations that could often be painful and might be both dangerous and unnecessary.

As the afternoon wore on, I was increasingly thankful for the appreciation I received from the patients, and impressed by their good nature and by the relentless conditions under which they often lived—between danger and survival.

Halfway through the afternoon Joan came in and asked, "How are things going?"

"Okay, as soon as I managed to work out the organization of the charts."

"The resident doctor had to leave for Repulse Bay this morning and there's a child here who I'm worried about. Would you mind having a look at him?"

"Not in the least, but it's been years since I've examined a child," I said. "What's the story?"

"The little boy's three years old. His mother says he developed a cold yesterday and is now having a lot of trouble breathing. He has a temperature and a slight rash. I think he may have pneumonia. He's also a bit blue so I've put him in the oxygen tent."

When we entered the emergency room I could see a worried-looking Inuit mother standing beside the cot with the plastic oxygen tent over it. In the cot the small boy was breathing rapidly, but he didn't seem in a great deal of distress. His mother looked up. "He better now," she said, her voice a mixture of forlorn optimism and disbelief.

"That's good," Joan said, trying to sound encouraging but clearly not convinced. "This is the doctor. He'll take a look at John."

There was no doubt the child was sick and short of breath. He had a rash and I agreed with Joan that he was slightly blue. I looked in his mouth. His tonsils were enlarged but not inflamed. They were not causing any obvious obstruction. None of the lymph nodes in his neck were enlarged. His lungs were moving equally and there was no dullness when I tapped his chest. But I could hear air bubbling through a fine fluid. Although it must have been fifteen years since I'd listened to a child's chest and heard these sounds, I remembered what they meant.

The rest of the examination did not reveal anything unusual. I concluded the boy had a lung infection with pneumonia. It was probably a viral infection which would account for the rash. The real issue was—what to do! I needed help.

"I think he has pneumonia. Probably due to a virus. But he should be on antibiotics." I paused. "What do you usually do in these cases?" I asked.

"When we think a patient has pneumonia we start them on antibiotics and then ship them off to Churchill as soon as we can," she replied.

"How long does that take?"

"If we charter for a Medevac and there's a plane here, it only takes an hour or so. If the plane has to come in from elsewhere, we may have to wait several hours. Sometimes, when there's a whiteout, we have to wait for the weather to break. That might take several days."

"How often does that happen?"

"About ten percent of the time. With medical cases we don't worry because time is less of an issue and besides, we can get advice over the phone. Often we'll wait for the next scheduled flight. But with surgical, trauma and obstetric emergencies, the situation can become very stressful. Even so, things are better here than at the other stations. At least there's a charter company based here. In more remote and smaller stations things are very different; it might take several hours if not days to get someone out.

"A few weeks ago there was a patient in shock in Baker Lake with a ruptured ectopic and it took five hours to get her to Churchill. She was lucky to survive. They told us that the blood they took from her, when she got there, was like pink water, it was so diluted with IV Ringers Lactate. When we evacuate patients a nurse or doctor has to go with them. This can cause problems at a station when they are short-staffed. We also get fed up with travelling back and forth across the Keewatin in all kinds of bad weather.

"I'll get an IV started and get things organized for John. Thanks for having a look at him."

At the end of the day I went back to the hotel. After dinner I wandered into the "common" room and asked the bartender for a beer. He said the bar didn't open for another half-hour, so I settled into one of the stuffed sofas to watch TV. The image was black and white, the picture snowy, and there was only one station. With nothing else to do and no one to talk to, I wondered what it would be like to live in the North for long periods of time. One would need to be self-sufficient. And perhaps take up old-fashioned hobbies like reading, painting, photography, and crafts. Or, better still, play bridge, if one could find a foursome.

At coffee break the next day I asked Joan what people did in their spare time.

"There's lots to do if you get involved with the community," she said.

"Such as?" I asked.

"Fishing. In the summer, most people go fishing. Or watch whales and other sea life. A lot go birdwatching. All manner of migratory birds come up here to nest. The tundra is covered in magnificent ground cover. People come from all over the world to look at the flowers and take photographs. If you're more adventurous you can go on canoe trips or hunting trips with the locals.

"In winter there are the usual winter activities. Ice hockey, ice fishing and Ski-dooing. Some people even go winter camping. You might have noticed that there are several churches in town. They organize a variety of social activities. Some people do volunteer work. In fact, a person can always find something to do. We socialize a lot and some of us even end up learning how to cook! For readers, there's a library. The new school has a gym where we can play badminton or basketball. Unfortunately, not everyone gets involved. Those people who don't can become lonely and depressed. The North's not for everyone. We are isolated. Some of us like that. Plus the slower pace of living, I suppose."

"How often do you get away?"

"We get three to four weeks' holiday and there are some update seminars and meetings we can attend. The trouble is that travelling out of the area is very expensive. We only go out when we get subsidized."

"What you're saying reminds me of Uganda. Most ex-pats thought of it as a hardship post but I liked it. Many of the problems are the same."

"That's why this is known as the Third World of the West!"

At four o'clock we gathered in the largest of the examination rooms for the in-service. There were three nurses, one interpreter, the X-ray taker and the resident family physician who had just returned from Repulse Bay on the Arctic Circle.

"How was the trip?" I asked her.

"Long and cold," she replied. "It's not one of my favourite places to visit. I often get stuck there for longer than I expect so I have to take food with me."

"How big is the community?"

"About five hundred people. I go up there once or twice a month. They usually have quite a few medical problems for me to deal with. We're concerned about the number of new TB cases diagnosed there recently. A team of doctors and nurses are coming up sometime in the next few weeks to see what's going on. They'll decide if it's an epidemic and what to do about it. It's a touchy situation, perhaps a political scandal. The population is supposed to have been vaccinated against

TB. There's a policy in effect that requires the TB vaccination for all Inuit newborns. And yet it appears they haven't received the shots. This is a problem few physicians in Winnipeg would be aware of."

"I saw many cases of TB when I was in Uganda. When I returned to Oxford and was working in the infertility clinic, we found that seven to ten percent of infertilities there were due to genital TB. And that was less than fifteen years ago. I gather TB is rare in southern Canada but more common amongst the First Nations and Inuit communities."

"True enough, but now it's affecting young children. Recently, a couple of cases of meningitis have been reported, which is very serious."

I found her story distressing. While these diseases were well-known to people in the Third World, for us they had become curable. Yet another sign of our prosperity and sense of entitlement.

When talking to small groups I've always felt it's important to find out what the group wants and what they already know. With a mixed group, like this one, I used a question-and-answer format. After a few questions it was obvious they were most interested in how to handle the acute emergencies with which they had to deal. Additionally they wanted to know how to handle problems related to sexually transmitted diseases, which they said were far too common in the region.

The most serious emergencies they encountered were in obstetrics. Changes for the worse could occur very rapidly and become life-threatening to both mother and baby. This was nothing new to physicians, but in the North it was much more frightening because of the lack of medical backup. In the stations the nurses had to make decisions and perform procedures that would normally be the responsibility of physicians. In obstetrics these emergencies could include recognizing high blood pressure problems, abnormal bleeding, early fetal distress, as well as diagnosing complications such as diabetes or ectopic pregnancy, and arriving at a correct estimate of an expected date of delivery. Even with modern technology and the use of ultrasound, it was still not possible to forecast when a mother would go into labour.

The nurses in these stations were also responsible for looking after the occasional patient in labour and judging if it were safe or possible to transfer the patient to Churchill before delivery occurred.

At the end of the session, Joan summarized the situation. "You know, Dr. Binns, you and your colleagues come up here once every few months. The family physicians based at Churchill come to the stations once or twice a month to see patients and to give us advice. We live here and have to run the station on a day-to-day basis. Our responsibilities are considerable and we seem to be a dying breed. Recruitment of nurses to the area is becoming more difficult, the qualifications of the applicants less, and their desire to stay in the North less. The result is that the nurses who are here are moved around more and more and don't get to know the communities. This results in lower standards of care, and poor communication with the local population. They in turn complain to the local and central government who then bring more pressure to bear on the nurses in the stations. On top of all this we're affected by financial restraints and budget cuts. Which just make things more difficult. This is obviously a vicious circle and I can't see how it can be broken."

As I was packing up another nurse thanked me and suggested I best get over to the hotel before I missed dinner.

I got into my heavy winter parka and boots and walked briskly back to the hotel under a starry sky. The evening meal was the usual fare, as much as you could eat. All of it was likely flown in and presumably accounted for the high cost of staying in the hotel.

During the night I woke up and heard the wind howling outside. I didn't pay much attention to it at the time and drifted off to sleep again. When I woke up in the morning my roommate, who was an Inuit counsellor from Baker Lake, said, "A blizzard's blown in. No planes will make it. We'll have to stay. How long you here for?"

"I was supposed to catch the eleven-thirty flight today. But I think the nurses have some more patients for me to see, so I won't be idle."

"Getting back to Winnipeg depends on how long the storm lasts," he said. "Sometimes they last for three or four days."

I realized that if the blizzard went on for more than twelve hours

I'd have to cancel my office appointments in Winnipeg as well as my three surgical cases booked for the rest of this week. I could imagine the consternation and annoyance this was going to cause the nurses, patients and the operating room staff at the two hospitals. In the future, when I was going North, I'd have to make certain I had no surgical cases booked.

After breakfast I fought my way through the strong winds and blowing snow to the nursing station. To my surprise I saw several other people struggling against the wind. In Winnipeg, when a blizzard blew in, the streets were deserted. Traffic stopped and people stayed indoors, except for those in essential services. Police, doctors and nurses.

When I arrived at reception, six patients were waiting to see me.

"I see you've managed to find some work for me this morning. When will we know if there'll be a flight out today?" I asked Joan.

"We won't know until shortly before the plane is due, but if this keeps up for more than an hour or so you'll be out of luck. Chances are you could be here for a couple of days at least. If you don't make it out by tomorrow you may have to stay until next week. There are no flights out of Churchill over the weekend."

I was lucky. Although the scheduled flight did not make it that day the winds dropped and there was a Medevac for a young man with a broken leg that evening. I went to Churchill with him as his medical attendant. This saved one of the nurses having to go.

The next day I was on a jet back to Winnipeg and home.

Over the next twenty years I continued to go to the North. I loved the Arctic and its people. While my visits remained a constant many things changed during that time—people, places and government policy.

I was often asked if I liked going up north. My answer was simple: If I didn't enjoy it, I wouldn't have gone—even though leaving Elaine and the family for days at a time and sometimes longer was difficult.

An experience similar to my first visit to Churchill and Rankin

Inlet would have been enough to put most people off. Some of the visiting consultants only went up in the summer months. Even then they encountered problems with mosquitoes and black flies and fog delays. The lifestyle was different, some of the medical problems horrendous.

But I liked to travel and found that going north gave me a break from the city and the frustrations of working in the Health Sciences Centre. Also, I felt strongly that we had a responsibility to care for people in their own communities. There was a tendency for the medical profession and politicians from Winnipeg to ignore the northerners and their problems. It was much easier to ship patients south whenever there was an emergency. This was the simple solution. This attitude left the nurses and doctors in the North feeling isolated and ignored, which was bad for morale. In my view, maintaining direct contact with the people working in the North was the only way to understand their problems.

For various reasons, younger physicians tended to criticize the standards of care in the North. They, too, supported the philosophy that northern patients would be better served in larger urban hospitals or clinics. Such views were often unfair and aggravated the situation. Also, I felt it was better to meet the nurses on their own turf for small group in-services, than for them to come to Winnipeg twice a year for refresher courses. These courses were frequently run by people who had never been up North so they couldn't fathom what it was like to cope with the complications of an ectopic pregnancy in a snowstorm. Visiting locals *in situ* gave them needed moral support and gave us the opportunity to meet them face-to-face where they lived.

Another dramatic change that occurred was the accelerated pace of staff turnover. Nearly all the nurses and doctors were replaced at least once every year or so. In fact, all the nurses I met on my last four trips were new to the Keewatin.

At the same time, connections with the North were improving. The air service to Churchill was better and more frequent. Yet north of Churchill the number of commercial flights didn't change. The planes rattled as much as ever and still felt like taking a spin on a roulette wheel. For political reasons the service to Rankin Inlet had been increased by NWT Air. Flights now crossed east-west and stopped at Rankin once or twice a week. In addition, a direct flight from Winnipeg serviced Rankin once a week on Thursdays. After much debate the emergency ambulance jet, based in Winnipeg, extended its service to Churchill, but would not go out of province.

Churchill received a small ultrasound machine for use by visiting University doctors. Ironically there was much resistance to training a local technician to operate it. Even the local medical practitioners were prohibited from using it. Again the reasons seemed to be political and economic. The University appeared to be more concerned with the potential loss of revenue than with providing adequate health care. To me this was short-sighted and could only harm the image of the departments concerned. The people who suffered most from this bickering were the patients. However, having the use of the machine when we were there saved many patient-trips to Winnipeg for the dating of pregnancies and other diagnoses.

During this period I was often asked if there had been any major improvements in the standards of care the northern patients received. My answers were always ambivalent. In the first place, I could only speak for my own specialty. We had improved our medical standards in Winnipeg and this quality of service was available to northern patients, once we got them to the city. It was a catch-22 situation. We had refined the mechanisms for evacuating patients, and we had introduced policies that had reduced the number of deliveries in the settlements. This, we assumed, had improved the standard of care that the patients received. However, the communities were concerned that these protocols might be causing more problems than they cured.

Inuit women were upset because they were forced to go to Winnipeg to have their babies. Many women concealed their pregnancies from the nurses or hid when they were scheduled to be evacuated south. I could sympathize with their behaviour and tactics.

The women were simply protecting their cultural heritage. They felt they were losing their independence and their ability to look after their own maternity needs because of policies forced upon them by southern governments. As the medical service providers, we were one of the causes of this ill feeling. When we said that all births should be in Churchill or Winnipeg we did not consider the fact that all the children would have Manitoba birth certificates and be labelled as Manitobans for the rest of their lives. This was an insult to the Inuit. They wanted their children to be born in the lands of their ancestors.

Another worry was the negative impact the evacuation policy had on families while the mothers were away. Everyone was concerned about potential bonding problems. And what repercussions would this separation have on future labour choices?

A few years after I had stopped going north, I talked to one of my colleagues who still visited there. He pointed out that Rankin Inlet was now much larger with a population of over 2,500 and had become the administrative hub for the region. A large medical centre had been built that was serviced by local doctors and midwives. This meant that women could have their babies in town. The concern about being born in Manitoba was no longer a worry. Emergencies were still transferred to Winnipeg or Edmonton. The town council of Rankin Inlet had taken over many of the responsibilities that had been handled by Churchill. Both Arviat and Baker Lake had also increased in size and the tourist industry was prospering. Polar bears sitting on ice floes were often sighted by visitors at the end of a lens.

Another service the department provided was to the Outpatients Department in the Women's Centre at the Health Sciences Centre. Unfortunately the facility was archaic. The physical layout prevented patient privacy. Interviewing a patient without others overhearing what was being said was impossible. The examining tables were only separated by flimsy curtains and the environment for the patients was not conducive to a comfortable clinical experience.

The majority of patients we saw in this clinic came from Winnipeg's inner city. Many did not have their own doctors, others were transient. Some had been referred to the full-time consultants working in the clinic by private doctors or colleagues. We ran clinics Monday through Friday and we saw both obstetric and gynaecological patients.

Prior to 1988 and the landmark Supreme Court decision *R. v Morgentaler* which struck down the country's abortion law as unconstitutional, abortions were only legal if a panel of two physicians signed that it was necessary for the physical or mental health of the mother.

For various reasons, the Women's Health Clinic became the primary referral clinic for women seeking abortions. Some were done by private physicians at peripheral hospitals but the majority of abortion services in Manitoba were done through our clinic at the Health Sciences Centre. We became extremely busy. Regrettably only some physicians and nurses were willing to participate. Occasionally newspaper publicity and anti-abortionist picketing interfered with the running of all the clinics. In the mid-eighties one of our obstetricians, Dr. Fainman, was shot in the shoulder at his home by a man with a rifle. Fortunately Dr. Fainman was not hurt badly but due to this life-threatening incident he and several others gave up doing abortions.

As we got busier it was obvious that our facility needed to be upgraded if we were to provide a safe and more holistic clinical service for women. After discussions with Professor Manning and the Hospital administration we obtained funds to review and plan some major structural changes. I spent several hours with the hospital architects and financiers and we eventually came up with plans for some major renovations. Work went ahead. The new renovations included five examining cubicles, an adequate waiting area, and a separate area where staff could talk to students and residents.

Most of the clinicians working at the Women's Clinic were full-time associate or assistant professors. As time progressed, the number of patients seen in the therapeutic abortion clinic grew so large we had to ask private physicians to come and assist us. I assumed responsibility for this program.

Therapeutic abortions were a quick procedure and not terribly risky, but they did not provide suitable clinical teaching for our students. On the other hand, the majority of our other patients presented excellent teaching experiences for our residents, interns and students. Perhaps the most valuable aspect of these clinics was the research projects Dr. Brunham and I organised in the areas of vaginitis, cervisitis, and methods of detecting chlamydia infections. Another colleague, Dr. Guigon, began his important research into the human papilloma virus (HPV) and cervical cancer in our clinic. When the project grew too large for our facility, it was moved to the Clinical Practice Unit.

Most of my time was spent overseeing the renovations to the Outpatients' Clinic, organizing and running the abortion clinics, and organizing the student undergraduate and clinical teaching. I continued to initiate research projects that focused on chlamydia disease in women, research which lasted for the next four years.

Dr. Tyson's second term as Head of the Department came to an early end in 1984 due to political pressures. People were apprehensive about the direction in which he was leading the Department. Perhaps this was the result of the rapid expansion of the department, coupled with the erosion of the practices of private physicians working in peripheral hospitals. University funding was slashed. The federal government argued that there were too many doctors being produced across the country. Consequently, student intake was reduced by five percent with the same reduction in funding.

The open position was awarded to Dr. Frank Manning who was well qualified to take the role. He headed the ultrasound/fetal maternal health unit and had published a number of important research papers.

I soon learned there were major challenges ahead but I settled in to a changing position with enthusiasm and trepidation. It was immediately clear that the University faculty was worried about the performance of students in Obstetrics and Gynaecology. In the first and second year our students (ninety per year) received several hours of lectures and their first patient contact. In the third year they received some clinical lectures and in the fourth year they received two weeks of clinical gynaecology and four weeks of obstetrics. Unfortunately, the two weeks of gynaecology and four weeks of obstetrics were separated by several months. This meant that their gynaecological experience varied making assessment of their performance almost impossible. Consistency was a huge issue.

The obstetric portion of their clinical training also varied because it was done at peripheral hospitals where their experience depended on the number of patients who were having babies when they were there.

During the next year I interviewed all the students who went through our department. Two things became obvious. First, they were uncomfortable with our specialty and second, they had problems with some of our instructors. Additionally, our students did not perform well in the national (LMCC) examinations. Also, few were interested in taking up obstetrics and gynaecology as a speciality after graduation.

In an attempt to remedy some of these problems I made presentations to the faculty and ran Saturday morning workshops. In these workshops I emphasized ways in which the faculty could improve their clinical teaching. I was keen to generate some enthusiasm within the faculty about education. Many of the part-time faculty felt that having students in their offices reduced the volume of patients that they could see in an afternoon. One of the part-timers commented that teaching students was a very expensive hobby!

In time my philosophical and financial differences with Dr. Manning reached an impasse. I was especially aggrieved to be losing contact with some of my students. I had now been on the University faculty for over eight years and I was being paid less than when I had started. I enquired about taking a six-month sabbatical leave. I proposed to spend time looking into medical education and the ways in which we could improve our teaching methodology. Dr. Manning agreed. Dr. Brunham confirmed that our research projects on infectious diseases would continue.

Beginning in March of 1989, I spent my sabbatical attending seminars and workshops in Canada and around the world. These workshops were usually held over three to five days and covered the following topics: medical education; oral communication; planning and evaluation of courses; teaching techniques; new concepts in education and audio/visual presentations; and medical student and faculty evaluations. At the University of Dundee I learned there was an entire faculty dedicated to medical education. Each year, they hosted several longer workshops, ten to fourteen days, and I attended two of these.

Wherever possible I made a point of contacting the senior obstetrics and gynaecology faculty members in the schools where these workshops were being held: Seattle and San Francisco in the States; Hamilton, London and Winnipeg in Canada; and Guy's, Oxford and Dundee in the UK. I asked them what they did to produce successful medical school graduates in my discipline.

Following my sabbatical, I put my findings into a report and submitted it to Dr. Manning. My research highlighted the fact that the University of Manitoba's Medical School needed to offer its undergraduate students more coordinated and combined clinical time in the Obstetrics and Gynaecology Department. Dr. Manning never replied to my summary, and I concluded my position in the University was becoming untenable.

In the end, Elaine and I decided I should resign from my full-time position and become a part-time faculty member. Since part-time positions had a reduced teaching commitment, this gave me the opportunity to do some work with outpatients, gynaecologic patients and the abortion clinic.

Importantly, Elaine was working full-time and was happy in her career.

At this time, we also discussed retirement and decided that, while a change was in order, retirement was not yet an option. After all, I was only fifty-eight.

My colleague and mentor Dr. McCord had had a stroke shortly after his wife died. He suggested that Winnipeg was not the place in which to live with any sort of serious disability. Navigating the icy sidewalks in winter was hard enough for the able-bodied. On a visit to Vancouver Island in 1989, Elaine and I purchased a lot on a golf course where we would ultimately retire.

Eighteen months later Elaine and I decided that the time had come for us to work less and explore the world more by doing some short-term locum work. We hired an architect and built a house on the West Coast into which we moved in 1992. While house plans took shape on the drawing board, I looked for work in the medical journals and contacted an agency that helped match doctors with vacancies. Eventually I settled for a consultant obstetrician and gynaecologist locum in Whakatane, on the east coast of the North Island of New Zealand. I signed on for six months. Elaine continued to work in Winnipeg until the early part of the following year, when she joined me "down-under" to do a locum in anaesthesia.

In retrospect, I enjoyed the ten years I spent as an assistant professor in the University. I accomplished a few important things during my time as a teacher and researcher. First, after my sabbatical I convinced the University to revamp the obstetrics and gynaecology undergraduate program and to combine the gynaecology clinical rotation with clinical obstetrics. The department then had the students for six weeks, allowing them to look at our speciality as a whole. Surveys done after this change showed that the students' interest in our department markedly improved.

My infectious diseases research initiated a better understanding of pelvic inflammatory disease, sexually transmitted diseases, obstructive infertility, and the use of prophylactic antibiotics in our specialty. This was precious time well spent with enthusiastic and respected researchers.

Perhaps immersing myself in the culture and problems of the people in the Keewatin area brought me the greatest joy. I felt and still feel I contributed something to the care of Inuit patients who favoured me with their insight and good humour. Song, story and family were the antidote to ever-drifting snow.

My failure to get the two departments to understand each other reminded me of what had happened in Uganda after I returned to the UK. Improvements to patient care always seemed the first casualty of conflict.

Fundamental philosophies shape our goals and focus. In medicine, should we value the hands-on apprenticeship model of teaching, where students spend time with patients, learning to understand and value their case histories; or do we diagnose and interpret illness from what we glean primarily from technology, textbooks and lectures? Do we need to ask if we are treating the disease, and not the patient?

When my father was working in Medical Headquarters in the Northern region of Nigeria he was responsible for the recruitment of staff and assigning them to their posts. He said that young doctors from schools that encouraged patient contact were by far the best for his purposes—they adapted to the Third World environment with ease. They listened. This was certainly my observation when I was in Uganda.

I was always grateful for the patient contact I had in my medical schooling. While it is doubtful if medical schools will ever return to the teaching methods of fifty years ago, I feel we need to find some way of increasing patient contact, of listening to and appreciating the power of story, if we are to produce physicians who are comfortable and compassionate when they go out into the world to practice.

Coda

Since my retirement I have stood with a foot in each hemisphere, in a curious way returning to the hemisphere of my birth while still maintaining residence in my adopted country of Canada. During these twenty years I have watched the practice of medicine become increasingly expedient. Or perhaps the word utilitarian would be more apt. I have observed disturbing trends in the way in which medical care is taught and administered. Economics and bottom-line policies increasingly trump all other concerns. Physicians in much of the developed world now appear to treat the diagnosis, not the patient. Diagnosis has become more important than the patient's story and history; the patient is consulted less and less, machines relied on more and more.

Perhaps this is why practicing medicine in New Zealand over the past two decades has been a blessing for both Elaine and me, for here the patient's story remains a critical part of the diagnostic process and treatment, reminiscent of our training and early practice in the UK. We both embraced the familiar with exuberance. And yet I've sometimes wondered if we were too content with the tried and true. But I don't think so. Medicine is still a relationship, an art, practiced between people, people who trust and depend on each other in a community of peers.

Elaine and I consider ourselves fortunate to have found locums and full-time work in Whakatane. We purchased a small house with a beautiful garden in a town that reminds us of an English village. We now divide our time between Canada and New Zealand. We tramp about the countryside, play golf, and travel extensively.

We have indeed been lucky.

Acknowledgements

I'm indebted to both of my parents for their kindness and inspiration. Although my mother died long before I dreamt of writing a book about my travels and career, her stories told before a fire or around the kitchen table about our early lives in the Falkland Islands, India and Kashgar undoubtedly planted the seed. Father, who died a year or so after I started scribbling, was a major influence in my life and on the direction it took.

Thanks to Elaine who has always been supportive and my beloved friend and companion down the years.

And thanks to Kathryn who has been patient and read and advised me; and Helen and Patrick who have given me encouragement.

And thanks to Pat Smith who took on the challenge of copyediting a manuscript that had swelled to over eight hundred pages.

Many friends read drafts of the expanding text and offered helpful comments. These include Mike Boundy in Adelaide, Australia, Ali Pirani for his input on both Uganda and Winnipeg, and Mike Yip, Bob Thompson, Jocelyn Ponanga, Mike O'Rouke, Ian Finch, David and Bonny Nunwick, Margaret Thompson, Laurel Daly, David Finn, Roger Miners, Beverly Graham, my cousin, Anne Binns, Barry Newport, and Garnet and Barb Hunt.

I owe much to my teachers at Nottingham. Without them I would not have even begun the journeys I took; and likewise the faculty at Guy's. Many others are acknowledged in the narrative. Those I've missed know who they are. Thanks to all.

I'm grateful to David Stover at Rock's Mills Press for liking the manuscript enough to make it a book.

And, finally, thanks to Ron Smith, my neighbour, who became my co-author when I needed reining in and the text needed shaping.

About the Authors

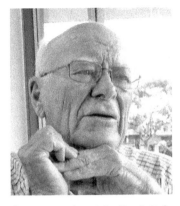

After a disruptive childhood and early schooling in India and Chinese Turkestan, **Dr. Bernard A.O. Binns** graduated from Guy's Hospital Medical School in London, specializing in Obstetrics and Gynaecology before practicing in the UK, Uganda, Canada and New Zealand. Following a long and distinguished career, he added infectious diseases to his résumé and worked as an assistant professor in the Medical School at the University of Manitoba, Canada. He now lives with his wife, also a physician, in Nanoose Bay, B.C. and Whakatane, New Zealand.

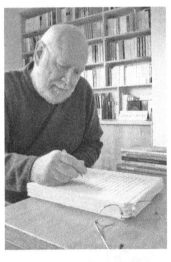

Ron Smith is the author and editor of several books. His most recent book, *The Defiant Mind: Living Inside a Stroke*, was long-listed for the George Ryga Prize and won the Independent Publishers IPPY gold medal for memoir. For close to forty years he taught at universities in Canada, Italy, the States and the UK. In 2002 he received an honorary doctorate from the University of British Columbia and in 2005 he was the inaugural Fulbright Chair in Creative Writing at Arizona State University. In 2011 he was awarded the Gray Campbell Award for distinguished service to the British Columbia publishing industry. He now lives with his wife, Patricia Jean Smith, also a writer, in Nanoose Bay, B.C.

CPSIA information can be obtained
at www.ICGtesting.com
Printed in the USA
BVHW031542200821
614044BV00001B/1

9 781772 441932